Nutrition for Top Performance in Soccer

PROFESSOR MICHAEL GLEESON

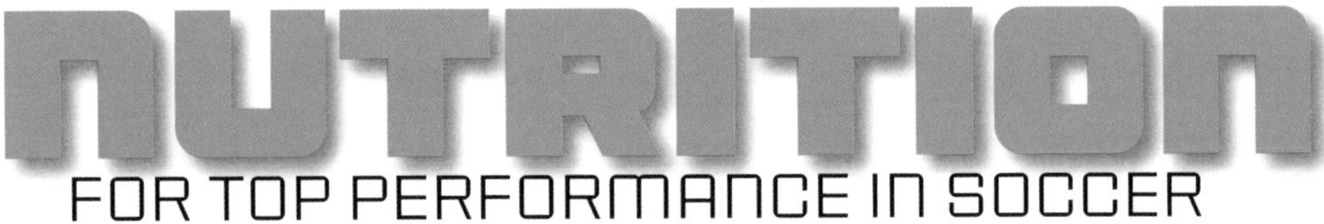

NUTRITION FOR TOP PERFORMANCE IN SOCCER

FOREWORD BY **BRENDAN RODGERS**

EAT LIKE THE PROS AND TAKE YOUR GAME TO THE NEXT LEVEL

Meyer & Meyer Sport

British Library of Cataloguing in Publication Data
A catalogue record for this book is available from the British Library

Nutrition for Top Performance in Soccer
Maidenhead: Meyer & Meyer Sport (UK) Ltd., 2022
ISBN: 978-1-78255-230-7

Aachen, Auckland, Beirut, Dubai, Hägendorf, Hong Kong, Indianapolis, Cairo, Cape Town, Manila, Maidenhead, New Delhi, Singapore, Sydney, Tehran, Vienna

Credits
Cover design: Isabella Frangenberg
Interior design: Anja Elsen
Layout: DiTech Publishing Services, www.ditechpubs.com
Cover photos: © AdobeStock
Interior photos: © AdobeStock, unless otherwise noted
Interior figures: © Michael Gleeson, unless otherwise noted
Managing editor: Elizabeth Evans
Copyeditor: Sarah Tomblin, www.sarahtomblinediting.com

 Member of the World Sport Publishers' Association (WSPA), www.w-s-p-a.org

Printed by Print Consult GmbH, Munich, Germany
Printed in Slovakia

ISBN: 978-1-78255-230-7
Email: info@m-m-sports.com
www.thesportspublisher.com

CONTENTS

FOREWORD

While the fundamentals remain the same, football has changed dramatically in recent years. The modern game is an exciting spectacle with supporters across the world fanatically cheering on their team and many young children dreaming of becoming the next superstar. In truth, to get to the top takes a lot of hard work, dedication, and do not forget talent. Not only is the intensity of matches higher than ever before but teams are required to compete more regularly due to extremely congested fixture schedules. I pride myself on leading a team that plays with a high energy level, the ability to make continuous high-speed running actions and to a high technical level; all of which require the highest levels of football and physical fitness possible.

Given the increased demands placed upon the modern player, where possible, clubs seek to invest in Medical and Sports Science expertise while also developing cutting-edge facilities in an attempt to maximise the potential of their playing squad. It is of course my role to ensure that each department and individual brings a passion to their work, an expertise and knowledge of the subject that allows us to progress, an ability to communicate with the players in order to improve them and a persistence to ensure not only short but long-term development. I am continually looking to evolve in an attempt to ensure no stone is left unturned when it comes to the preparation of my players. Undoubtedly, nutritional support is a very important aspect for players to get right, which is why we must ensure high standards at the training ground day in and day out. First and foremost, the food we provide must meet the needs of the players and should be tailored to the demands of training and match play. However, this doesn't mean it has to be boring; of course not. It is the role of the team chef to utilise healthy, lean produce to create exciting dishes bursting with flavour which will aid performance.

Historically, players may have only considered nutrition to be the measure of their percentage body fat, a crude marker of whether they were in appropriate shape or not. However, nutritional support is now so much more than that. Body composition is important in order to be strong, athletic and robust on the pitch and so, for many emerging talents, improving muscle mass and ensuring they are eating enough is important for their development. It is about educating the players in the hope that we can inform their decision making when it comes to food choices. It is now widely accepted that nutrition plays a very important role in performance. Players must fuel their bodies to perform at the highest intensity throughout the full 90 minutes. This doesn't just mean having a bowl of pasta three hours before kick-off; it is instead about the choices that are made and strategies that are in place throughout the days leading into a match. The need to fuel is just as important throughout the training week, with it being essential before tough training sessions when the squad are put through their paces. For me I expect the starting point to be the player's work ethic. Before strategy, tactics, theories, managing, organising, philosophy, methodology, talent or even experience you are dead in the water without this significant attribute.

Nutrition also plays a vital role after competitive matches and heavy training sessions, aiding recovery and supporting the body as it attempts to repair and adapt to the workload undertaken. This is important for not only reducing the risk of injury among the squad, but also helps speed up the turnaround so I can safely work with the players on technical and tactical aspects on the pitch. Given the busy fixture schedule teams often face when competing in European competitions, it is important to identify windows of opportunity when the science can help accelerate the recovery process. Despite our best efforts, the stresses and strains of competition may take their toll on the body; however, clean, lean, healthy food can be a powerful medicine when it comes to reducing risk of illness and boosting player health. We should never underestimate the power that a nice meal has in improving our mood, boosting our energy levels, and helping support our immune system. Professional clubs tend to support their players by providing breakfast and lunch either side of training; however, the decisions which players make away from the training facility are just as important. Through this relentless pursuit of excellence, players begin to understand the level that they need to operate at and in time they change their habits, behaviours and ultimately expectations of the food they eat.

As you can tell, I see the importance of putting in place good nutritional support and that is why I entrust nutritionists and sports science staff to implement strategies which they deem appropriate. When it comes to experts on this specific area, Professor Michael Gleeson is a leader in the field. He has immersed himself in the science and literature throughout his career, sharing his insights and theoretical knowledge along the way which I know has helped shape the careers of so many practitioners working in sport today. Nutrition for Top Performance in Football is a fantastic resource for anyone looking to improve their knowledge and understand the effect that nutrition can have on performance. It doesn't matter what age you are or what level you play at, this book is a great read for anyone who is interested in improving their performance. It will also be of interest for anyone wanting to begin a career working in football as it provides valuable insight into how evidence-based guidelines are put into practice within the professional game. Enjoy the read and good luck in your pursuit of continued improvement, whatever your individual goal may be.

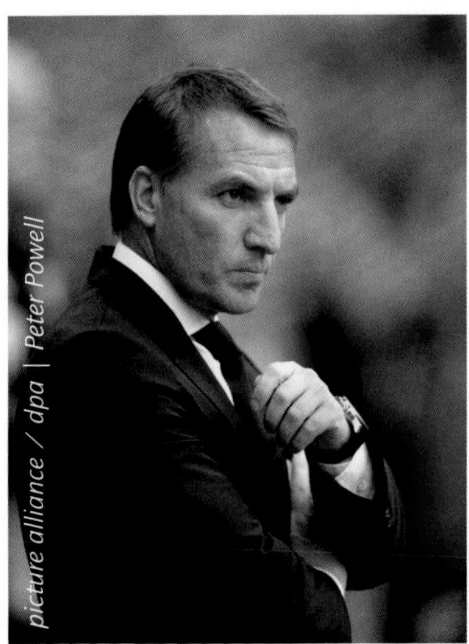
picture alliance / dpa | Peter Powell

–Brendan Rodgers, Leicester City FC manager

ACKNOWLEDGEMENTS

Many people have helped me to write this book and I am indebted to them for the helpful information, advice, insights and quotes they have provided me with. I have tried to list as many of them as I can remember here and I apologise if I have omitted anyone. Any mistakes you find in this book are unintentional and entirely my own. I particularly want to thank all the co-authors of the 2020 UEFA Expert Group Statement on Nutrition in Elite Football, namely (in the order in which they are listed in the paper): James Collins, Ronald Maughan, Johann Bilsborough, Asker Jeukendrup, James Morton, Stuart Phillips, Lawrence Armstrong, Louise Burke, Graeme Close, Rob Duffield, Enette Larson-Meyer, Julien Louis, Daniel Medina, Flavia Meyer, Ian Rollo, Jorunn Sundgot-Borgen, Benjamin Wall, Beatriz Boullosa, Gregory Dupont, Antonia Lizarraga, Peter Res, Mario Bizzini, Carlo Castagna, Charlotte Cowie, Michel D'Hooghe, Hans Geyer, Tim Meyer, Niki Papadimitriou, Marc Vouillamoz and Alan McCall. I am also extremely grateful to Brendan Rodgers for writing the foreword to this book and explaining the importance of nutrition in elite football from an expert manager's perspective. My grateful thanks for anecdotes, quotes (in person or from books and media articles), edits and/or comments also go to: the late George Best and Nick Broad, James Collins, Julian Dowe, Becky Dowst, Sam Erith, Sir Alex Ferguson, Pep Guardiola, Ilkay Gundogan, Harry Kane, Trevor Lea, Don Maclaren, Ron Maughan, Alan McCall, Brian McClair, James Morton, Jordan Nobbs, Tom Parry, Matt Reeves, Alex Savva, James Sinclair, Jamie Vardy, Neil Warnock and Arsène Wenger. Thanks also to Ron Maughan and Matt Reeves for supplying me with some of their own photos and giving me permission to use them in this book. My special thanks go to my friends and superbly talented, world-renowned, elite performance chefs Rachel Muse and Bruno Cirillo who have provided many of the meal plans, recipes and accompanying photos in chapter 12. I also want to extend my grateful thanks to my fantastic editor Liz Evans and the wonderful Sarah Pursey for her assistance with the promotion of the book. Finally, and undoubtedly most important, thanks and lots of love to my lovely wife Laura for your love and support, putting up with all the time I spend researching and writing, for just being there for me and for helping to promote my books. Without you, life would not be worth living.

CHAPTER 1

Does Nutrition Really Matter in Football?

- Why Nutrition Is Important for Football Performance
- Who am I?
- What Is Different About This Book?
- A Brief History of Nutrition for Football
- The Role of the Performance Chef
- Demons and Wizards
- Some of the More Surprising Nutrition Choices Players Have Made

Firstly, I want to thank you for buying *Nutrition for Top Performance in Football*, or if you're from across the pond, *Nutrition for Top Performance in Soccer,* and congratulate you on your decision. The aim of this book is to provide you with an insight into nutrition for football (or soccer as the game is called in some parts of the world, such as in North America, Australasia and the Pacific Islands). In other words, I will describe what elite football players eat and drink and explain some of the science that underpins the current recommendations made by nutrition experts. If you are an amateur player at any level – from national amateur leagues to pub teams – you can use the same nutritional strategies as the top professional players to improve your own game, increase your endurance, recover more quickly and avoid illness. This book is aimed primarily at the amateur player, but it will also be of interest to professional players, academy players (and their parents), nutritional, medical and sport science support staff, football coaches, managers, match officials and frankly anyone who is a fan of the beautiful game. For secondary school, college and university students studying physical education, sport science or sports nutrition this book will provide a useful resource and an understanding of how nutrition research can be applied in a real-world sport setting.

Nutrition is an important issue in many sports and football is no exception because it plays a crucial role in the health of the individual, in adaptations to exercise training, in weight maintenance and in match performance, whether by professional players or by those who play the game for fun or for health reasons. Indeed, nutrition influences nearly every process in the body involved in energy production, adaptation to training and recovery from exercise. If we look back 30 years or more, nutrition was largely ignored by those involved in professional football. Nowadays, it is seen as an essential component to maximise player performance, health and recovery as outlined in the foreword by Brendan Rodgers.

WHY NUTRITION IS IMPORTANT FOR FOOTBALL PERFORMANCE

Pep Guardiola, current manager of Manchester City and one of the most successful managers in club football, puts it very simply: 'For me the food is so important in football.'

So why exactly is nutrition considered to be so important for football performance now, when quite frankly, it wasn't only some 30 or so years ago? A good place to start is by quoting Arsène Wenger, the former Arsenal manager who was tasked by the Union of European Football Associations (UEFA) with writing an editorial in 2020 about his perception of the role of nutrition in football. He stated: 'The goal of any elite team is performance – to win as many matches as possible over the duration of the season. To achieve this performance there are myriad factors that are involved including technical, tactical, mental and physical qualities. One area that I have advocated for many years (as early as the 1980s) that can help us achieve our performance goals is "nutrition", an area which has grown in importance within the game.'

For the manager or coach, according to Mr Wenger, nutrition has the following objectives (figure 1.1) within the performance model: '(1) To ensure that players are in the best physical condition for the match: with an optimal level of body fat and muscle mass; (2) to accelerate their recovery from the previous match or from hard training sessions; (3) that players are fuelled and have the energy to sustain the intensity for 90 minutes or even more if called upon; and (4) to support an overall healthy, balanced lifestyle both inside and outside of the club environment.'

Playing football involves lots of running with repeated, high-intensity actions interspersed by periods of less-intense physical activity over the course of a 90-minute picture alliance / Marius Becker/dpa | Marius Becker

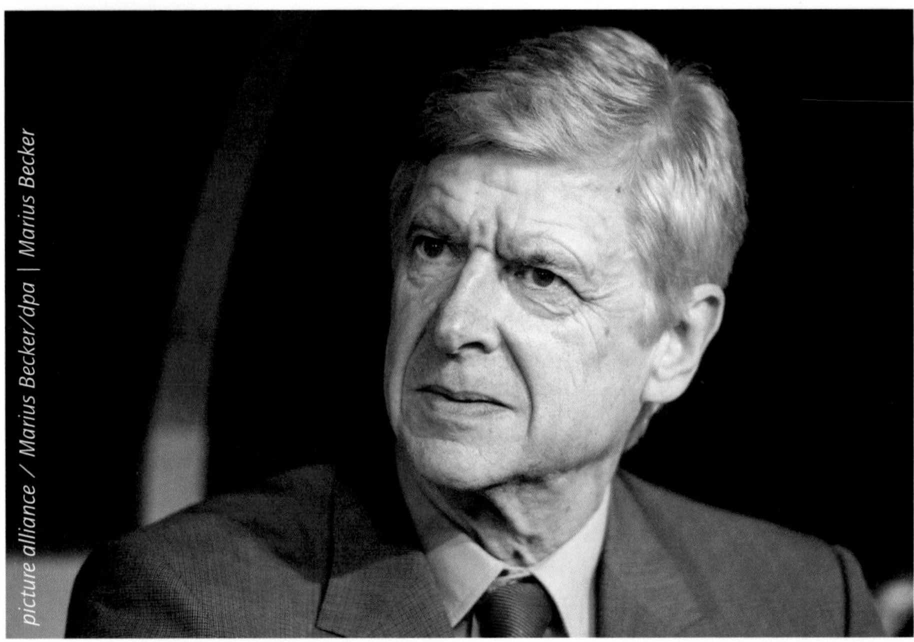

Photo 1.1 Arsène Wenger, one the first top managers to appreciate the importance of nutrition for the performance, recovery and health of footballers.

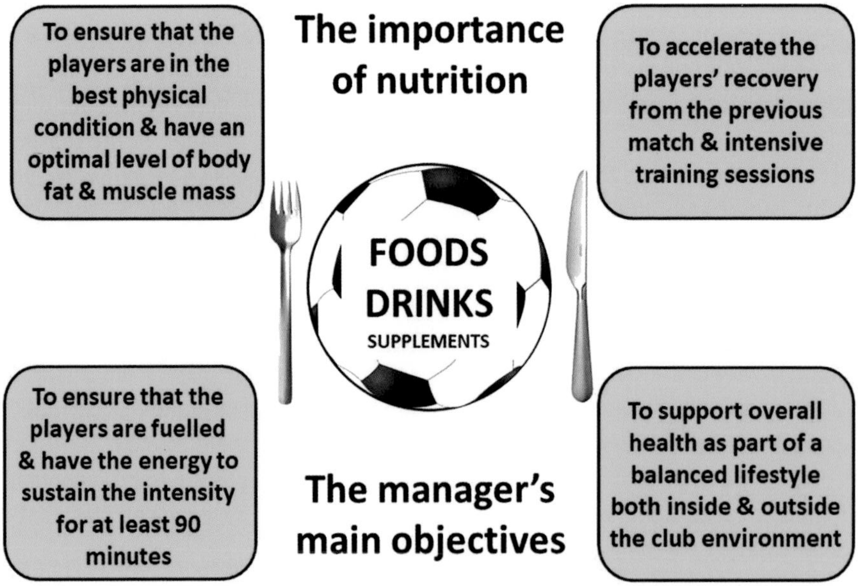

To ensure that the players are in the best physical condition & have an optimal level of body fat & muscle mass
The importance of nutrition
To accelerate the players' recovery from the previous match & intensive training sessions
FOODS
DRINKS
SUPPLEMENTS
To ensure that the players are fuelled & have the energy to sustain the intensity for at least 90 minutes
The manager's main objectives
To support overall health as part of a balanced lifestyle both inside & outside the club environment

Figure 1.1 The coach's perception of the importance of nutrition in the club's football performance model (according to Arsène Wenger).

match. An elite soccer player typically covers at least 10 km (6 miles) in a 90-minute match with about 600 metres covered at full sprint speed. Heart rate is maintained at about 85% of maximum and the total amount of energy expended by players who complete the full 90 minutes is about 1,600 kilocalories (kcal) with around 60–70% of that energy coming from carbohydrate. Match play involves not only running but also various in-play actions, such as jumping, tackling, passing the ball, dribbling and shooting. In addition, mental functioning is important for the timing of ball strikes and tackles, quick reactions, passing accuracy, decision making and staying concentrated. All of these are affected by fatigue. Minimising fatigue relative to the opposing team is an important strategy in football, because most goals are conceded in the last few minutes of each half (figure 1.2) and are commonly attributed to fatigue. Appropriate nutrition can address two of the major contributors to the development of fatigue, namely carbohydrate depletion and dehydration. In addition, some dietary supplements such as creatine, beetroot juice and caffeine can produce small improvements in performance in some players. Recovery starts immediately after the match ends, and nutrition is crucially important at this time for muscle repair and refuelling, particularly

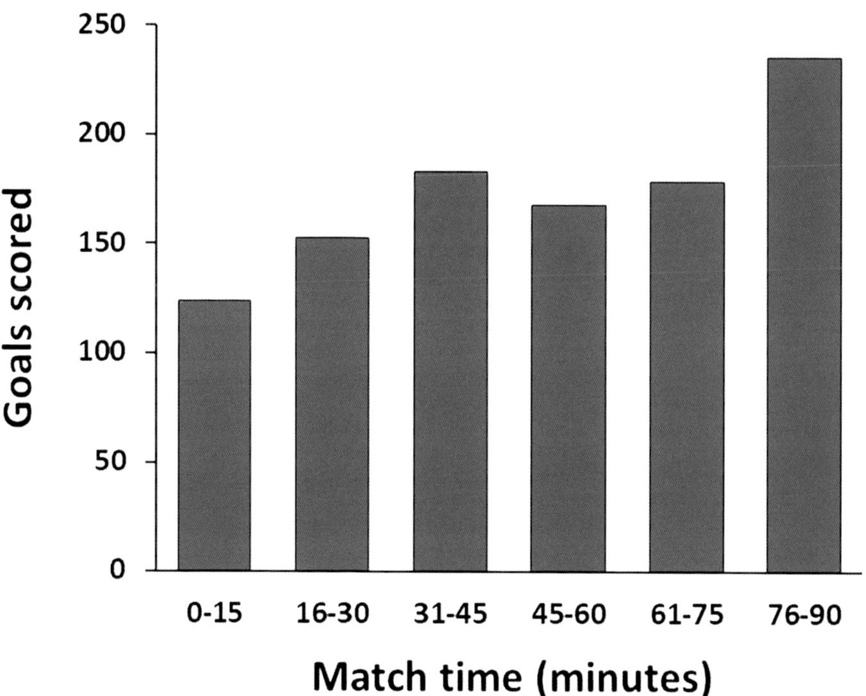

Figure 1.2 Average number of total goals scored in the English Premier League in the five full seasons from 2015–2016 to 2019–2020 during different periods of a match. The values for periods 31–45 and 76–90 minutes include added time.

in congested fixture periods when the next match can be less than 72 hours away. Appropriate food choices and timing are also important to allow a player to perform hard training, avoid illness, reduce injury risk, maintain mental concentration, sleep well, maintain an appropriate body weight and composition, and recuperate from injury (see the infographic at the end of this chapter).

It is important to appreciate that the amount and type of physical activity that a player does varies from day-to-day and that nutrition in football is what scientists call 'periodised' meaning that the diet changes to suit the players' specific training and match schedule. The concept of periodised nutrition is fully embraced by all top football clubs and, although every club will do things a little differently, the core elements of a nutrition plan will be essentially the same. Each player will receive a nutrition plan in the form of a day-by-day calendar that is tailored to their individual needs, which will depend on their body size, body composition, playing position, training load and training goals, their involvement in match play and their health status (by that I mean that the plan will change drastically if a player cannot play or train due to injury or illness, or is undergoing a period of recuperation from injury). Table 1.1 provides an example of a typical weekly periodised nutrition plan for a healthy player who plays one match per week. Note that the percentage contribution of protein to daily energy intake remains relatively constant, but the relative contributions of carbohydrate and fat vary more widely from day-to-day to accommodate pre-match carbohydrate loading and post-match carbohydrate replenishment.

So, the answer to the question 'does nutrition really matter in football?' is yes, it does. It matters very much indeed. Good nutrition may not make a footballer with average talent into a world-class player, but it can improve endurance, delay both physical and mental fatigue and speed up recovery – an important consideration not only for the professionals but also for many amateur players who may have a tiring match on a Sunday morning and have to go to work on Monday. It is also true that a poor choice of food and beverages can make an elite footballer become a pretty average player.

WHO AM I?

I am a recently retired university professor who has spent the last 45 years of his life teaching, researching and writing in the field of exercise physiology, metabolism, immunology and health with a particular interest in sport nutrition and a love of watching football. My last two academic positions were at the University of Birmingham and Loughborough University, two of the top universities in the world for sport and exercise

Table 1.1 A typical weekly nutrition calendar showing daily needs for a professional player

Day	MD-4	MD-3	MD-2	MD-1	MD	MD+1	MD+2
Main activity	Intense training	Moderate training	Intense training	Light training	Match play	Recovery	Light training
Energy (kcal)	3,300	3,000	3,300	2,800	3,500	2,500	2,800
Carbohydrate (g/kg BM)	6.0	5.5	6.0	6.5	7.5	6.0	5.7
Carbohydrate (g)	440	405	440	488	562	453	430
Carbohydrate (%EI)	53	54	53	70	64	72	61
Protein (g/kg BM)	1.8	1.6	1.8	1.4	1.8	1.4	1.5
Protein (g)	135	120	135	105	135	105	113
Protein (%EI)	16.4	16.0	16.4	15.0	15.4	16.8	16.1
Fat (g/kg BM)	1.5	1.3	1.5	0.6	1.0	0.4	0.9
Fat (g)	110	100	110	48	78	30	70
Fat (%EI)	30	30	30	15	20	11	22

MD = match day. %EI = percentage of total daily dietary energy intake. g/kg BM = grams per kilogram body mass. The daily energy expenditure and amounts of carbohydrate, protein and fat are based on a player weighing 75 kg and playing a full match on one day per week with weekly energy intake sufficient to match weekly energy expenditure.

science. I have authored several books on the biochemistry of exercise and training, immune function in sport and exercise, nutrition for sport, a trilogy of healthy lifestyle guidebooks and contributed chapters to more than 30 other books. I have published over 250 research papers in scientific and medical journals, and much of this was focused on the well-being of athletes, including footballers, and the factors influencing their performance.

My longstanding interest in football began when my father took me to watch my first live match in 1961. It was at Boundary Park, home of Oldham Athletic, my hometown team that I have supported ever since. I was only five years old and would not have been able to see anything with the supporters standing all around us, but my dad perched me on his shoulders and as he was 6 ft 4 in (1.93 m) tall I probably had the best view in the ground! Oldham beat Mansfield Town 3–1 that day and I was hooked. I have loved the game from that day onwards. Oldham may not be the most fashionable or successful team in England, but in my lifetime, they have had their moments including beating the likes of Manchester United, Liverpool and Chelsea when, for a few years in the early 1990s, they made it into the Premier League. Currently they are back in the same division as when I saw them first play; so is Mansfield Town.

Many of my former university students now work in sport science support roles at major football clubs including several in the English Premier League and the North American Major Soccer League (MLS). I occasionally provide nutrition advice to Leicester City FC, who became the Premier League Champions in 2016 as 5,000–1 outsiders and won the FA Cup for the first time in their history in 2021. Leicester is the other team I support, having lived not far from the city for the past 35 years. Plus, Matt Reeves, who is the Head of Fitness and Conditioning at the club, is a past student and a friend of mine.

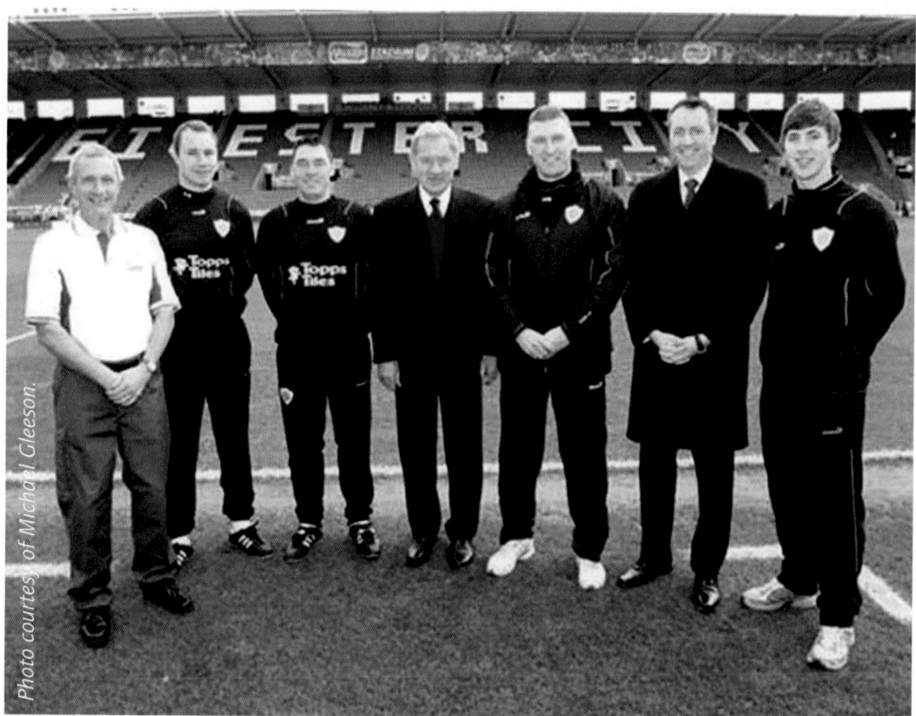

Photo 1.2 The author (far left) with members of the Leicester City FC team support and management staff at the King Power Stadium in 2009. A very young Matt Reeves is on the far right.

WHAT IS DIFFERENT ABOUT THIS BOOK?

This book is unique as it provides useful and (hopefully) interesting information about what footballers eat and drink and – more importantly – explains what they are recommended to eat and drink (and when) by football nutrition experts. This information is based on the 'UEFA expert group statement on nutrition in elite football', which was first published online in October 2020 in the *British Journal of Sports Medicine*. The authors of the paper were experts in applied sports nutrition research as well as practitioners working with elite clubs and national associations and were asked to issue a statement on a range of topics highly relevant to elite football nutrition. These topics included match-day nutrition (e.g. what to eat and drink on match day), training nutrition (e.g. what to eat and drink on training days), body composition (e.g. what is the desired body composition of a player and how it can be changed), stressful environments and travel (e.g. the influence of playing in the heat or cold or at altitude as well as long-distance travel challenges), cultural diversity and dietary differences (e.g. the implications of things like Ramadan and vegan diets), dietary supplements (e.g. which supplements might improve performance or training adaptation), rehabilitation (e.g. what can be done to optimise the rehabilitation from injury process and accelerate return to play), the specific nutritional needs of referees and junior high-level players and differences between the needs of elite male and female players (figure 1.3). I contributed to the writing and editing of this landmark paper – the first one of its kind since 2006 – but I have attempted to explain it all in simpler terms in this book – at least in a way that any reasonably intelligent person can understand.

As well as giving evidence-based guidelines to optimise football performance through appropriate nutrition, the book also provides some amusing anecdotes about the history of football nutrition, comments from people that I have worked with in the professional game, and some of the obscure, and even absurd, food and beverage choices that professional footballers have made over the years, including right up to the present day. It also provides numerous meal plans and recipes to allow anyone to emulate exactly what the professional players are eating.

Football nowadays is a truly global game that is constantly evolving. Over the past decade, there have been substantial increases in the physical and technical demands of match play. Now, players do more high-intensity actions, more sprinting and more tracking back. Some teams adopt what is called a pressing style of play, meaning the forwards and attacking midfielders, in particular, are expected to put pressure on opposition defenders who have the ball in an attempt to regain possession while still in the attacking third of the pitch. This, of course, requires more running and tackling from those attacking players. In order to cope with these increased demands, teams' training

JUNIOR HIGH-LEVEL PLAYERS
MATCH-DAY NUTRITION
REFEREES
UEFA
TRAINING NUTRITION
REHABILITATION
BODY COMPOSITION
DIETARY SUPPLEMENTS
ENVIRONMENT AND TRAVEL
CULTURE

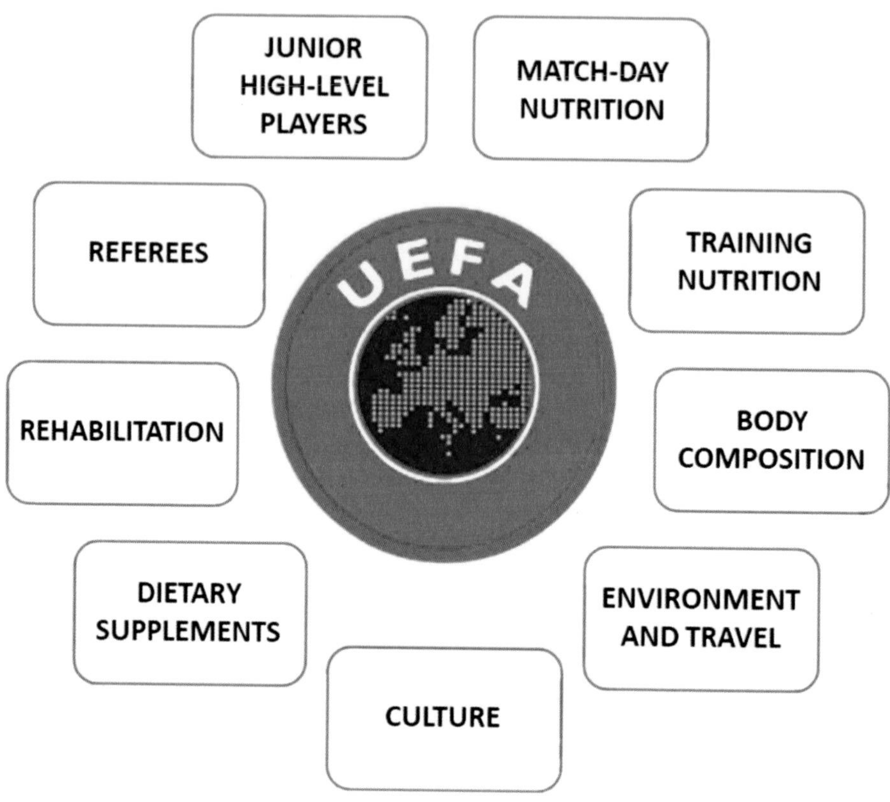

Figure 1.3 Nutrition-related aspects of football that were considered in the '2020 UEFA Expert Group Statement on Nutrition in Elite Football' by Collins et al. (2021).

regimens have become more multidimensional, in an attempt to prepare players optimally to cope with such evolutions and to address individual player needs. As part of this multidimensional approach, nutrition can play a valuable integrated role in optimising the performance of elite players during training and match play, and in maintaining their overall health throughout a long season. An evidence-based approach to nutrition that emphasises, a 'food first' philosophy (i.e. prioritising food over supplements to meet nutrient requirements) is fundamental to ensure effective player support. This requires relevant scientific evidence to be applied according to the constraints of what is practical and feasible in the football setting.

There is obviously little opportunity for nutrition during actual match play, and this is usually limited to taking a drink during breaks in play when a player is being treated for an injury by the physio on the pitch or when a substitution is being made. But what a player eats and drinks before a match, during the half-time interval and after a match can have important consequences for their match performance and subsequent recovery. The science underpinning sports nutrition is evolving at a fast pace, and practitioners must be alert to new developments. Knowing what the top professional players are doing in terms of their nutrition can help amateur players improve their own performance. To understand and apply the principles of sport nutrition in football, some basic understanding of nutrition is necessary, as is some fundamental knowledge of metabolism and the physiological and technical demands of the game itself. The first few chapters of the book provide all this basic background information.

The book provides the very latest comprehensive information on nutrition guidelines for professional players. The needs of adolescent and female players, as well as match officials, are also covered. Relevant issues such as eating and drinking during travel, food hygiene and the influence of cultural and religious beliefs are also considered. Most of these issues are also very relevant to the amateur player who wants to be able to perform to the best of their ability. People who engage in similar team sports to football in terms of physical, energy and mental demands, such as rugby, hockey, basketball and netball can also benefit from the information about nutrition provided in this book. The book contains numerous tables and figures that are used to illustrate important data and information. At the end of each chapter, there is an infographic that summarises the most important take-home messages from the chapter. The final chapter provides some example meal plans and snacks for training days and match days. For this final chapter of the book, I am joined by two of the best performance chefs in the world, Rachel Muse and Bruno Cirillo, who prepare meals for several English Premier League and Danish Superliga players, respectively.

A BRIEF HISTORY OF NUTRITION FOR FOOTBALL

Football was, for a long time, classed as just another endurance sport akin to long-distance running or cycling largely because a football match lasted at least 90 minutes. Therefore, 30 years ago, much of our understanding of the nutritional requirements of football players was simply extrapolated from early scientific research carried out in relation to these other endurance sports. However, the training loads associated with these sports are vastly different from those in football. A closer inspection of the energy demands makes it abundantly clear that daily energy expenditure of professional football players may not be particularly high compared with, for example, an athlete training for a marathon race or an elite cyclist training for the Tour de France. Football players are generally pretty inactive when not directly involved in match play or training, and their training load will vary depending on factors such as the stage of the season, or whether tactical or fitness drills predominate in training.

Professor Ron Maughan, a colleague and friend of mine, who worked at the University of Aberdeen, was the first British scientist to assess the dietary intakes of top professional footballers. In 1997, he managed to get 51 players from two Scottish Premier League clubs to perform seven-day weighed food intakes and found their average daily energy intake to be approximately 2,840 kcal, which was considerably lower than the reported intakes of most other endurance athletes, which were typically 3,500–5,500 kcal/day. If football players were to consume 7–10 g of carbohydrate per kilogram (kg) body mass each day (a common recommendation both then and now for athletes in endurance sports) then a quick calculation that included reasonable amounts of protein and fat would generate a daily energy intake closer to 4,200 kcal. Clearly, the early dietary recommendations for professional football players had been slightly misjudged. One potential problem is that this dietary energy excess would likely lead to weight gain if maintained for more than a month or two. That could be one of the reasons why you can remember (if you are over 40 years of age) that prior to the 1980s there were a few seemingly somewhat overweight players in your favourite team. Another reason was that players were generally less fit, the game was played at a less frantic pace, and most players were ignorant of the need for good nutrition.

When finally the importance of nutrition for performance in football was actually properly recognised, a number of other problems developed and persisted in the delivery of nutritional support in football. In many teams, the responsibility of implementing a nutritional support strategy was given to the strength and conditioning coach, physiotherapist or sport scientist. From the early 1990s, football started to attempt to apply scientific analytical techniques, and experts employed by clubs tended to adopt a 'measure everything' approach, in part because they didn't want to be seen to be missing anything of potential importance, but also because nobody at the time actually knew what was most important. Hence, blood, saliva, urine, sweat and expired air were all being indiscriminately extracted from players, often with very little feedback offered in return. In the world of nutrition and football, at first, science was calling the shots, although in a rather haphazard way, until a more discriminatory approach was adopted, discarding what was found to be not useful and a better understanding was gained of what really needed to be known.

Nowadays, football has caught up with science and now dictates where most efforts are directed. For example, rather than just recommending a high-carbohydrate, low-fat diet with sufficient protein and micronutrients all the time, emphasis is now placed more on achieving optimum carbohydrate intake before matches, and during the recovery period after matches, particularly when some clubs find themselves involved in up to three games per week in the busiest parts of the season. The importance of the amount, timing and quality of protein consumed on training adaptation and recovery is now recognised, as are the roles of certain micronutrients, such as vitamin D and iron, and the potential value of performance-enhancing dietary supplements, such as creatine, caffeine and nitrate. The role of the sport nutritionist in professional football is now seen as one of manipulating carbohydrate, protein, fat, fibre, fluid and micronutrient intake through diet, and the occasional use of supplements to maintain health, promote adaptation to training, speed recovery and ultimately enhance performance or at least help to maintain performance over the course of a season. Also, a more personalised approach to nutrition advice for individual players has been adopted rather than a 'one-size-fits-all' strategy.

It has taken rather a long time for good nutrition to be accepted in professional football, and one of the main reasons is that the game is steeped in tradition, with many coaches and support staff employed from within who have not been educated in sport science or nutrition and have not taken on what other sports have been doing. Having mentioned that, it is also true that these people know the sport and its peculiarities better than anyone. Furthermore, the practice of employment from within, and improved coach education in tandem with the recruitment of expert nutritionists to the support staff of professional clubs, has spawned a new breed of coaches that now have a far better understanding of the value of sport nutrition.

Another issue has been the power of the players and the desire of managers, coaches and support staff to try to keep them happy at all times, or at least most of the time. However, letting players eat and drink what they want, when they want, is not usually the best strategy to achieve their best performance on the pitch. Given a choice, many players would choose to eat fish and chips, pies, burgers, hot dogs or pizza after a game (no doubt washed down with a few beers), and only 20 to 30 years ago it would not be unusual to see a team bus parked outside a fish and chip shop or even a pub when travelling home on the coach from an away match! Before a match, many players opted for some crisps and chocolate an hour or two before kick-off rather than a nutritious, high-carbohydrate meal a little earlier than that. When Arsène Wenger arrived in England in 1996 he was alarmed at the diet – or more accurately, the lack of any scientifically-led, performance-enhancing diet – among his Arsenal players. Wenger banned chocolate immediately, causing several senior members of the squad to bristle with resentment. He recalls the resistance en route to his first game: 'We were travelling to Blackburn and the players were at the back of the bus chanting: "We want our Mars bars!"' Now, some 25 years later, the landscape has changed dramatically in English football. Clubs now provide detailed nutritional advice to their players, with pretty much all top clubs employing their own full-time nutritionists and chefs. The same is true of other top clubs in Europe and in the MLS. Many elite players now employ their own personal performance chefs to prepare and cook their food when they are at home (i.e. on their days off and for evening meals on training days).

In the past, nutritional support was brought in as and when needed, rather than being a service that was required on a day-to-day basis, but the modern attitude is to take a more holistic approach and be open to anything that can be done – nutritionally or otherwise – to help players from both a performance and recovery perspective. Nowadays, players are so much more receptive and open-minded than they used to be, and they have come to realise what an impact good nutrition can have on their performance, recovery and injury/ illness prevention, and will act upon it accordingly. Eating together has always been an important part of bonding as a team. To quote Arsène Wenger again: 'Previously food was provided at the training ground and players were educated on how to eat at home. We are now witnessing clubs managing every aspect of nutrition, such as preparation of meals, and the use of chefs to deliver club guidelines, away from the training ground.'

The technology available to nutritionists has also improved, with everything from heart rate, distance covered in training (using GPS devices), body mass and body-fat percentages checked and monitored on a regular basis. There are even occasional blood tests on the players that can help to detect deficiencies in certain nutrients such as iron or vitamin D, and which can be used as a basis to target a correctional nutrition intervention by modifying the diet or providing supplements. The role of the nutritionist has also become more complex as professional clubs now have more players from all over the world. Not only does the nutritionist have to understand the technical side of their subject area, but also the foods, culture and religious practices that influence individual player food preferences in order to build trust and work effectively with players of different nationalities.

Educating all the players themselves is key to the successful implementation of desired nutritional strategies, and the nutritionist has the important role of engaging all players and taking them on a journey to understand the use of food for fuel, performance, recovery and overall health. This will include advising not only the current first team squad but also the under-23 squad, youth players within the academy and all new signings. Some players know quite a lot about nutrition and the macronutrient contents of different foods but it is probably true to say that most do not, so even relatively simple terms such as 'legume' need to be explained to them. I was told by a club nutritionist that one player (whom I will not name to avoid embarrassing him) was asked if he knew what a legume was. He said he did not have a clue, so the nutritionist asked him if he knew the difference between a parsnip and a chickpea. After a little thought, the player laughed and replied 'Not really but I know I would not pay £200 to have a parsnip on my face'. A little crude, I know, but I assume you get the point.

In the past – and we are only talking about 25–30 years ago – players ate just to satisfy their hunger and remain weight stable. Now, after just a few decades of the application of science in professional football, we know that what a player eats before, during and after training or a competitive match can have huge implications on how they perform, how they recover and how they feel. That is why, in modern-day football, nutrition is no longer overlooked or viewed as just a treatment or basic necessity but very much as a performance and recovery enhancer.

Other advances in nutrition provision and means of influencing players' food choices have been introduced in recent years. As James Collins, lead author of the UEFA expert group statement on nutrition in elite football and former head nutritionist at Arsenal FC explains: 'We used to have a lot of information on the walls. We've moved away from that because the messages became like wallpaper and they weren't changing the players' behaviour. Today, whether downstairs in the changing room or upstairs in the restaurant, we believe in simple signposting. In the restaurants we may use colour-coded containers for the proteins, carbohydrates, healthy fats and vegetables. We also look at the flow and set up easy access around restaurants so that food is labelled and the players can build their plates. The priority now is to send digital information direct to their mobile phones. Their physical activity loading changes from day to day, so what we're asking them to eat on each day must also change as well. We can send them their plans and supporting educational information about their nutrition for the day. The engagement is far higher.'

At some of the top clubs in Europe, nutrition provision for players has gone beyond even this to the next level as Sam Erith, head of sport science at Manchester City FC has revealed: 'Nutrition has taken huge steps forward for us in recent years; we now employ full-time nutritionists. Their role is so much more practically based, with presence at all meals offering advice to players in the here and now rather than just more "clinical" reviews periodically. The food has also become incredibly more adventurous and tasty! Very different to the days of pasta, chicken and tomato sauce!' This reflects the increasing involvement of the performance chef, a person who is expert in cookery and who has a good understanding of nutrition, who can provide delicious meals for players that are tailored to the nutritionist's plans for daily energy and macronutrient intakes for individual players while at the same time taking on board each player's personal food preferences.

THE ROLE OF THE PERFORMANCE CHEF

Some players have now taken to hiring their own personal chefs. Matt Reeves is a key member of the sport science support team at Leicester City FC and liaises with the club's nutritionist, the medical staff and performance chefs to ensure that players get the nutrition that is right for them. He recently told me 'Clearly in the last five to ten years there has been a big shift in the nutritional mindset within the professional game, with players focused not just on what they eat but how food is prepared. In the past couple of years, we have seen more players investing their money in having a private chef at home which reflects the importance they place on fuelling and recovering appropriately.' Harry Kane, the Tottenham Hotspur and England striker (who also had a loan spell at Leicester in his younger days) started working with his own chef a few years ago. A newspaper article in 2017 quoted him as saying 'It kind of clicked in my head that a football career is so short. It goes so quickly, you have to make every day count. I have a chef at home to eat the right food, helping recovery. You can't train as hard as you'd like when you have so many games, so you have to make the little gains elsewhere, like with food. He's there every day, Monday to Saturday, and leaves it in the fridge for Sunday. I hardly ever see him because I'm at training, but he'll cook the food and leave it in the fridge. We've got a good plan going.'

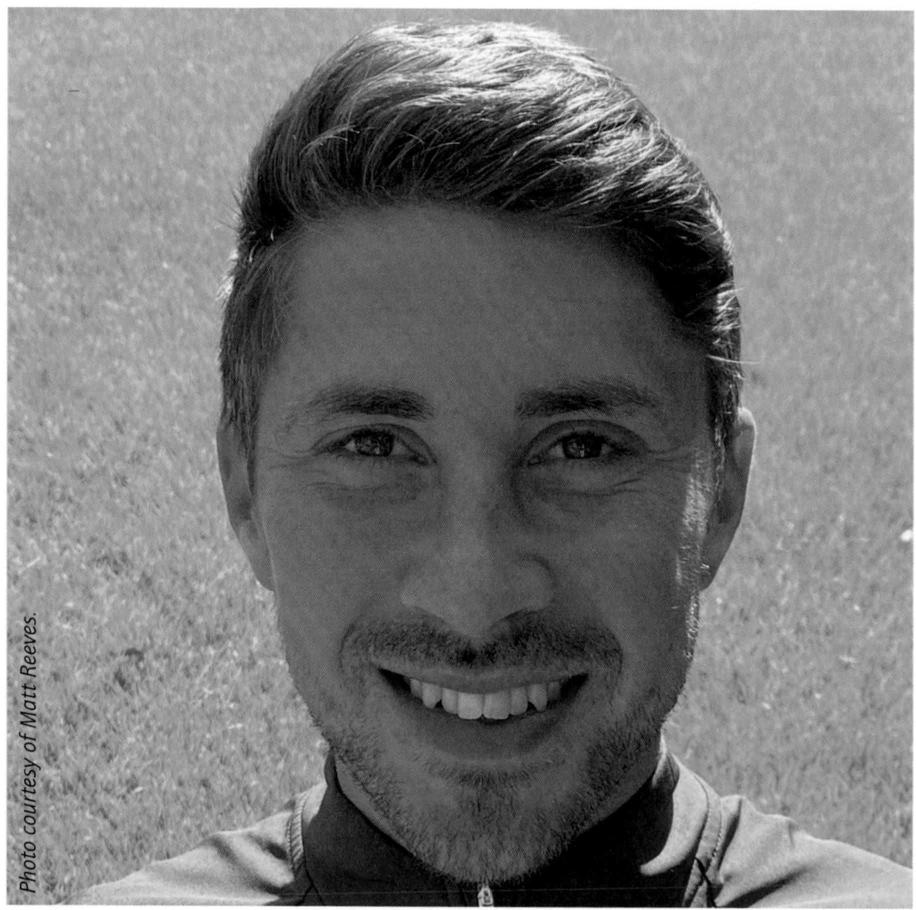
Photo courtesy of Matt Reeves.

Photo 1.3 Matt Reeves, head of fitness and conditioning at Leicester City, liaises with the club's nutritionist, the medical staff and performance chefs to ensure that the players in the first team squad get the nutrition that is right for them.

Having a personal chef is commonplace among top players now, and several businesses have developed to help arrange and manage this union of footballers and expert cooks. The chefs will usually liaise closely with the club nutritionist to ensure menus are tailored specifically towards the players' requirements and tastes. Nutritional advice will differ depending on the individual player's age, metabolism, position, training or recovery demands, as well as their cultural background and food preferences. Chefs need to be able to prepare a variety of menus suitable for a Mediterranean, Scandinavian, African, Asian or South American diet, as well as English or Scottish ones. Sometimes chefs may cook in the players' homes, but more often the meals will be prepared for the week ahead and then be delivered all over the country to the players.

Rachel Muse is one of the top performance chefs in the world, and she cooks meals for many English Premier League players. Here she shares her experience of working with club nutritionists and the players themselves: 'As a private performance chef my team and I cook for one particular player (and their family or the friends they live with) in their own home. On training days, the football club provides breakfast and lunch (plus snacks) at the club's training ground. On match days the club will provide a pre-match meal for their players. In my experience all Premier League clubs take nutrition seriously, they all have an individual who is responsible for nutrition, either a member of the in-house team or a consultant. The club will have great kitchens with knowledgeable chefs who, together with the nutritionist, design menus. The food provided on training days and match days is always fresh, colourful and packed with nutrition. At the training ground food and nutrition are treated seriously and the player has no choice but to eat well. However, outside of the training ground players are left to their own devices when it comes to nutrition. A player will be given guidance by the club's nutritionist for the food that should be eaten when the player isn't being catered for by the club. However, the player may not understand this information, may not have the cooking skills to follow the advice or may simply not be interested in following the guidance. This is where a private performance chef steps in.'

Now Rachel explains how she interacts with the club nutritionist and the player to come up with suitable meals that the player will enjoy. After all, eating good food is part of the enjoyment of life and there is no point in preparing a wonderfully nutritious meal if it is made with some foods that the player does not like. The chef wants the player to really enjoy their food and eat everything that is served on the plate to achieve the nutrition goals provided by the nutritionist. She continues: 'When I work with a player, I will first receive instructions from the player's nutritionist. The nutritionist is almost always employed by the club the player is currently playing for. Very occasionally the player will use the nutritionist they have worked with before arriving at their current club. On the rare occasions this happens, the current club agrees that the player should continue to use the advice from the previous nutritionist. My belief is that it is a personal

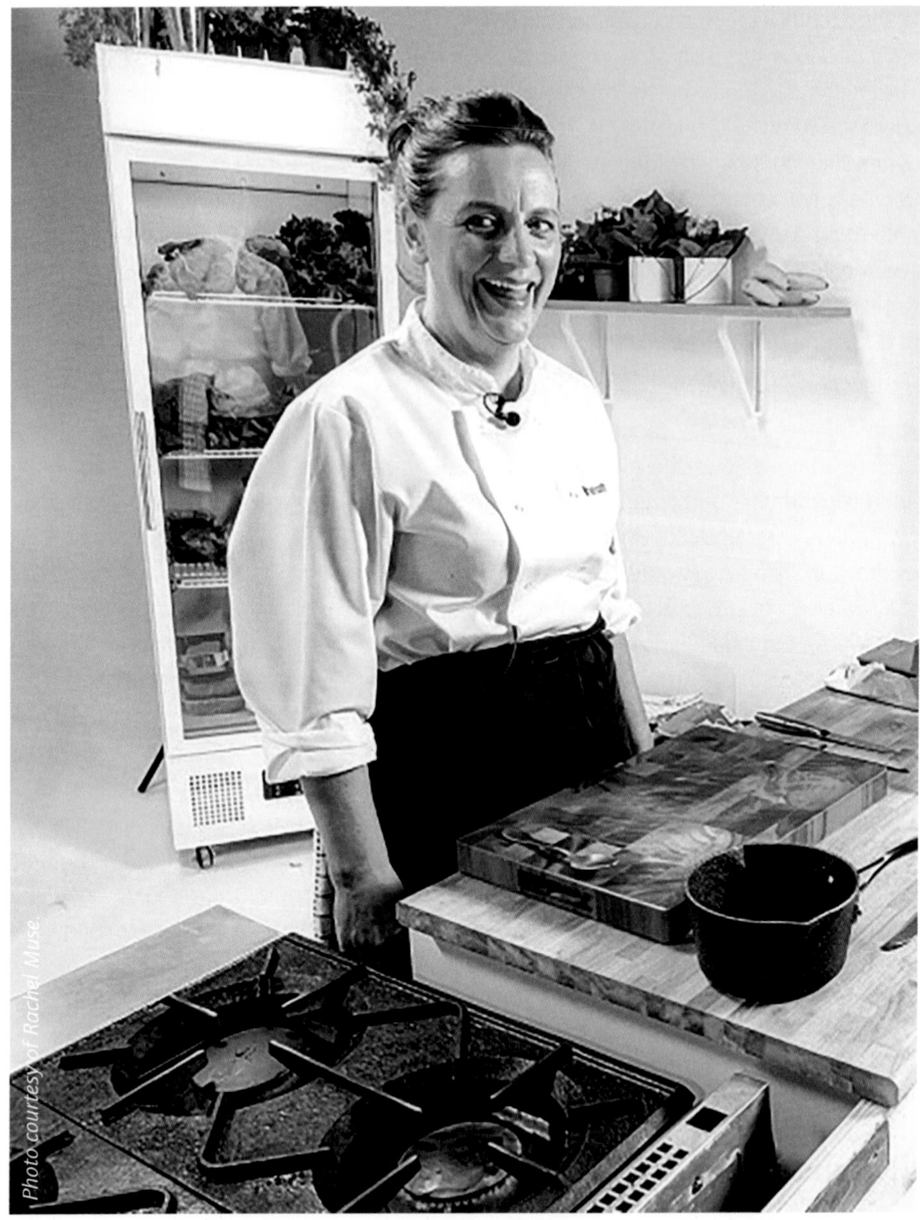

Photo 1.4 Rachel Muse is one of the top performance chefs in the world, and she cooks meals for many English Premier League players. She runs a business that provides well-trained performance chefs for many professional players in the UK.

preference based on a cultural tie or a language tie that keeps the player attached to their previous nutritionist. When I talk to the nutritionist, I will receive the nutritional advice for the individual player and I'll ask about body composition. What are the targets for the individual player? The player will know exactly what the nutritionist has told me and will often be present when this happens: either at a face-to-face meeting or a three-way telephone call. We are all working together towards the common goal of a happy, well-fuelled, relaxed player. We (nutritionist, private chef and player) all need to know exactly the same things about the player's diet and be able to communicate clearly within this group. So it begins with the club nutritionist (in the presence of the player) giving the performance chef the body composition target and the daily macronutrients required to achieve that target. The performance chef asks about anything that's unclear or they don't understand.'

Note that when Rachel mentions 'body composition targets' she does not simply mean body weight or percentage body fat. Nutrition requirements for evening meals will depend on many factors including the player's body size and the physical demands of training on that particular day and whether the food to be consumed is intended for match preparation or recovery from a hard training session. The main purpose of the meals is to provide the desired macronutrients (i.e. carbohydrate, protein and fat) and usually the nutritionist will give the chef a simple list of the number of grams of carbohydrate, protein and fat a player should be eating for their evening meal. If the protein is given as 30 g then that is the actual amount of protein in the protein source (meat, fish, beans, tofu, etc.), not the weight of the protein source. So for example, 30 g of protein would be found in 100 g of chicken, 100 g of lean beef, 150 g of sea bass, 185 g of tofu or 330 g of chickpeas. These macronutrients, specifically designed by the nutritionist to achieve the target for the individual, can potentially be 'built' into thousands of different meals, so it may as well be the meal the player actually wants to eat for their dinner that evening. That is just what Rachel does: she asks the player what they would like to eat. This can become an interesting discussion as she explains: 'Often the player doesn't have a great knowledge of cuisine and their vocabulary for describing food is somewhat limited. That's absolutely fine, we can always find a way to communicate. The player might take photos of things they have liked eating in the past or show things they have seen on social media that they would like to try. Or a player may mention foods from their childhood that the chef isn't familiar with. In that case the chef "googles" the food the player has mentioned, and then shows what they have found to the player. When the exact childhood dish has been found, the chef works out how to cook that particular meal in a way that will provide the desired macronutrient content. The chef can then write the menu. The next steps are to shop, prepare and cook the food for the menu. The food must always be "built" accordingly the nutritionist's instructions. This invariably involves "monkeying" with the ingredients and how the dish would be cooked if nutrition (the macronutrients) were not a vital element of the food.'

DEMONS AND WIZARDS

From a nutritional perspective, undoubtedly the biggest 'demon' for footballers is drinking alcohol. Older readers will no doubt recall the issues with alcohol that have blighted the career and health of some of the world's top players including George Best, Paul Gascoigne, Tony Adams and Paul Merson. For a long time, and indeed right up to the present day, alcohol has been part of the fabric of football culture: having a drink after a match with teammates, parties at Christmas, birthday and wedding celebrations, with family or friends, relaxing on days off or on pre-season tours. And we have all read some stories in the newspapers about players behaving badly on some occasions when they have had a few too many drinks.

Other potential nutrition-related 'demons' are contaminated dietary supplements, which if ingested by players can lead to a positive doping test and a lengthy ban from playing in competitive fixtures; another is taking orally administered psychoactive recreational drugs or substances (i.e. chemicals that alter brain function to produce temporary changes in perception, mood, consciousness or behaviour). Some examples include snus (a form of oral chewing tobacco), cannabis cakes, ecstasy, psilocybin and amphetamines. Some of these can lead to a doping violation as well as being damaging to dental and mental health.

Another nutrition-related 'demon' that players and support staff need to be aware of is poor food hygiene that can result in 'food poisoning' (in other words a bacterial infection of the gut), which can result in symptoms such as nausea, abdominal pain and diarrhoea, which could impair players' performance or even prevent them from playing. Some of these issues will be revisited in the later chapters of this book. Of course, there can be other 'demons' in a player's life that can affect their physical and mental health, or both, including smoking tobacco products or marijuana, inhaling nitrous oxide, insufflating (snorting) drugs such as cocaine and addiction to gambling, but these are beyond the scope of this book.

The wizards, from a nutritional perspective, are the managers who first had the foresight and intelligence to understand the importance of what players eat and drink and the effect it could have on their performance, and proactively did something about it. I am thinking of past managers like Arsène Wenger at Arsenal and Sir Alex Ferguson at Aberdeen and Manchester United.

Ferguson was one of the first top managers to employ a full-time nutritionist when Trevor Lea was appointed to the Manchester United support staff in 1992. One of the first things Lea did was to confiscate the custard creams, bourbons and chocolate digestives that were staple favourites of the players. He replaced those biscuits with jaffa cakes which have a light spongy base with an orange-flavoured jelly above that is covered in thin layer of dark chocolate. Each 12.2 g jaffa cake contains around 46 kcal, 8.5 g of carbohydrate, 1.0 g of fat and 0.6 g of protein. According to Brian McClair, the Scottish forward who was one of Ferguson's first major signings in 1987, the squad were ordered to eat 'five jaffas on training days and three before games', meaning players consumed 230 kcal before training and 138 kcal before games with 75% of the energy content from carbohydrate. Lea later weaned the players onto other high-carbohydrate foods before training and matches and recommended meals such as cereal and milk, spaghetti or baked beans on toasted granary bread, cottage pie (oven-baked, low-fat beef mince with a mashed potato topping, apparently a real favourite of Wayne Rooney) or light pasta dishes with salmon or chicken. These dietary changes he introduced seemed to work for United's players, as they went on to win 13 Premier League titles, four FA Cups, four League Cups, two Champions Leagues, and the FIFA Club World Cup under Ferguson from 1992.

Other wizards worthy of mention are the scientists who pioneered the first experimental and observational studies on the physiological demands of football match play, the impact of hydration, diet and supplements on player performance, and the prevailing nutritional choices of elite footballers. These scientists also often worked with athletes and games players in other sports (e.g. athletics, marathon running, cycling, American football) and were mostly academics working in British, European and North American universities in the 1970s, 80s and 90s whose research focused on human metabolism and nutrition in relation to exercise. They include Lawrence Armstrong, Jens Bangsbo, George Brooks, David Costill, Edward Coyle, Björn Ekblom, Paul Greenhaff, Mark Hargreaves, Eric Hultman, Don Maclaren, Ron Maughan, Tom Reilly, Bengt Saltin, Lawrence Spriet and Clyde Williams. These have been followed by others who have subsequently engaged in football-specific research and the importance of nutrition; notable examples include Graeme Close, Barry Drust, Asker Jeukendrup, Peter Krustrup, Magni Mohr, James Morton and Susan Shirreffs, to name just a few. I was lucky enough in my career to have met most of them and worked with some of them. You will find many journal papers that they have authored in the list of reference sources I have compiled at the end of this book.

In addition, of course, there are the nutritionists who work with the players at professional football clubs. James Collins has recently summarised their important role as follows: 'Fundamentally, the nutritionist determines the overall sports nutrition philosophy at the club, which supports the club's training and performance outcomes. From a team perspective, nutrition strategy encompasses match or training day preparation and recovery, hydration, body composition, travel, food service and supplementation. On an individual level the sports nutritionist consults with players, working to shape their diet to support their health and performance. Primarily, this involves educating and up-skilling players to understand the science behind their dietary strategies (for example, the timing, type and quantity of food). As part of the ongoing support with players, effective monitoring of outcomes of dietary status is crucial. This is because any ongoing issues in these areas such as nutrient status, recovery, body composition and hydration can negatively impact a player's training adaptation or match performance.' To this end, *Nutrition for Top Performance in Football* aims to provide the reader with an insight into how sports nutrition is used to improve football performance in the professional game. But first let me finish this chapter by letting you in on some of the more unusual food choices that some players have made.

SOME OF THE MORE SURPRISING NUTRITION CHOICES PLAYERS HAVE MADE

Footballers, of course, are people and like many other people they have their own particular likes and dislikes when it comes to food and drink. Often, their food choices may not make the best sense nutritionally speaking, but many will stick with a certain routine, particularly in the last meal or two they may consume before playing a match. For example, Alan Shearer, the centre-forward who played for Southampton, Blackburn, Newcastle and England from 1988 to 2006 had a favourite pre-match meal of chicken and beans. This would not be considered a particularly good choice nowadays as his meal did not contain much carbohydrate, but at the time it did not seem to do him any harm as he scored an average of a goal every other game. In the 1980s and 90s, not many other players paid much attention to their diet so it was a pretty even playing field in that sense in those days.

Another prolific goal-scoring striker, Jamie Vardy of Leicester City and England writes in his 2016 biography *From Nowhere, My Story* that in his nonleague playing days he did not worry too much about what he was eating and drinking, and that fast food (burgers, fried chicken etc.) was part of his staple diet, even as a pre-match meal for weekday evening games. Partly this was due to his circumstances – he worked at a factory during the day – he just needed to get some food eaten quickly after work, which would only be a couple of hours before kick-off. Indeed, that situation may sound familiar to many other current amateur footballers. When he moved to Fleetwood Town FC, a nonleague club with big ambitions to get into the Football League, and started being a full-time player with daily training, he took to drinking three cans of Monster Energy drink every day. When he got his big-money move to Leicester City in 2012, his pre-match nutrition habits did not change that much. He didn't eat breakfast but drank a can of Red Bull just after waking up; his pre-match meal (eaten at 11:30am for a 3:00pm kick-off) consisted of cheese and ham omelette with baked beans, washed down with another Red Bull. A little later after arriving at the stadium, he would have a double espresso coffee. When he got into the dressing room at the King Power Stadium, he opened his third can of Red Bull and sipped it until it was time to go out on the pitch for the warm-up. So now you know it's all that caffeine that helps him to 'run around like a nutjob on match day'; his words, not mine! Well, this routine still seems to work for him as he won the English Premier League title with Leicester in 2015/16 and was the league's leading goal scorer in 2019/20.

James Sinclair, who has only recently retired after playing professional football for 17 years in several countries and on continents around the world (his last club was Swedish Division 1 side Oskarshamns) and is also a qualified sport nutritionist, told me about a nutritional strategy that he began by chance. He was feeling hungry on the night before a big match and ended up buying a large (600 g) bag of pick 'n mix candy and ate the whole bagful while watching a movie. At the match the next day, he said he 'felt amazing' and could have played another game straight after! James felt that he had gears six and seven in his engine, whilst everybody else in the game faded away, which he attributed to the large amount of the carbohydrate in the candy he consumed. He tried the same routine for the next couple of games and got the same result and not too surprisingly half the players in his team started the same routine! Although this 'diet' could not be recommended for more than one occasion per week it did supply him with a large amount (over 500 g, equivalent to more than 2,000 kcal) of carbohydrate. When it comes to decisions about what is the best nutrition for match-day performance of players in football, quite a lot of trial and error can be involved as every player will have different preferences, and what works for one player may not suit all of his or her teammates. Dele Alli, the Tottenham and England attacking midfielder is another player who likes his candy and always brings his own pick 'n mix sweets and dairy milk chocolate buttons for snacking on match days. He apparently has always enjoyed a McDonalds after a game and rarely eats the food provided to his teammates.

James also told me about another English player who played for Östersunds FK, in Sweden who was a very picky eater, one who couldn't or wouldn't eat any jam on his toast if it contained any bits of fruit (raspberry or strawberry), and insisted on essentially only eating the cheapest, most refined jam that you could buy. He had a similar issue with peas, which he would only eat as mushy or mashed, and he disliked any form of onion. During a meal out, if he had ordered spaghetti bolognese and it arrived at the table with some onion in it, he would pick out all the bits of onion.

A current South Korean national team player who, despite only being 5 ft 6 in tall, probably has the biggest appetite I have heard of in professional football. He basically had the same evening meal at home every night: essentially it consists of a large pack of Korean spicy ramen noodles, with a large bowl of steamed rice served with a couple of boiled eggs on top and a dolloping of hot Sriracha sauce (made from a paste of chilli peppers, distilled vinegar, garlic, sugar and salt) over the whole thing. All eaten whilst he played online computer gaming. For lunch, he had pretty much the same thing, plus a separate plate filled with just pan-fried chicken, sometimes up to four chicken breasts. With these meal choices, he was getting lots of carbohydrate and protein, but his diet was certainly lacking in fruit and vegetables, so was not the healthiest choice.

At LA Galaxy in the MLS, the players would always have cupcakes with the dinner meal the night before a game, and for Irish striker Robbie Keane's birthday and St Patrick's Day there would be special chocolate ones with green icing! Robbie always ate the same pre-match meal during his whole career: chicken with pasta, which is actually a very good choice.

Ashley Cole, who played for Arsenal and Chelsea and was considered to be one of the best full-backs to play for England, never had breakfast until he moved to the Italian club Roma late in his career where he enjoyed an Italian espresso and then started to incorporate a banana with a coffee when he moved to the MLS to play for LA Galaxy.

Finally, I will mention a tale I was told by a Premier League club nutritionist just a few years ago. A player came to him with a query about bulls' testicles. Apparently, he had been told by some of his fellow professionals that eating bulls' testicles would increase his testosterone and aggression and he wanted to know if this was true. The nutritionist, of course, recognised that the other players had been pulling his leg and informed the quizzical player that such a suggestion 'was pure bull-sh*t'.

THE IMPORTANCE OF NUTRITION

Fuelling

Match Performance

Recovery

Health

Training Adaptation

Sleep

Body Composition

Immune Function

Injury Risk

Cognitive Function

Hydration

Rehabilitation

Infographic 1 The importance of nutrition for a player's health and performance.

CHAPTER 2

Some Things You Need to Know About Nutrition and Nutrients

- What Are Nutrients?
- The Need for Energy
- The Major Classes of Nutrients

In order to understand how nutrition can influence football performance and recovery, it helps to know something about the different types of nutrients and the roles that they play in various bodily processes, including energy supply for exercise. That is what this chapter is all about and it should be particularly helpful to the reader who is not too familiar with the sources, properties and roles of various nutrients.

WHAT ARE NUTRIENTS?

Let's begin by learning exactly what nutrients are: a nutrient is a substance found in food that performs one or more specific functions in the body. Nutrients are usually divided into six different categories: carbohydrates, fats, proteins, vitamins, minerals and water. Functions of nutrients include promotion of growth and development, provision of energy and control of metabolism. Nutrition is often defined as the total of the processes of ingestion (eating and drinking), digestion (breaking down), absorption (moving nutrients from the gut into the blood) and metabolism (processing) of food, and the subsequent assimilation of nutrient materials into the tissues and organs. The energy we obtain from food is mainly supplied in the form of carbohydrates and fats. These are two of the macronutrients (nutrients that are ingested in relatively large – more than 10 g/day – quantities) in our diet; the other two macronutrients are protein and water (table 2.1). All other nutrients that are needed in quantities of less than 10 g/day are classed as micronutrients and they include vitamins, phytonutrients and minerals. All vitamins, and many minerals, are essential for health but are only needed in relatively small amounts; in fact, many are needed in only milligram quantities on a daily basis. Phytonutrients are not considered to be essential but they are needed if you want your health to be optimal – in other words as good as it can be.

THE NEED FOR ENERGY

Our bodies need to take in energy in the form of food regularly in order to be able to expend energy to do useful work, which includes muscle contractions to allow us to move, sending messages via nerves to allow us to sense changes, to react and think, or biosynthetic processes to produce new molecules and cells. Without an input of food energy, we would wither away and die. Energy is expressed in calories (the imperial system) or joules (the metric system). One calorie represents the quantity of heat energy needed to raise the temperature of 1 g (1 mL) of water by 1°C (1.8°F). Thus, food containing 1,000 calories (1 kcal) has enough energy potential to raise the temperature of 1 L of water by 1°C (1.8°F). In everyday language, kilocalories are often referred to as Calories (written with a capital C, although on many food items this is not done, and the energy is listed as calories). Because this may be a source of confusion, the term kilocalorie (abbreviated kcal) is used in this book. The SI (International System of Units) unit for energy is the joule (J), named after the British scientist Sir Prescott Joule (1818–1889). One joule of energy moves a mass of 1 g at a velocity of 1 metre per second (m/s). A joule is not a large amount of energy; therefore, kilojoules are more often used; one kilojoule (kJ) equals 1,000 joules. To convert calories to joules or kilocalories to kilojoules, the calorie value must be multiplied by 4.184. Nowadays, food packaging labels indicate the energy content in both kcal and kJ, but most people still talk in terms of calories although it really should be kcal.

THE MAJOR CLASSES OF NUTRIENTS

In the remainder of this chapter, I will briefly describe the characteristics, roles and sources of the major classes of nutrients. These include the macronutrients (carbohydrate, fat, protein and water), the essential micronutrients (vitamins, minerals and trace elements) and some of the nonessential nutrients including phytonutrients, dietary fibre and alcohol.

Table 2.1 The major classes of nutrients

Macronutrients	Subclasses	Examples	Food sources
Carbohydrate	Simple sugars	Glucose, fructose, sucrose	Fruit, soft drinks, sugars
	Starches	Amylose, amylopectin	Sweets, honey, vegetables, cereals,
	Fibre	Pectin, cellulose, lignin	Bread, corn, pasta, baked goods
Fat	Simple	Triglyceride	Fatty meats, poultry,
	Compound	Phospholipids, glycolipids	Oily fish, vegetable oils, nuts, avocado,
	Derived	Fatty acids, steroids, hydrocarbons	Egg yolk, dairy products
Protein	Complete	Most animal proteins	Animal products
	Incomplete	Several plant proteins	Some fruits, vegetables
Water			Tap water and bottled or canned beverages but also many natural foods including fruits, vegetables and lean meats are at least 50% water by weight
Micronutrients	**Subclasses**	**Examples**	**Food sources**
Vitamins	Water-soluble	C, B1-B9	Fruits, vegetables, animals
	Fat-soluble	A, D, E, K	Liver, eggs, dairy, fats, oils
Minerals	Macrominerals	Sodium, potassium, calcium, magnesium	Fruits, vegetables, animals
	Trace elements	Copper, iron, zinc	
Phytonutrients	Carotenoids	β-carotene, lycopene	Fruits and vegetables
	Flavonoids	Anthocyanins, catechins, flavones	

CARBOHYDRATES

Carbohydrates include sugars, starches and fibre, and we get almost all of our dietary carbohydrate from plants (photo 2.1). Carbohydrates provide 4 kcal of energy per gram (kcal/g) and they are the main source of energy for football match play and intense training. Common food sources of carbohydrate in the form of starch (a large molecule composed of many thousands of linked glucose molecules known as a polysaccharide) include cereal products, corn, potatoes, sweet potatoes, pasta, rice and bread. Sugars (also known as saccharides) are found in fruit juices, fruits, sweetened cereals, baked goods, candy, sweets, soft drinks, energy drinks, sports drinks, milk, beet and cane sugar, brown sugar, table sugar, maple syrup, honey and treacle. Also, many processed foods, including ready meals and sauces, tend to have high sugar content. Sugars in our diet include glucose, fructose, galactose, maltose, lactose and sucrose.

Fibre is another form of carbohydrate and much of it cannot be digested in the human gut so it has a much lower energy value than starches and sugars. Sources of fibre include whole-grain cereals and breads, oats, fruits, beans and peas, and other vegetables such as cabbage, courgette (zucchini), celery, spinach and salad leaves (photo 2.2). Fibre cannot

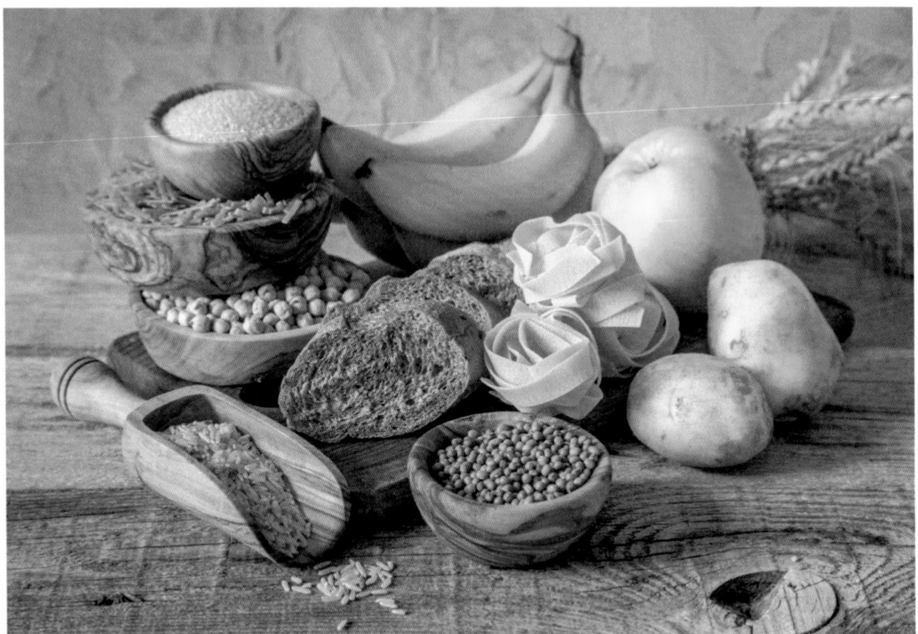

Photo 2.1 A variety of high-carbohydrate foods.

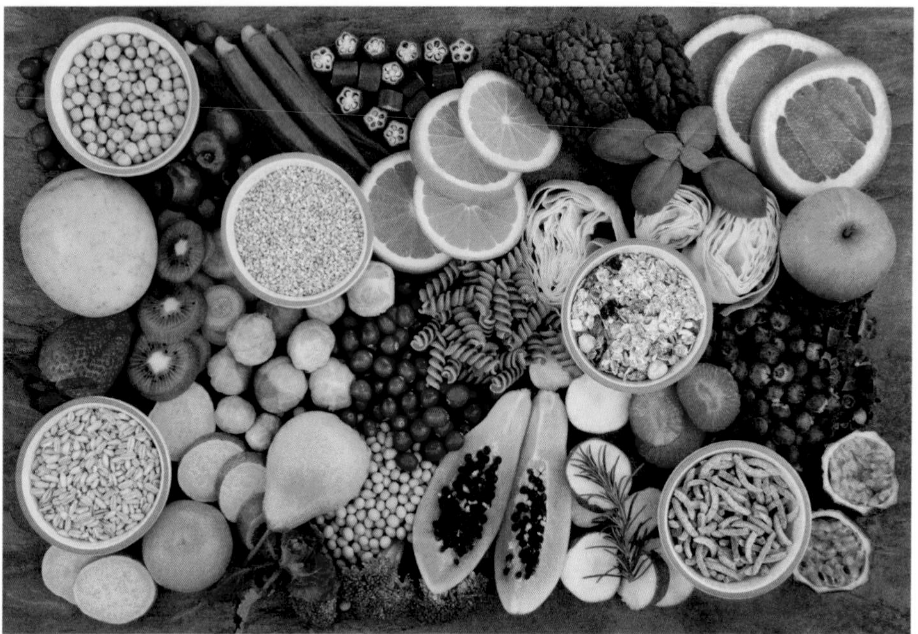

Photo 2.2 A variety of high-fibre foods.

be digested by enzymes in the human stomach and small intestine, and so it passes into the large intestine (colon) largely unchanged. In the large intestine, most soluble fibre (fibre that dissolves in water) can be broken down into sugars by the resident population of bacteria (in total there is about 1 kg of bacteria in our colon) known as the gut microbiota. The bacteria rapidly ferment these sugars to produce short-chain fatty acids such as butyric acid, which can be used as an energy source by both the bacteria themselves and the human cells that line the colon. Soluble fibre makes up about 70% of the fibre in our diet and has an energy value of about 1.5 kcal/g. Most insoluble fibres (e.g. cellulose and lignins that form the structure of plant cell walls) are not digested or fermented at all and are excreted unchanged in the faeces and hence have zero energy value to humans.

FATS

Fats, also known as lipids, are compounds that are soluble in organic liquids such as acetone, ether and chloroform but have very poor solubility in water. The term *lipid,* derived from the Greek word *lipos* (meaning fat), is a general name for oils, fats, waxes and related compounds. Oils are liquid at room temperature, whereas fats are solid. For simplicity, and to avoid confusion, the term 'fat' is used throughout this book. Fats provide more than twice the amount of energy as carbohydrates at 9 kcal/g and are an important energy source at rest and during light- to moderate-intensity exercise. Fat in the diet also aids the absorption of the four essential fat-soluble vitamins: A, D, E and K. There are several classes of fats, including fatty acids, triglycerides, lipoproteins, cholesterol and phospholipids. The latter are an important constituent of all cell membranes and intracellular organelles including the cell nucleus and mitochondria. Triglyceride (also known as triacylglycerol) is the main storage form of fat in the body and is also the most abundant form of dietary fat. If we consume more carbohydrate and fat than we need to meet our energy requirements, the excess is mostly stored as triglyceride in adipose tissue. Most sportspeople, including footballers, do not want too much of this in their body as it adds weight, which can slow a player down; however, some body fat is essential (about 3–5% of body mass for men and 10–12% for women). Most professional male outfield players have about 7–15% body fat. We'll look at the issue of body composition in more detail in chapter 8.

Common food sources of fat include fatty cuts of meat (e.g. beef, pork, lamb) and poultry (e.g. chicken, duck, turkey), animal liver, oily fish such as mackerel, salmon and sardines, egg yolk, cream, cheese, butter, margarine, oils, nuts and avocado (photos 2.3 and 2.4). Many processed foods including ready meals and creamy sauces, plus any foods cooked in oil such as French fries and fish in batter tend to be high in fat.

Triglycerides are made up of a glycerol molecule linked to three long-chain fatty acids. The chains are formed from repeating hydrocarbon units. Fatty acids can be either saturated (meaning they contain only single bonds between the carbon atoms in the

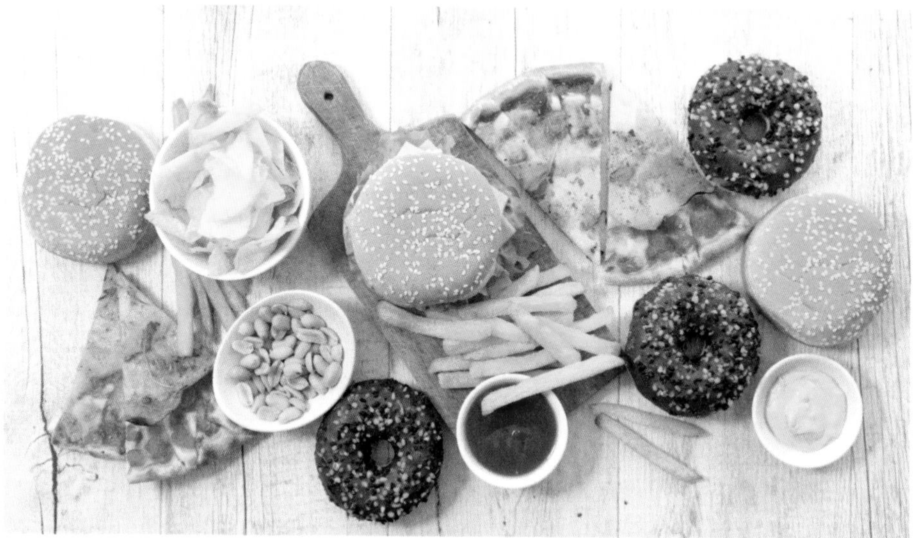

Photo 2.3 A variety of not-so-healthy high-fat foods (junk foods).

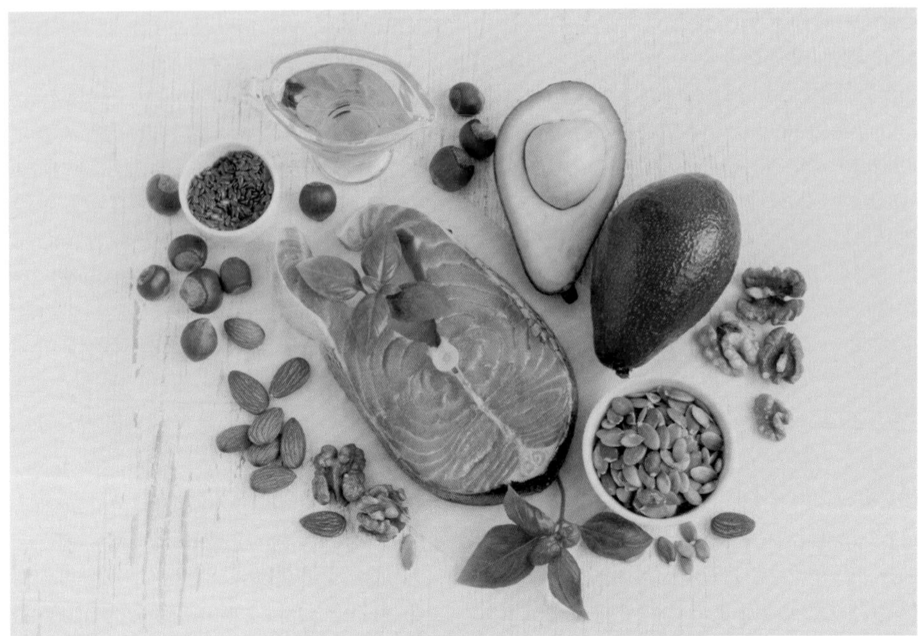

Photo 2.4 A variety of healthier sources of dietary fat.

chain) or unsaturated (meaning they contain at least one double bond between the carbon atoms in the chain). Monounsaturated fatty acids contain just one double bond in their hydrocarbon chain, whereas polyunsaturated fatty acids (PUFA), including omega-3 and omega-6 fatty acids, contain two or more double bonds. Two of the PUFAs, linoleic acid and alpha-linolenic acid, are essential nutrients for humans. The intake of monounsaturated fats and PUFAs should be prioritised as they support cognitive function, heart health and muscle recovery. Good food sources of PUFAs include oily fish like salmon, tuna and mackerel; vegetable oils like sunflower and rapeseed; and walnuts and seeds like flax, sunflower and chia. Soy products such as soy bean oil and tofu are also high in PUFAs. Olive oil and avocados are high in monounsaturated fats.

Saturated fat comes from animal products in our diet, whereas most of our unsaturated fat comes from plants. Saturated fat is considered to be less healthy than unsaturated fat and generally people are advised to have no more than 10% of their dietary energy in the form of saturated fat. Another form of fat that has harmful effects on health are trans fats which are found in some margarines and some products made using margarine such as biscuits, pastries, pies and some processed foods such as french fries. It is best to avoid trans fats altogether as they can raise harmful LDL cholesterol and cause inflammation.

PROTEINS

Proteins are composed of one or more chains of linked amino acids. Of the 20 amino acids normally found in dietary protein, humans can synthesise 11. Those that can be synthesised in the body are called nonessential amino acids. The nine amino acids that cannot be synthesised and must be derived from the diet are called the essential amino acids. Proteins that contain all the essential amino acids are called high-quality proteins or complete proteins. Proteins that are deficient in one or more essential amino acids are called low-quality proteins or incomplete proteins. Most animal food products contain high-quality protein, whereas several plant foods contain low-quality proteins. In order to produce new protein in our bodies, we require the presence of all the essential amino acids in the foods we eat.

Proteins provide structure to all cells in the human body. They are an integral part of the cell membrane, the cytoplasm and the organelles. Muscle, skin and hair are composed largely of protein. Bones and teeth are composed of minerals embedded in a protein framework. When a diet is deficient in protein, these structures break down, resulting in reduced muscle mass, loss of skin elasticity, weakened bones and thinning hair. Many proteins are enzymes that increase the rate of metabolic reactions; others act as transporters to help molecules such as glucose move across cell membranes. Some proteins are hormones such as insulin, there are receptors for hormones and neurotransmitters, antibodies that are important for immune function, and molecules involved in oxygen transport (haemoglobin) and its utilisation in energy metabolism (cytochromes).

Protein contains 5 kcal/g of energy, but after digestion, absorption and metabolism only about 3 kcal/g is available to use in the body, and it is not normally used as an energy source except when the body's carbohydrate stores become depleted or during periods of starvation. Unlike fat and carbohydrate, a high intake of protein is not usually linked with diseases such as cancer, tooth decay, Type 2 diabetes, atherosclerosis or coronary heart disease. Prolonged deficiencies of dietary protein, however, have devastating consequences for health that result in severely impaired immunity with a high risk of infection, fluid accumulation in the abdomen and limb extremities (known as oedema), and muscle wasting; ultimately, organ failure or severe infection will result in death. The recommended daily protein intake is usually a minimum of 0.8 g protein per kilogram of body mass (kg BM) which is about 60 g for a person weighing 75 kg – the average body mass of a professional male football player – with slightly higher requirements for growing children and pregnant or lactating women. Protein intake in the Western world is usually well in excess of the recommendations, averaging about 1.0–1.4 g/kg BM/day (i.e. about 70–100 g/day) with protein providing 10–15% of the total daily energy intake. Even so, somewhat higher protein intakes are recommended for sportspeople, including footballers, mainly due to their increased needs for muscle training adaptation, recovery and repair.

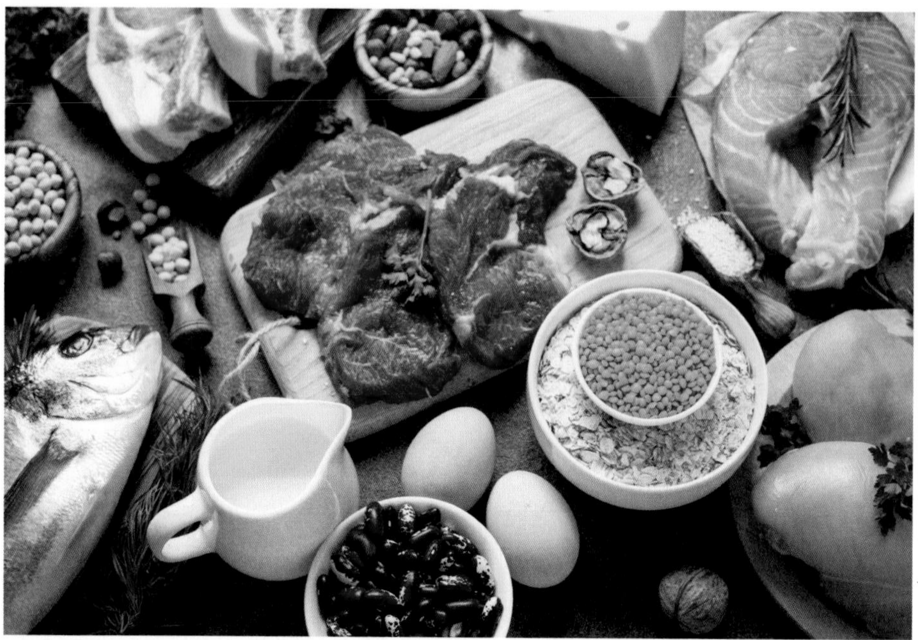

Photo 2.5 A variety of high-protein foods.

Several foods with high-protein content include meat, poultry, fish, eggs and dairy produce (photo 2.5). Because animal products are the most common sources of protein, vegetarians and vegans could be at risk for marginal protein intake. Vegetarians often compensate by eating more grains (e.g. wheat, rice, oats, cornmeal, barley) and legumes (e.g. peas, beans, chickpeas, lentils), which are both excellent protein sources (photo 2.6). Any missing essential amino acid in one particular plant food can be compensated for by eating other plants that do contain it, and there are plenty of plant-based foods (e.g. lentils, chickpeas, beans, quinoa, nuts and soy products such as tofu) that do contain high-quality protein with all the essential amino acids.

WATER

Water (H_2O) is also classed as a macronutrient, although, of course it does not supply any energy. However, it is an extremely important essential nutrient. Usually going without any water for more than three days will result in death. The adult body is about 60% water by weight. Two-thirds of the body water content is inside cells (intracellular fluid), and the remaining one-third is found outside cells (extracellular fluid) and includes the blood plasma, cerebrospinal fluid and lymph. Most sedentary people consume about 2 litres (L) of water per day with 1.2 L from drinks and 0.8 L from solid foods. On most

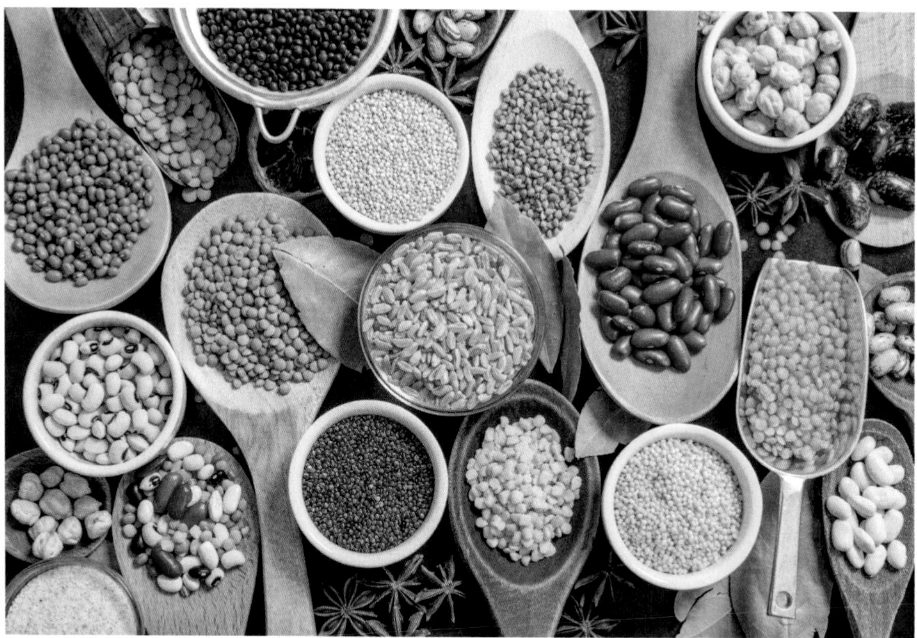

Photo 2.6 A variety of legumes (e.g. peas, beans, chickpeas, lentils) that are among the best sources of protein from plants.

days, footballers will need more than this as water is lost in sweat, which helps to cool the body during exercise. When the muscles are contracting, they produce more heat than at rest and this would result in a potentially fatal rise in core body temperature if it were not prevented by increasing blood flow to the skin and increased sweating. As the sweat evaporates from the skin surface it exerts a cooling effect. Even so, on a hot day, a higher than usual core temperature will occur and induce an earlier onset of fatigue in footballers as the brain needs to protect itself from becoming too hot.

ESSENTIAL NUTRIENTS

Some nutrients cannot be synthesised in the body but are needed for some critical functions throughout life, so they must be provided by the diet. These are called essential nutrients. Many are required for growth, health and survival, and their absence from the diet or inadequate intake results in characteristic signs of a deficiency, disease and ultimately death. Humans have an essential requirement for at least 46 nutrients. The essential nutrients include nine essential amino acids, two essential fatty acids (linoleic acid and alpha-linolenic acid), 13 vitamins, water and several minerals and trace elements. Vitamins, minerals and trace elements are collectively known as the micronutrients.

Vitamins

Vitamins are organic compounds, whereas minerals and trace elements are inorganic compounds. Many micronutrients are needed for the function of various enzymes and other functional proteins, including those involved in oxygen transport and energy metabolism. Any sustained deficiency of an essential vitamin or mineral will cause ill health.

All of the 13 known vitamins that are essential for human health have important functions in most metabolic processes in the body. Vitamins must be obtained from the diet, except vitamin D, which can also be synthesised in the skin from sunlight, and vitamin K, which is synthesised by the bacteria resident in the large intestine. When a vitamin becomes unavailable in the diet, a deficiency may develop within 3–4 weeks. Vitamins are either water-soluble or fat-soluble (see tables 2.2 and 2.3). Water-soluble vitamins dissolve in water; fat-soluble vitamins dissolve in organic solvents and are usually ingested with dietary fats.

Although vitamins do not directly contribute to energy supply, they play an important role in regulating metabolism, acting as reusable coenzymes (or cofactors) and are essential for the proper functioning of some important enzymes in metabolism. A deficiency of some of the B-group vitamins, which act as cofactors of enzymes in carbohydrate metabolism (e.g. niacin [B3], pyridoxine [B6] and thiamin [B1]), fat metabolism (e.g. riboflavin [B2], thiamin [B1], pantothenic acid [B5] and biotin [B7]), and protein metabolism (pyridoxine [B6]), results in feelings of tiredness and an inability to sustain exercise (table 2.2). Other vitamins play a role

Table 2.2 Major functions of water-soluble vitamins, effects of dietary deficiency and main food sources

Vitamin	Major roles in body	Effects of deficiency	Main food sources
B1 (thiamin)	Forms coenzyme involved in carbohydrate metabolism and central nervous system function	Loss of appetite, apathy, depression, beriberi and pain in calf muscles	Whole-grain cereal products, fortified bread, pulses, potatoes, legumes, nuts, pork, ham and liver
B2 (riboflavin)	Forms coenzymes involved in carbohydrate and fat oxidation; maintains healthy skin	Dermatitis, lip and tongue sores, and damage to cornea of eyes	Dairy products, meat, liver, eggs, green leafy vegetables and beans
B3 (niacin)	Forms coenzymes involved in glycolysis, carbohydrate and fat oxidation, and fat synthesis; maintains healthy skin	Weakness, loss of appetite, skin lesions, gut and skin problems, and pellegra	Meat, liver, poultry, fish, whole-grain cereal products, lentils and nuts

Vitamin	Major roles in body	Effects of deficiency	Main food sources
B5 (pantothenic acid)	Forms coenzyme A needed for energy metabolism, carbohydrate and fat oxidation, and fat synthesis	Nausea, fatigue, depression and loss of appetite	Liver, meat, dairy products, eggs, whole-grain cereal products, legumes and most vegetables
B6 (pyridoxine)	Forms coenzyme involved in protein metabolism, formation of haemoglobin and red blood cells, and glycogen breakdown	Irritability, convulsions, anaemia, dermatitis and tongue sores	Meat, liver, poultry, fish, whole-grain cereal products, potatoes, legumes, green leafy vegetables, dairy products, bananas and nuts
B7 (biotin)	Forms coenzyme involved in carbohydrate, fat, and protein metabolism	Nausea, fatigue and skin rashes	Meat, milk, egg yolk, whole-grain cereal products, legumes and most vegetables
B9 (folic acid)	Forms coenzyme involved in production of DNA and RNA; promotes formation of haemoglobin and red and white blood cells; maintains gut health	Anaemia, fatigue, diarrhoea, gut disorders, and infections	Meat, liver, green leafy vegetables, whole-grain cereal products, potatoes, legumes, nuts and fruit
B12 (cobalamin)	Forms coenzyme involved in production of DNA and RNA; promotes formation of red and white blood cells; maintains nerve, gut and skin tissue	Pernicious anaemia, fatigue, nerve damage, paralysis and infections	Meat, fish, shellfish, poultry, liver, eggs, dairy products and fortified breakfast cereals
C (ascorbic acid)	Antioxidant; promotes collagen formation and development of connective tissue. Also promotes catecholamine and steroid hormone synthesis and iron absorption	Weakness, slow wound healing, infections, bleeding gums, anaemia, scurvy	Citrus fruits, green leafy vegetables, blackcurrants, broccoli, kiwi fruit, melon, papaya, potatoes, peppers and strawberries

Table 2.3 Major functions of fat-soluble vitamins, the effects of dietary deficiency and main food sources

Vitamin	Major roles in body	Effects of deficiency	Main food sources
A (retinol)	Maintains epithelial tissues in skin, mucous membranes, and visual pigments of eye; promotes bone development and immune function	Night blindness, infections, impaired growth and impaired wound healing	Liver, fish, dairy products, eggs, margarine; formed in body from carotenoids in carrots, dark green leafy vegetables, tomatoes and oranges
D (calciferol)	Increases calcium absorption in gut and promotes bone formation. Also important for muscle and immune function	Weak bones (rickets in children and osteomalacia in adults). Sub-optimal muscle function. Increased susceptibility to infections	Liver, fish, eggs, fortified dairy products, oils, and margarine; formed by action of sunlight on the skin
E (α-tocopherol)	Defends against free radicals; protects cell membranes	Haemolysis and anaemia	Liver, eggs, whole-grain cereal products, vegetable oils, seed oils, margarine and butter
K (menadione)	Forms blood-clotting factors	Bleeding and haemorrhage	Liver, eggs, green leafy vegetables, cheese and butter; formed in large intestine by bacteria

in red and white blood cell production (folic acid [B9] and cobalamin [B12]) or assist in the formation of bones, connective tissue and cartilage (e.g. vitamins C and D). Vitamin C is also an antioxidant. The fat-soluble vitamins are A (retinol), D (calciferol), E (α-tocopherol) and K (menadione). Of these vitamins, only vitamin E has a probable role in energy metabolism but the other three have other important functions (table 2.3). In addition, β-carotene (provitamin A) and vitamin E have antioxidant properties. Vitamin K is required for the addition of sugar molecules to proteins to form glycoproteins and is essential for normal blood clotting.

Minerals and Trace Elements

Minerals can be divided into macrominerals and trace elements (also known as microminerals). Macrominerals are required in daily intakes of more than 100 mg, or are present in the body in amounts greater than 0.01% of the body weight. The macrominerals include calcium, chlorine, magnesium, potassium, phosphorus and sodium and, just like the vitamins, they play important roles in bodily functions (table 2.4). Several of the macrominerals are

Table 2.4 Major functions of macrominerals, effects of dietary deficiency, and main food sources

Macromineral	Major roles in the body	Effects of deficiency	Main food sources
Calcium	Promotes bone and teeth formation, muscle contraction and nerve impulse transmission; regulates enzyme activity	Osteoporosis, brittle bones, impaired muscle contraction and muscle cramps	Dairy products, egg yolk, beans and peas, dark green vegetables and cauliflower
Chlorine	Promotes nerve impulse conduction and hydrochloric acid formation in the stomach	Convulsions	Meat, fish, bread, canned foods, table salt, beans and milk
Magnesium	Promotes protein synthesis and cofactor for important enzymes involved in muscle contraction and is a component of bone	Muscle weakness, fatigue, apathy, muscle tremor and cramps	Seafood, nuts, green leafy vegetables, fruits, whole-grain products, milk and yoghurt
Potassium	Promotes nerve impulse generation, muscle contraction and acid-base balance	Muscle cramps, apathy, loss of appetite and irregular heart beat	Meat, fish, milk, yoghurt, fruit, vegetables and bread
Phosphorus	Promotes bone formation; buffer in muscle contraction; component of ATP, DNA, RNA and cell membranes	Osteoporosis, brittle bones, muscle weakness and muscle cramps	Meat, eggs, fish, milk, cheese, beans, peas, whole-grain products and soft drinks
Sodium	Maintenance of blood volume, nerve impulse generation, muscle contraction, acid-base balance	Dizziness, coma, muscle cramps, nausea, vomiting, loss of appetite and seizures	Meat, fish, bread, canned foods, table salt, sauces and pickles
Sulphur	Acid-base balance; liver function	Unknown and extremely unlikely to occur	Bok choy, broccoli, cabbage, cauliflower, horseradish, kale, kohlrabi, mustard leaves, radish, turnips, watercress, coconut milk, milk, eggs, legumes and beans, meat and fish, nuts, onions, leeks, wine and grape juice

classed as electrolytes, which are minerals that can conduct electrical impulses in the body. Common electrolytes are calcium, chloride, potassium and sodium. Electrolytes control the fluid balance of the body and are important in muscle contraction, nerve impulses, energy generation and many biochemical reactions in the body. The trace elements are required in daily intakes of less than 100 mg or are present in the body in amounts less than 0.01% of body weight. Despite the small amounts needed, they play essential roles in a variety of bodily functions (table 2.5). The trace elements include cobalt, copper, fluorine, iodine, iron, manganese, molybdenum, selenium and zinc. Some of the trace elements such as iron and zinc form part of metalloenzymes, which are enzymes in which the metal is bonded within the protein structure and functions as a cofactor, which is necessary for the action of the enzyme.

Table 2.5 Major functions of trace elements (microminerals), effects of dietary deficiency and main food sources

Trace element	Major roles in body	Effects of deficiency	Main food sources
Chromium	Increases insulin action	Glucose intolerance and impaired fat metabolism	Liver, kidney, meat, oysters, cheese, whole-grain products, beer, asparagus, mushrooms, nuts and stainless-steel cookware
Cobalt	Forms component of vitamin B12 needed for red blood cell development	Pernicious anaemia	Meat, liver and milk
Copper	Promotes normal iron absorption, oxidative metabolism, connective tissue formation, and haemoglobin synthesis	Anaemia, impaired immune function and bone demineralisation	Liver, kidney, shellfish, meat, fish, poultry, eggs, bran cereals, nuts, legumes, broccoli, banana, avocado and chocolate
Fluorine	Promotes bone and teeth formation	Dental caries (tooth decay)	Milk, egg yolk, seafood and drinking water
Iodine	Forms component of thyroid hormones	Goitre and reduced metabolic rate	Iodised salt, seafood and vegetables

Trace element	Major roles in body	Effects of deficiency	Main food sources
Iron	Transports oxygen as haemoglobin and myoglobin; forms cytochromes and metalloenzymes; promotes immune function	Anaemia, fatigue, and increased infections	Liver, kidney, eggs, red meats, seafood, oysters, bread, flour, molasses, dried legumes, nuts, leafy green vegetables, broccoli, figs, raisins and cocoa
Manganese	Forms cofactor with energy metabolism enzymes; promotes bone formation and fat synthesis	Poor growth	Whole grains, peas and beans, leafy vegetables and bananas
Molybdenum	Forms cofactor with riboflavin in carbohydrate and fat metabolism enzymes	No known deficiency effects	Liver, kidney, whole-grain products, beans and peas
Selenium	Forms cofactor with glutathione peroxidase an important antioxidant enzyme	Cardiomyopathy, cancer, heart disease, impaired immune function and red blood cell fragility	Meat, liver, kidney, poultry, fish, dairy products, seafood, whole grains and nuts
Zinc	Forms metalloenzymes; promotes protein synthesis, immune function, tissue repair, energy metabolism and antioxidant activity	Impaired growth, impaired healing, and increased number of infections	Oysters, shellfish, beef, liver, poultry, dairy products, whole grains, vegetables, asparagus and spinach

The following table provides a list of the recommended daily intakes for selected vitamins, minerals and trace elements in the UK. There are a few notable differences between men and women and for adolescents compared with adults. Values may differ slightly in some other countries, including the US and Australia. The values are based on the needs of healthy people who are sedentary or recreationally active. For football players and athletes in other sports, the recommended intakes of some of the micronutrients are higher and the reasons for this will be discussed in the chapters that follow.

Table 2.6 Recommended daily intakes for selected vitamins, minerals and trace elements in the UK

	MEN			WOMEN		
	11–14 years	15–18 years	19–50 years	11–14 years	15–18 years	19–50 years
Folate (µg)	200	200	200	200	200	200
Niacin (mg)	15	18	17	12	14	13
Riboflavin (mg)	1.2	1.3	1.3	1.1	1.1	1.1
Thiamin (mg)	0.9	1.1	1.0	0.7	0.8	0.8
Vitamin B6 (mg)	1.2	1.5	1.4	1.0	1.2	1.2
Vitamin B12 (µg)	1.2	1.5	1.5	1.2	1.5	1.5
Vitamin A (µg)	600	700	700	600	600	600
Vitamin C (mg)	35	40	40	35	40	40
Vitamin D (µg)	10	10	10	10	10	10
Calcium (mg)	1,000	1,000	700	800	800	700
Chloride (g)	2.5	2.5	2.5	2.5	2.5	2.5
Copper (mg)	0.8	1.0	1.2	0.8	1.0	1.2
Iodine (µg)	130	140	140	130	140	140
Iron (mg)	11.3	11.3	8.7	14.8	14.8	14.8
Magnesium (mg)	280	300	300	280	300	270
Phosphorus (mg)	775	775	550	625	625	550
Potassium (g)	3.1	3.5	3.5	3.1	3.5	3.5
Selenium (µg)	45	70	75	45	60	60
Sodium (g)	1.6	1.6	1.6	1.6	1.6	1.6
Zinc (mg)	9.0	9.5	9.5	9.0	7.0	7.0

Data from Dietary Reference Values for Food Energy and Nutrients in the United Kingdom: Report of the Panel on Dietary Reference Values of the Committee on Medical Aspects of Food Policy, *London: Her Majesty's Stationary Office, 1991. One milligram (mg) is one thousandth of a gram and one microgram (µg) is one millionth of a gram.*

NONESSENTIAL NUTRIENTS

Deficiencies of some nonessential nutrients such as phytonutrients and fibre will not cause symptoms of disease, but they are required for optimal health.

Phytonutrients

Phytonutrients are certain organic components of plants, which are thought to promote human health but are not considered to be essential nutrients. Examples include carotenoids, catechins and flavonoids. They differ from vitamins in that respect because a lack of phytonutrients will not cause a deficiency disease, but they are needed in the diet for health to be optimal – that is as good as it can possibly be. Many phytonutrients have antioxidant, anti-inflammatory or anti-viral effects.

Fibre

Fibre is another nonessential nutrient; it used to be known as roughage. It comprises the edible parts of plants that are not broken down and absorbed in the human gastrointestinal tract. As mentioned previously, the human stomach and small intestine have no enzymes to break down fibre, but some can be digested and fermented by bacteria in the colon producing short-chain fatty acids that can be absorbed and have broad, significant health effects. Fibre adds bulk and helps to retain water in the colon, resulting in a softer and larger stool. Fibre also speeds up the movement of faecal matter through the intestines and helps to prevent constipation and promotes bowel regularity. A diet high in fibre also helps to lower blood cholesterol concentrations and normalises blood glucose, and both of these actions are good for our health. Several scientific studies have shown that diets high in fibre are associated with a lower risk of cardiovascular and metabolic diseases, as well as a reduced risk of colon cancer.

Alcohol

Alcohol is a common constituent of the Western diet but is not an essential nutrient and excessive intakes can be very harmful to health. An alcohol intake in excess of one glass of wine or bottle of beer per day increases the risk of many diseases, and alcohol contains 7 kcal per gram and for many people, it can be an important contributor to weight gain. There is certainly some truth in the notion of a 'beer belly' in people who regularly drink substantial volumes of beer, cider or wine. One 750 mL bottle of wine contains about 600 kcal (that's equivalent to two standard McDonald cheeseburgers) and a 330 mL bottle of beer contains about 150 kcal. Note that many food and health agencies report intakes as units of alcohol. One unit of alcohol is equivalent to 8 g or 10 mL of pure alcohol, so a 175 mL glass of wine or a 330 mL bottle of beer both contain just over two units of alcohol, and the maximum recommended intake for adults is 14 units per week. You will not be surprised to learn that drinking alcohol is discouraged for footballers. As well as providing useless excess calories (alcohol cannot be used as a fuel by the muscles) that can lead to weight gain, it impairs mental function, which can lead to inappropriate behaviours. We have all heard some stories about professional footballers going on the occasional bender, doing things they shouldn't, being found out and getting into trouble with their managers and sometimes the law! What is perhaps less well known, is that binge alcohol drinking can impair immune function, delay wound healing and slow down recovery processes after exercise.

KNOW YOUR NUTRIENTS

MACRONUTRIENTS
Carbohydrate
Protein
Fat
Water

NON-ESSENTIAL
Phytonutrients
Fibre
Deficiency does not cause illness but they are needed for optimal health

ALCOHOL
Provides 7 kcal/g
Impairs cognitive function, adaptation & immune function
DON'T DRINK IT!

CARBOHYDRATE
Provides 4 kcal/g
Limited stores as muscle & liver glycogen.
The main fuel for football match-play & training

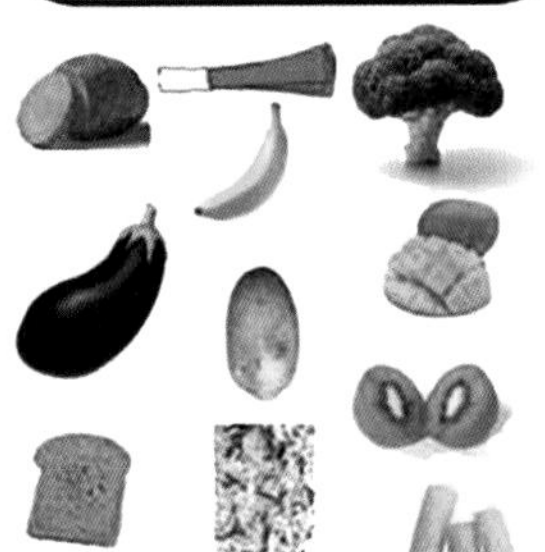

ESSENTIAL MICRONUTRIENTS
Vitamins/Minerals
Any deficiency can cause ill health & impair performance

PROTEIN
Provides 3 kcal/g
Contains 20 amino acids, 9 of which are essential. Important for muscle adaptation & repair

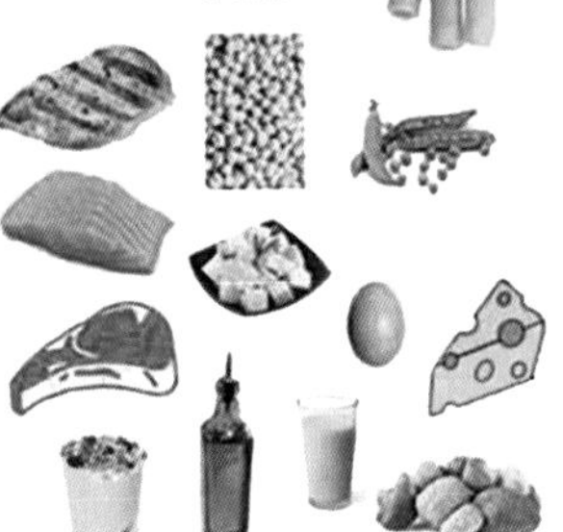

VITAMINS
13 essential organic compounds, 4 are fat-soluble (A, D, E, K) & 9 are water-soluble (B-complex, C). Many roles in energy metabolism

WATER
Essential for all cells, blood, lymph, urine. Body fluid losses are increased by sweating. Dehydration impairs performance

FAT
Provides 9 kcal/g
Contains 2 essential fatty acids and source of fat-soluble vitamins. Fat is the body's largest energy store

MINERALS
Essential for many body functions including oxygen transport (iron), healthy bones (calcium), & immunity (zinc)

Infographic 2 The major nutrients in a player's diet.

CHAPTER 3

Some Things You Need to Know About the Body's Metabolism

- What Happens to the Food Consumed After It Has Entered the Body?
- Some Basics of Energy Metabolism
- How We Get the Energy From Stored Fuels for Exercise and Other Energy-Requiring Processes
- Energy Stores in the Body
- Replenishing Energy Stores After Exercise
- Losing or Gaining Body Weight: The Energy Balance Concept

The description of nutrition and nutrients in the previous chapter only briefly mentioned how food is processed in our bodies. It is helpful to know something about the journey your food takes through your digestive tract after you have eaten it, so let me just explain here what happens after food enters your mouth and how, after its digestion and absorption, some of it gets deposited as energy reserves: muscle and liver glycogen for carbohydrates and adipose tissue triglyceride for fats and any excess carbohydrate we consume. After that I'll focus on describing how the body derives energy from the nutrients we have absorbed in the gut and stored in our muscles, liver and adipose (fat) tissue and how – by utilising those stores and various metabolic pathways – we can meet the high-energy demands of intense prolonged physical activities such as playing football.

WHAT HAPPENS TO THE FOOD CONSUMED AFTER IT HAS ENTERED THE BODY?

Obviously, the first thing you do after putting food in your mouth is that you chew it. By doing so, you are mechanically breaking up the food into smaller pieces and increasing the surface area of food for the benefit of digestive enzymes (a type of protein that helps to chemically break down your food into particles small enough to be absorbed in the gut and used by the body). Some of the carbohydrate in your meal starts to be broken down by enzymes contained in saliva, which is secreted in greater amounts in anticipation of eating and while you are chewing food. Saliva also lubricates the food particles making them easier to swallow. The mouth and tongue also contain receptors that send messages via nerves to the brain's pleasure and reward centres, which is one of the reasons we get pleasure from eating. In addition to the sensation of taste, some of those receptors can detect the presence of carbohydrate, and research has shown that endurance athletes can get a performance boost by simply swilling a carbohydrate beverage around their mouth for 5–10 seconds (like a mouthwash) and spitting it out, without needing to swallow, digest and absorb the nutrient in the usual way. Essentially, the brain is being tricked into assuming some carbohydrate energy is on its way. Nowadays, it is not uncommon to see some professional players using this carbohydrate mouth rinsing on the pitch when play has been interrupted and there is an opportunity for the provision of drinks by the support staff. I'll explain more about this in chapter 6.

After swallowing your food, it travels down the flexible tube known as the oesophagus and passes into the stomach, which releases hydrochloric acid and more digestive enzymes to help break down the food further and to help kill, at least, some of the germs that might be present in our food. The stomach acts as a temporary storage depot while the food is digested and mixed with secreted fluids until it becomes rather like a soup, which is called chyme. The chyme is then gradually released into the small intestine, where the digestive process will be completed. The small intestine is a long, coiled tube that is about six or seven metres long, and, together with some help from enzymes secreted from accessory digestive organs including the liver, gall bladder and pancreas, it finishes chemically breaking down the food, so that it's now made up of small molecules that can be absorbed by the cells lining the inner gut wall in both the small and large intestine. Many of the nutrients such as sugars, amino acids and fatty acids pass through the intestinal wall cells and into the blood where they are transported to the liver and then beyond to be taken up by the body tissues, such as the brain, muscles and heart, ready to be used as fuel or as building blocks for larger molecules. The remaining food material consists of the undigested components such as fibre, plus some minerals and water, and it proceeds to pass through the large intestine (colon), which is about one and a half metres long but considerably wider in diameter than the small intestine.

The main function of the large intestine is to absorb water and minerals including sodium, potassium and chloride. As mentioned previously, some of the fibre that could not be digested in the small intestine is broken down into sugars and then fermented by the large population of bacteria that are resident in the large intestine. The resulting short-chain fatty acids are used as fuel by both the bacteria themselves and the human cells that line the large intestine. Once the large intestine has finished this process, what is left passes through into the rectum where it is compacted to form the faeces. I'm sure you know what happens next ... when you get the urge to sit down on the toilet. The whole digestive system, from mouth to anus, is effectively a long single tubular structure and is called the gastrointestinal tract. It contains smooth muscle, which helps to propel the food materials along the oesophagus and intestines and churn the food in the stomach to give it a good mixing with the acid and enzymes. The journey your food takes through the gastrointestinal tract is illustrated in figure 3.1.

SOME BASICS OF ENERGY METABOLISM

The human body needs energy to survive and function. In fact, every single cell in the body needs energy to survive and carry out its various functions. For example, muscle fibres need energy to contract, nerves need energy to generate impulses, and energy is needed for the biosynthesis of large molecules such as proteins and nucleic acids (DNA and RNA). Heat energy is continuously generated from chemical reactions in the cells of the body, and this is used to maintain a normal body temperature of about 37°C. Although the human body has some stored energy reserves, most of its energy must be obtained from food and drink that are derived from animal or plant sources (figure 3.2). During exercise, energy requirements increase considerably above resting energy requirements, and energy provision can become critical to exercise performance. On average, during a football match, a player's rate of energy expenditure will be about 10 times higher than at rest, but for any given minute could vary between 2 and 20 times the resting value depending on an individual's involvement and the intensity of play. Other sports have different energy requirements, which depend on the mode, duration and intensity of exercise performed and on whether the exercise is continuous like in marathon running or intermittent like in games such as rugby, basketball and tennis.

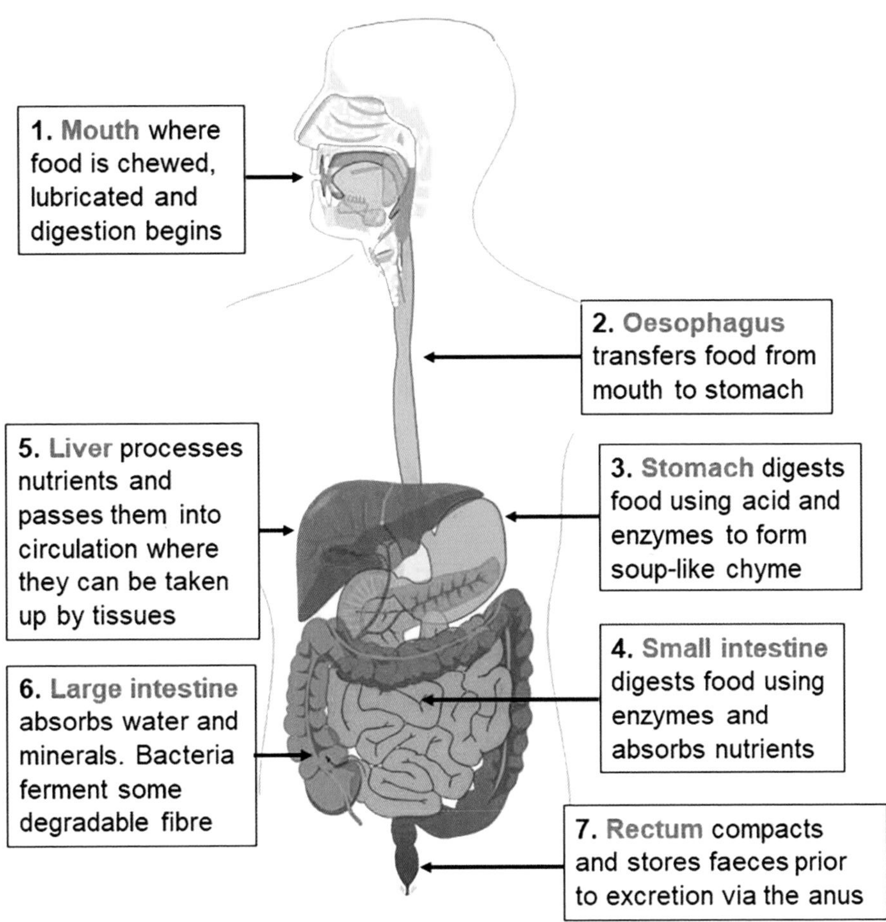

Figure 3.1 The gastrointestinal tract and the main processes that occur as your food passes through it to undergo digestion and absorption.

The energy in food is stored in the chemical bonds of various molecules, and so it is called 'potential chemical energy'. Breaking these bonds releases the energy, and it becomes available for conversion into other forms of energy. For instance, when glucose is broken down in the muscles during a sequence of reactions called glycolysis, chemical energy is converted to another form of chemical energy in the form of a very special molecule called adenosine triphosphate (ATP) and ultimately transformed into mechanical energy (muscle contraction) to generate movement. ATP is special because it is the only form of energy that can be used directly by the cells in the body to do any form of useful biological work. In addition to muscle contraction, ATP can be used for the transport of molecules across membranes, propagation of nerve impulses and in the synthesis of

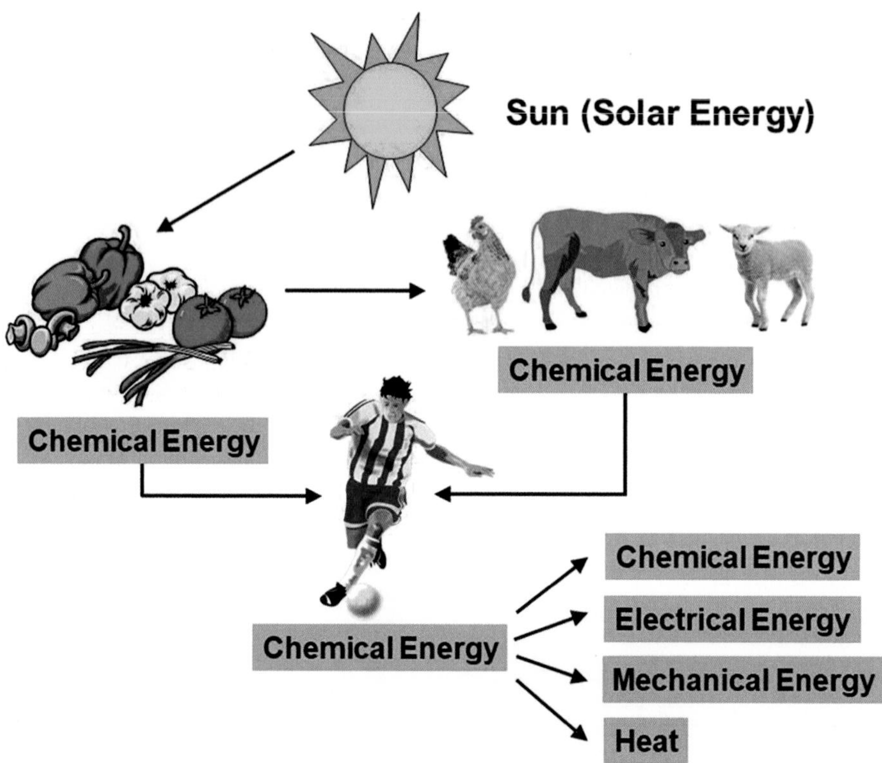

Figure 3.2 The energy we need comes from animal and plant food sources. Plants obtain their energy from sunlight.

large molecules such as proteins. None of these energy transfers or conversions are 100% efficient, and the 'waste' energy appears as heat, which allows us to maintain a body temperature of 37°C (98.6°F) and permits all the metabolic reactions in the body to occur at faster rates than they would at lower temperatures.

In physiology, energy represents the capacity to do work, which is often referred to as mechanical energy. Walking, running, throwing and jumping require the production of mechanical energy. Work (energy) is the product of force times the vertical distance covered:

Work = Force x distance, or W = F x d

If work is expressed per unit of time, the term power (P) is used:

Power = Work/time, or P = W/t

The rate of energy expenditure refers to the amount of energy used in kilocalories per unit of time to produce power. During conversion of one form of energy into another, no energy is lost. This is usually referred to as the first law of thermodynamics, also known as the Law of Conservation of Energy, which states that energy cannot be created or destroyed in an isolated system. For example, during the oxidation of carbohydrate and fat, chemical energy is converted into mechanical energy (muscle contraction) to perform movement, and some heat energy is released due the inefficiency of the process. The sum of the mechanical energy and heat energy produced will be the same as the amount of chemical energy used up.

The human body is not efficient in its use of energy from the breakdown of carbohydrate and fat. During running, for instance, only 15–20% of that chemical energy in those macronutrients is converted to power. The remainder of the energy becomes heat. This heat can be partly used to maintain normal body temperature at 37°C (98.6°F), but during intensive exercise, including football match play and training, heat production may be excessive, and body temperature usually rises by 1 or 2ºC. To prevent body temperature from rising too high, various heat-dissipating mechanisms such as increased skin blood flow and sweating must be activated.

The energy we need comes from food, mostly in the form of carbohydrate, fat and protein. Most of this is in the form of large molecules: plant starches for carbohydrate, triglyceride for fat and, to a much lesser degree, from whole proteins. As mentioned earlier in this chapter, these macronutrients are broken down into smaller molecules by enzymes in the gastrointestinal tract – glycerol and fatty acids for fats, sugars for carbohydrate and amino acids for proteins – and are absorbed in the small intestine. Fats are reassembled into triglyceride in the intestinal cells and pass into the blood via lymph vessels as particles called chylomicrons. These are further processed in the liver to form lipoproteins and enter the circulation. In this form, fats can be transported in the blood and taken up by adipose tissue for storage as triglyceride. Amino acids that pass into the blood from the gut are taken up by tissues and converted into tissue proteins and other compounds such as nucleic acids, creatine and neurotransmitters. Most excess amino acids are oxidised although some can be converted into glucose or fat.

Glucose that passes into the blood from the gut is taken up by tissues to be used as fuel or is converted into the polysaccharide glycogen (the body's principal store of carbohydrate) in the liver and muscles. Some of the excess glucose is taken up by adipose tissue where it is converted into fat. Glucose in the blood is also important for the brain and its concentration in the blood is normally maintained at about 5 millimoles per litre (mM or mmol/L) or 0.9 grams per litre (g/L) by the actions of two hormones: insulin, which promotes glucose uptake into the tissues when the blood-glucose concentration is higher than normal (e.g. after consuming a meal) and glucagon, which stimulates the breakdown of liver glycogen and the release of the liberated glucose into the blood when the blood-glucose concentration falls below normal (e.g. during fasting). The triglyceride in chylomicrons and lipoproteins are also added to the fat stores in adipose tissue. The synthesis of glycogen and triglyceride is energetically cheap, but the synthesis of proteins is far costlier. Proteins serve useful functions in the body as structural components, enzymes, transporters, etc. and are only a minor fuel for both resting and exercising energy requirements.

HOW WE GET THE ENERGY FROM STORED FUELS FOR EXERCISE AND OTHER ENERGY-REQUIRING PROCESSES

When we need energy (e.g. for exercise), some of the stored glycogen and triglycerides are broken down in a process that requires oxygen and generates carbon dioxide (CO_2) and water (H_2O). Carbohydrate in the form of glycogen or glucose is first converted to pyruvate in the cytoplasm of the cell in an anaerobic series of reactions that are known collectively as glycolysis. Anaerobic metabolism does not use oxygen. The oxidation of pyruvate, fatty acids and some amino acids takes place in the intracellular organelles called mitochondria, and is generally referred to as aerobic metabolism, or in simpler terms, the burning of fuel.

AEROBIC METABOLISM

Oxidation is an oxygen-requiring (aerobic) process. Fatty acids and pyruvate can both be completely oxidised to carbon dioxide (CO_2) and water (H_2O). The carbon and hydrogen atoms in some amino acids can also be completely oxidised, but the nitrogen atoms cannot. For amino acids, the amino groups (NH_2) are first removed, then converted into ammonia (NH_3) and urea ($CO(NH_2)_2$), and subsequently excreted in urine that is formed in the kidneys. The energy released in the oxidation of pyruvate, fatty acids and amino acids is used to convert adenosine diphosphate (ADP) to ATP, which is the energy currency of the cell. In fact, ATP is the only source of energy that can be used to drive energy-requiring reactions and processes in the body.

The mitochondria, where the oxidation of fuel takes place, are small organelles that are found inside most cells of the body (figure 3.3). Their most important role is to oxidise (burn) fuel obtained from the breakdown of fat and carbohydrate and use the energy released in this process to produce (or more accurately, resynthesise) ATP, via the addition of a phosphate group to ADP.

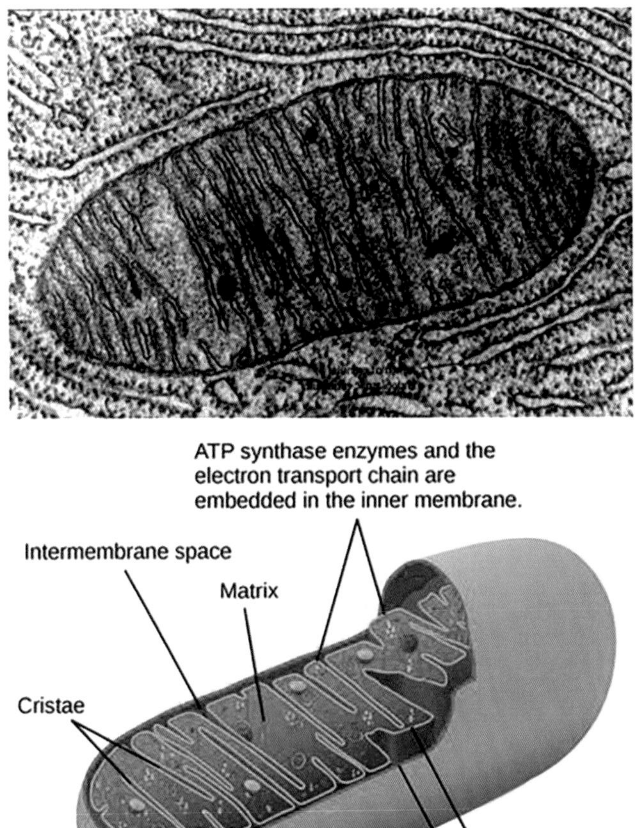

Figure 3.3 A single mitochondrion captured with the electron microscope and in diagrammatic form below.

All of the oxidation of fuels (carbohydrates, fats and amino acids) takes place in the mitochondria. At rest, they produce most of the ATP for energy-requiring processes such as membrane transport, nerve conduction and protein synthesis. During aerobic exercise, they produce most (more than 95%) of the ATP that is used to fuel muscle contraction. The reactions that result in ATP production take place in the inner matrix of the mitochondrion and are collectively known as the tricarboxylic acid (TCA) cycle, citric acid cycle or Krebs cycle after the German-born British biochemist, Sir Hans Adolf Krebs, who discovered it in the 1930s. Figure 3.4 summarises the metabolic pathways that result in the oxidation of fuels.

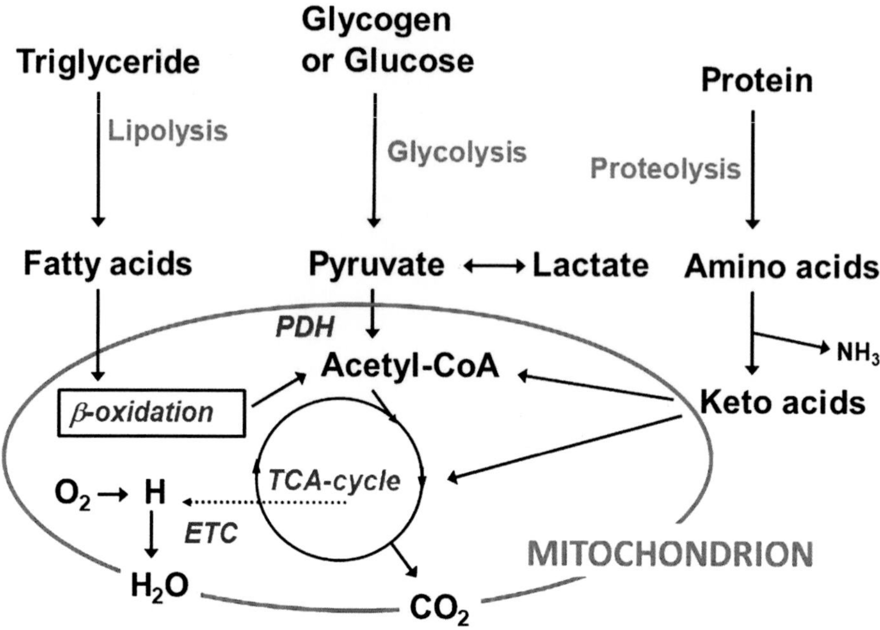

Figure 3.4 The metabolic pathways that result in the oxidation of fuels. CoA: coenzyme A; ETC: electron transport chain; NH_3: ammonia; PDH: pyruvate dehydrogenase; TCA: tricarboxylic acid.

ATP IS THE ENERGY CURRENCY OF THE CELL

The breakdown of ATP to ADP releases energy that is used to perform all forms of biological work: muscle contraction, membrane transport, synthesis of biomolecules, etc. Without a sufficient supply of ATP, our cells would not be able to function or survive. The structure of ATP is illustrated in figure 3.5. It is the process of breaking off the terminal phosphate (PO_4) group, which is commonly abbreviated as Pi, by various enzymes known as ATPases, which releases the energy that can be used to do biological work.

$$ATP + H_2O \rightarrow ADP + Pi + H^+$$

Although ATP is essential as the energy currency of the cell, the amount contained in cells, such as muscle cells, is rather small. In humans, the muscle ATP content is only about 2.5 g/kg of muscle which is only enough to last for 2–3 seconds of high-intensity exercise. Since depletion of ATP cannot be allowed to happen because it would be fatal to the cell, the ATP concentration is continuously maintained by resynthesis of ATP from ADP at essentially the same rate at which ATP is broken down. Three mechanisms are involved in the resynthesis of ATP for muscle force generation: (1) the breakdown of a compound called phosphocreatine (PCr); (2) glycolysis, which involves metabolism of muscle glycogen or blood-borne glucose

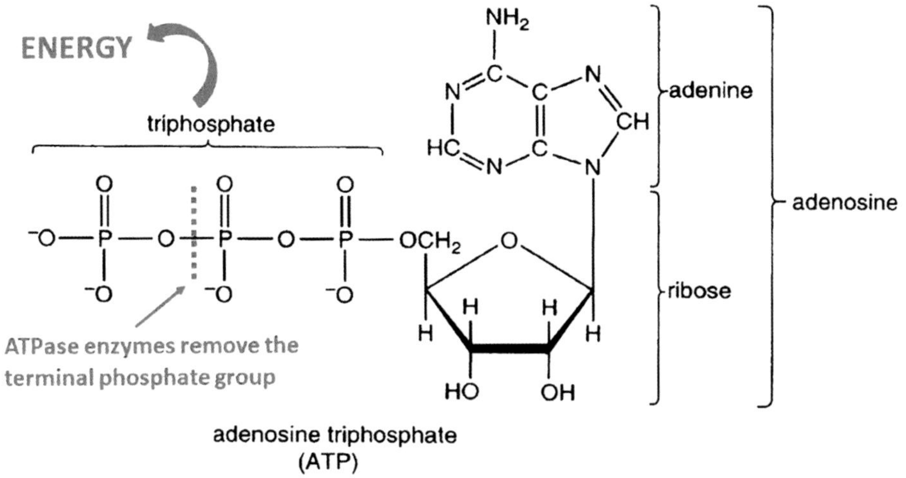

Figure 3.5 The structure of the ATP molecule indicating the action of ATPase enzymes to remove the terminal inorganic phosphate (Pi) group.

and produces ATP by several phosphorylation reactions in this metabolic pathway; and (3) oxidative phosphorylation, in which the products of carbohydrate, fat and, to a lesser extent, protein metabolism enter the TCA cycle in the mitochondria and are oxidised to carbon dioxide and water, which yields energy for the synthesis of ATP. The third mechanism has already been described and is an aerobic process meaning that it uses oxygen. The problem with aerobic metabolism is that it is a rather slow process and takes a while to get up to speed as breathing, heart rate and blood flow to the muscles all have to increase to supply the required amounts of oxygen. The other two mechanisms previously mentioned are anaerobic, which means they occur without the use of oxygen. They are both capable of regenerating ATP at much faster rates than aerobic metabolism so PCr breakdown and glycolysis are very important during the first few seconds and minutes of high-intensity exercise, respectively (table 3.1).

Table 3.1 Summary of the main pathways of energy metabolism that supply ATP for exercise

Pathway	Rate of ATP supply	Availability	Main role
Fat oxidation	Slow	Very large	Fuel for light–moderate exercise
Carbohydrate oxidation	Medium	Limited	Fuel for moderate- to high-intensity exercise
Glycolysis	Fast	Limited	High-intensity exercise
Phosphocreatine breakdown	Very fast	Very small	Exercise onset and short sprints

THE ROLE OF PHOSPHOCREATINE IN ANAEROBIC METABOLISM

Some of the energy for ATP resynthesis is supplied rapidly and without the need for oxygen by the breakdown of PCr. In human muscle, the concentration of PCr is three to four times greater than that of ATP. When PCr is broken down to creatine (Cr) and Pi by the action of the enzyme creatine kinase, the energy is released is used to donate the Pi group to ADP forming ATP:

$$ADP + PCr + H^+ \rightarrow ATP + Cr$$

As soon as the ATP content begins to fall during exercise, PCr is rapidly broken down by creatine kinase, releasing energy for restoration of ATP. Note also that the resynthesis of ATP through the breakdown of PCr mops up some of the hydrogen ions (H^+) formed as a result of ATP breakdown, which helps to prevent an increase in acidity in the muscle in the early stages of exercise. During high-speed running and all-out sprinting, the PCr concentration falls rapidly and can be depleted within 10–20 seconds. However, the reaction above is reversible, and when energy is readily available from aerobic metabolism, when resting or performing walking or jogging, Cr and phosphate can be rejoined to form PCr:

$$ATP + Cr \rightarrow ADP + PCr$$

The advantage of having PCr in muscle is that it is immediately available at the onset of exercise and can be used to resynthesise ATP very quickly, which is just what is needed when a football player suddenly has to run very fast. The major disadvantage of this process, compared with other means of regenerating ATP, is its limited capacity; the total amount of energy available is small.

THE ROLE OF GLYCOLYSIS IN ANAEROBIC METABOLISM

Of course, normally player's muscles do not become fatigued after only a few seconds of effort, so another rapidly accessible source of energy, other than ATP and PCr, must be available. This is a series of chemical reactions known as glycolysis (figure 3.6), which involves the breakdown of glucose (or glycogen) and ends with the formation of pyruvate. This process does not require oxygen but does result in ATP being available to the muscle from some of the reactions in the pathway where the energy released can be used to convert ADP into ATP. But the pyruvate must be removed as its accumulation would inhibit glycolysis. At rest, and in relatively low-intensity exercise such as walking or jogging, when adequate oxygen is available to the muscle, pyruvate is converted to carbon dioxide and water by oxidative metabolism in the mitochondria. In high-intensity exercise such as fast running and all-out sprinting when the rate of formation of pyruvate

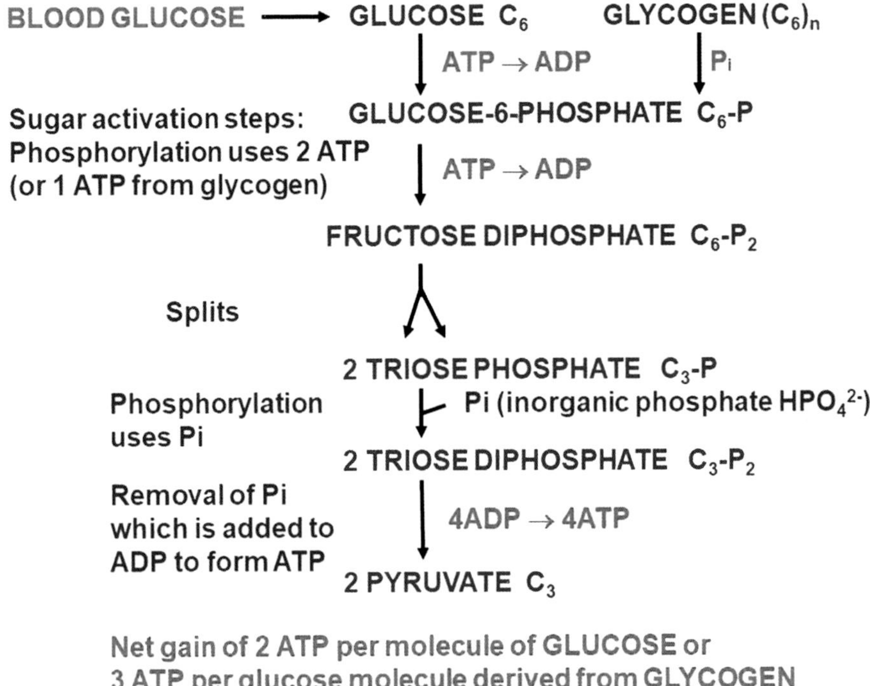

Figure 3.6 A much simplified illustration of glycolysis, which makes two molecules of ATP available for each molecule of glucose that passes through the pathway, or three molecules of ATP if muscle glycogen is the starting substrate.

is extremely high, the pyruvate can also be removed by conversion to lactate (more commonly known as lactic acid) in a reaction that does not involve oxygen. Because there are several reactions involved in glycolysis, it produces ATP at about half the maximal rate of PCr breakdown, but it is still a faster means of regenerating ATP than through aerobic metabolism. The main advantage of glycolysis is that it can be activated quickly within the first few seconds of exercise and be sustained for longer than PCr breakdown, which slows down as the availability of PCr in muscle rapidly declines.

ENERGY STORES IN THE BODY

Carbohydrate is the main fuel for football match play and intensive training sessions. Carbohydrate is stored in the muscles and the liver as glycogen, which is a polymer of glucose, but the total amount stored is usually no more than about 400 g (sufficient to

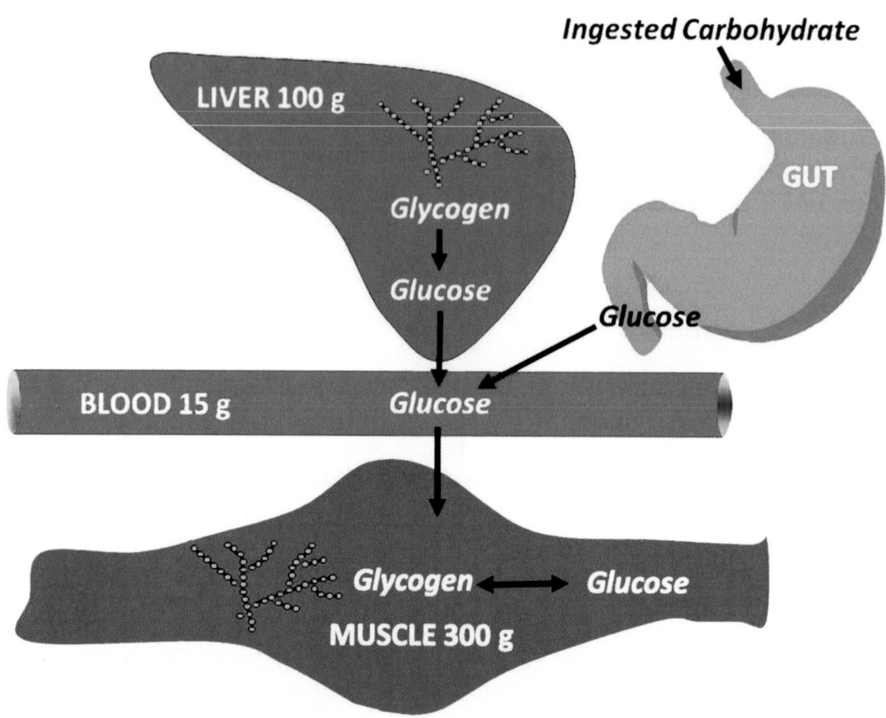

Figure 3.7 Carbohydrate availability in liver, blood (also including the other extracellular fluids) and leg muscles for running. Some glucose can also be provided from drinks or gels consumed just before or during exercise.

provide up to 1,600 kcal of energy for muscle contractions). Up to approximately 100 g of glycogen can be stored in the liver with the remainder in the muscles at a concentration of 10–20 g/kg. For running, a total of about 300 g of glycogen are available in the leg muscles (see figure 3.7). As mentioned previously, some glucose is also present in blood (at a concentration of about 0.9 g/L), which in the fasting state is derived from the release of glucose from the liver. Glucose can also be provided from drinks or gels consumed just before or during exercise with the rate of absorption from the gut and subsequent appearance in the blood limited to a maximum of about 1.0-1.5 g/minute. Fats are stored as triglyceride, mainly in white adipose tissue. Triglyceride molecules must be broken down by a lipase enzyme in a process called lipolysis (figure 3.4) to release fatty acids into the circulation for uptake by working muscle. Skeletal muscle also contains some triglyceride that can be used as an energy source during exercise after its breakdown to fatty acids by a similar lipase enzyme present in muscle.

Human skeletal muscle contains approximately 12 g/kg of triglyceride, and the total amount of muscle triglyceride available is thought to be around 300–500 g,

Table 3.2 Energy stores in an average male footballer

Fuel type	Amount (g)	Energy available (kcal)	Exercise time (min)
Liver glycogen	100	400	23
Leg muscle glycogen	300	1,200	71
Blood glucose	10	40	2
Fat	7,500	67,500	4,000
Protein	11,250	45,000	2,700

Assumes a body mass of 75 kg, a fat content of 10% of body mass and a protein content of about 15% of body mass. The value for blood glucose includes the glucose content of all other extracellular fluids. The exercise times are the approximate times that these stores would last if they were the only source of energy available during exercise at an energy expenditure of about 17 kcal/minute, which is typical for football match play.

equivalent to 2,700–4,500 kcal of chemical potential energy. In addition, a lean footballer weighing 75 kg with a body-fat percentage of 10% will have about 7 kg of triglyceride stored in his adipose tissue. Clearly, even in a slim person, fat stores in the body are far larger than carbohydrate stores, and fat is a more efficient form of energy storage, releasing 9 kcal/g compared with 4 kcal/g from carbohydrate. The total storage capacity for fat is extremely large, and for most practical purposes, the amount of energy stored in the form of fat far exceeds that required for any exercise task (see table 3.2).

During most forms of moderate-intensity exercise such as jogging, a mixture of fat and carbohydrate is oxidised to provide energy for muscular contraction. The main problem associated with the use of fat as a fuel for exercise is that the rate at which it can be taken up by muscle and oxidised to provide energy is limited. In fact, fat oxidation can only supply ATP at a rate sufficient to maintain exercise at an intensity of about 60% of aerobic capacity. To generate ATP to sustain higher exercise intensities (e.g. for football match play, the average relative exercise intensity is about 70% of a player's aerobic capacity), there is an increasing reliance on carbohydrate, as illustrated in figure 3.8, and the oxidation of carbohydrate will be the predominant fuel with fat contributing 20–30% or less. Both the aerobic oxidation of carbohydrate and the anaerobic pathway of glycolysis can supply ATP at a much faster rate than fat oxidation can, but using more fat allows greater sparing of the limited carbohydrate reserves. Regular exercise training increases aerobic capacity and the ability to use fat as a fuel, which is one of the reasons that good aerobic fitness improves endurance and is important for footballers.

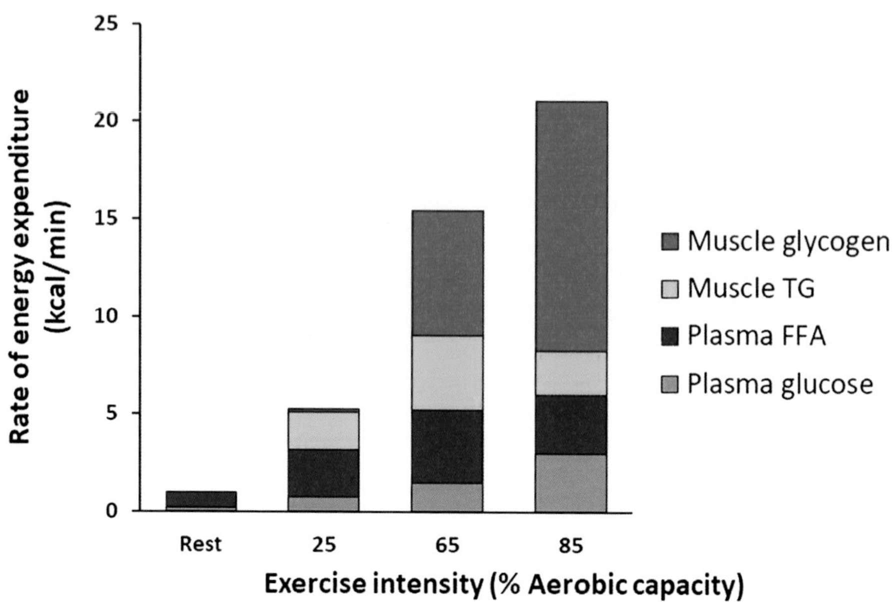

Figure 3.8 The contributions of carbohydrate (muscle glycogen and blood glucose) and fat (plasma free fatty acids and intramuscular triglyceride) fuel sources to energy expenditure at rest and different relative intensities of exercise. Data from Romijn et al. (1995). In football match play, the average intensity is about 70% of aerobic capacity.

Unlike carbohydrate (as glycogen) and fat (as triglyceride), protein is stored only as functionally important molecules (e.g. structural proteins, enzymes, membrane transporters, receptors and muscle contractile proteins), and availability of free amino acids in muscle and blood is quite low (e.g. the total amount of free amino acids in muscle is less than 3 g/kg). Hence, carbohydrate and fat are the preferred fuels for exercise, and the contribution of protein to energy expenditure in a 90-minute football match will likely not exceed a maximum of about 5% of total energy expenditure.

REPLENISHING ENERGY STORES AFTER EXERCISE

Playing 90 minutes of football will result in a substantial fall in the body's carbohydrate reserves with leg muscle glycogen content falling to 10–40% of pre-match levels. As carbohydrate is such an important fuel for football, it is important to replenish this before the next match, and it can only be achieved by consuming sufficient carbohydrate in the diet. How this is done will be described in subsequent chapters.

It is very important to understand that when muscle glycogen stores are depleted, only low-to-moderate intensity exercise is possible. The length of time that a fixed (i.e. constant) moderate exercise intensity (e.g. 75% of an individual's aerobic capacity, which is close to the average intensity of football match play) can be sustained is closely related to the size of the pre-exercise glycogen store (figure 3.9). The size of the store depends on the pattern of exercise and diet in the previous hours and days, so management of the timing and intensity of training sessions, as well as players' diets, are important considerations in football. If a player consumes a low-carbohydrate diet in the days following a match, the glycogen will not be fully restored, which will limit his or her ability to do intense training or perform at high intensity in a subsequent match. This is one of the reasons why very low-carbohydrate, or ketogenic, diets are discouraged in football.

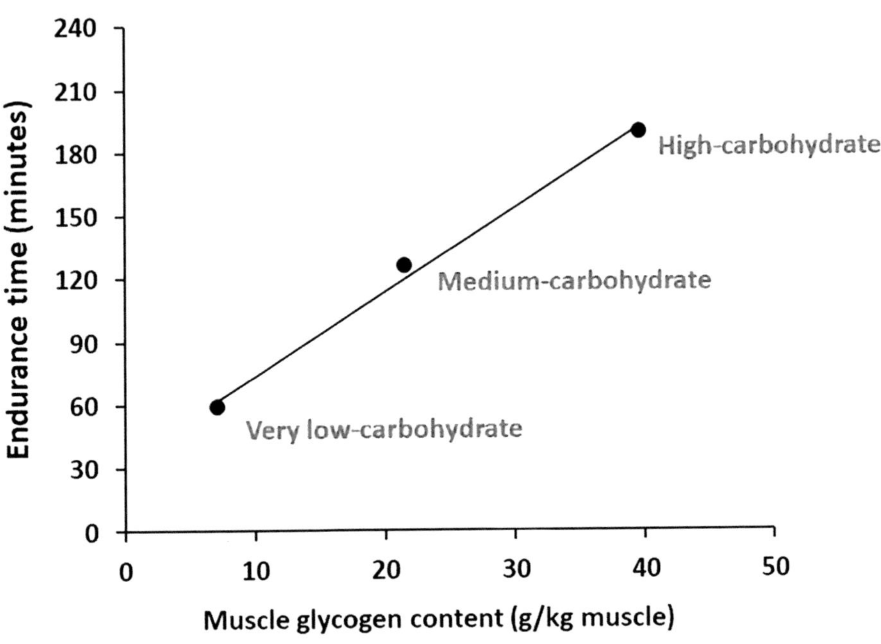

Figure 3.9 The effect of a very low-carbohydrate diet compared with moderate- and high-carbohydrate diets on leg muscle glycogen content and time to fatigue during cycling at 75% of aerobic capacity. The three data points in the graph represent the average values of nine participants in the study who performed the same exercise after first doing some hard exercise to deplete their glycogen stores, followed by three days on a very low-, moderate- or high-carbohydrate diet of equal total energy content. Data from Bergstrom et al. (1967).

LOSING OR GAINING BODY WEIGHT: THE ENERGY BALANCE CONCEPT

We all need food to survive, and we have evolved to be good at storing excess energy that we consume as fat, as this is our main storage form of energy and needed in times of starvation. The problem is if we overindulge and eat too much food over a prolonged period we become very fat, and this is bad for our health. While it is fine to have a certain amount of body fat (see chapter 8 for details), ideally, if we have a normal healthy body weight (or mass), we should just eat enough to supply our daily needs, not too little and not too much, which brings us to the concept of energy balance. Energy balance refers to the balance between energy intake and energy expenditure. Simply put, it is the difference between energy in and energy out. When energy intake is greater than energy expenditure (i.e. when more calories come in than go out), the energy balance is said to be positive, and weight gain will occur, as most of the excess energy gets converted into body fat. When energy intake is below energy expenditure, the energy balance is negative, and weight loss will result. Therefore, to maintain energy balance and a stable body weight, energy expenditure must closely match energy intake (see figure 3.10).

Over the long term, energy balance is maintained in weight-stable individuals even though this balance may be either positive or negative on a day-to-day basis. Over 24 hours, a person's energy intake is simply the sum of all the energy consumed in food and drink. Daily energy expenditure is the sum of the basal metabolic rate (BMR) (which is approximately 1,700 kcal/day for men and 1,600 kcal/day for women), plus the thermic effect of food, plus energy used in physical activity. The thermic effect of food (also known as diet-induced thermogenesis, DIT) is the increase in metabolic rate that occurs after eating food and represents the energy needed to digest, absorb and store the nutrients. In the average mixed Western diet (which consists of 50% carbohydrate, 35% fat and 15% protein), this adds about 10% to the metabolic rate; in other words about 170 kcal per day. Even a sedentary person does some physical activity to carry out the normal tasks of daily living, such as getting dressed, cooking food, going to the toilet and walking around the home, and this amounts to about 100 kcal per day. So, the typical daily energy requirements of a sedentary man are about 2,000 kcal and about 1,900 kcal for a sedentary woman. For footballers who participate in regular training sessions and play competitive matches, the average daily energy expenditure is higher than this – typically 1,000–1,500 kcal more – due to the additional energy expended in exercise. To achieve energy balance over a period of time (say weeks or months) and remain at a stable weight – whether you are sedentary person or an active footballer – your daily energy intake has to match your daily energy requirement.

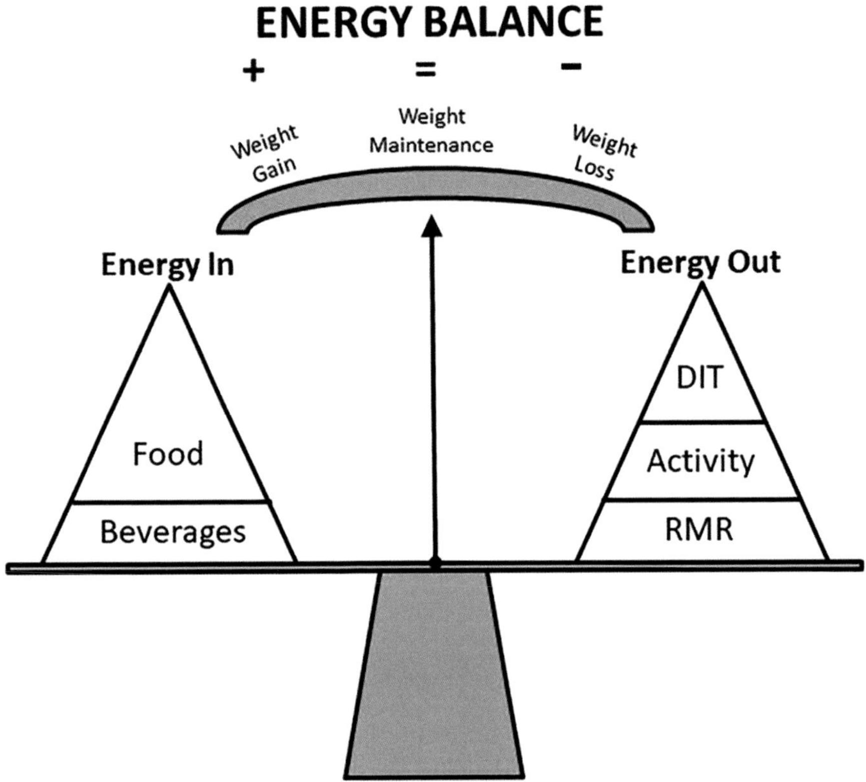

Figure 3.10 The concept of energy balance. DIT: diet-induced thermogenesis; RMR: resting metabolic rate.

You can estimate your own BMR from your sex, weight, height and age using the Mifflin-St Jeor equation, which was introduced in 1990. This equation is currently considered to be the best for estimating BMR.

Mifflin-St Jeor equation:

For men: RMR (kcal/day) = 10 x weight (kg) + 6.25 x height (cm) – 5 x age (years) + 5

For women: RMR (kcal/day) = 10 x weight (kg) + 6.25 x height (cm) – 5 x age (years) – 161

The BMR will be about 5–10% higher for a man than a woman of the same age and body weight because body composition (ratios of lean muscle, bone and fat) differ between men and women. The heavier you are, the more energy you need to sustain the larger muscle mass and larger organs, which is why heavier and taller individuals have a higher BMR. The other important factor age, because BMR decreases as you get older as muscle mass declines by 5–10% each decade after the age of 30, unless that is, you participate in regular resistance training to prevent this (and believe me, it is preventable). Nowadays, many apps on mobile devices can be used to calculate BMR or RMR, so if you don't like doing the maths calculations yourself you can use an app or an online BMR or RMR calculator that utilises the Mifflin-St Jeor equation. A suitable one can be found at this website: https://www.calculator.net/bmr-calculator.html

After calculating your own BMR, add an extra 10% to it to account for DIT. Now, to this value, add another 100 kcal to cover the energy expended in essential daily physical activities such as getting dressed, moving around the house, keeping an upright posture when seated or standing and doing a few household chores. This value will now be a reasonable estimate of your personal resting daily energy expenditure.

Here is an example calculation for a 30-year-old male, who is 178 cm tall and weighs 75 kg. The appropriate equation is:

For men: RMR (kcal/day) = 10 x weight (kg) + 6.25 x height (cm) – 5 x age (years) + 5

Inputting this man's weight, height, and age gives:

RMR (kcal/day) = 10 x 75 (kg) + 6.25 x 178 (cm) – 5 x 30 (years) + 5

= 750 + 1,113 – 150 + 5

= 1,718

Now we add 10% of 1,718 (172) to this value to account for DIT, which gives us 1,890 kcal/day and then add a further 100 kcal to account for energy expended in essential daily physical activity, giving us 1,990 kcal/day.

People who want to lose weight should increase their energy expenditure relative to their energy intake, which can be achieved either by increasing energy expenditure (by exercising more), reducing energy intake (by eating less) or a combination of both. There is no escaping this fact, and there are no quick-fix solutions to losing excess weight after it has been gained over a period of positive energy balance. If anyone tells you anything different from this simple truth, they are lying and you should ignore them.

As stated previously, weight gain will occur when a person is in positive energy balance and most of that excess weight will be body fat. Sometimes a footballer may want to gain more muscle but avoid putting on fat. Weight and strength gain through building bigger muscles can be achieved while maintaining energy balance by doing regular resistance exercise and consuming a relatively high-protein diet. This stimulates the growth of the muscles (commonly known as muscle hypertrophy) that are exercised but only occurs with resistance exercise such as weight lifting. More details about this can be found in chapter 8. Muscle hypertrophy will not occur with aerobic (cardio) exercise such as running or cycling and will not occur just by eating more protein.

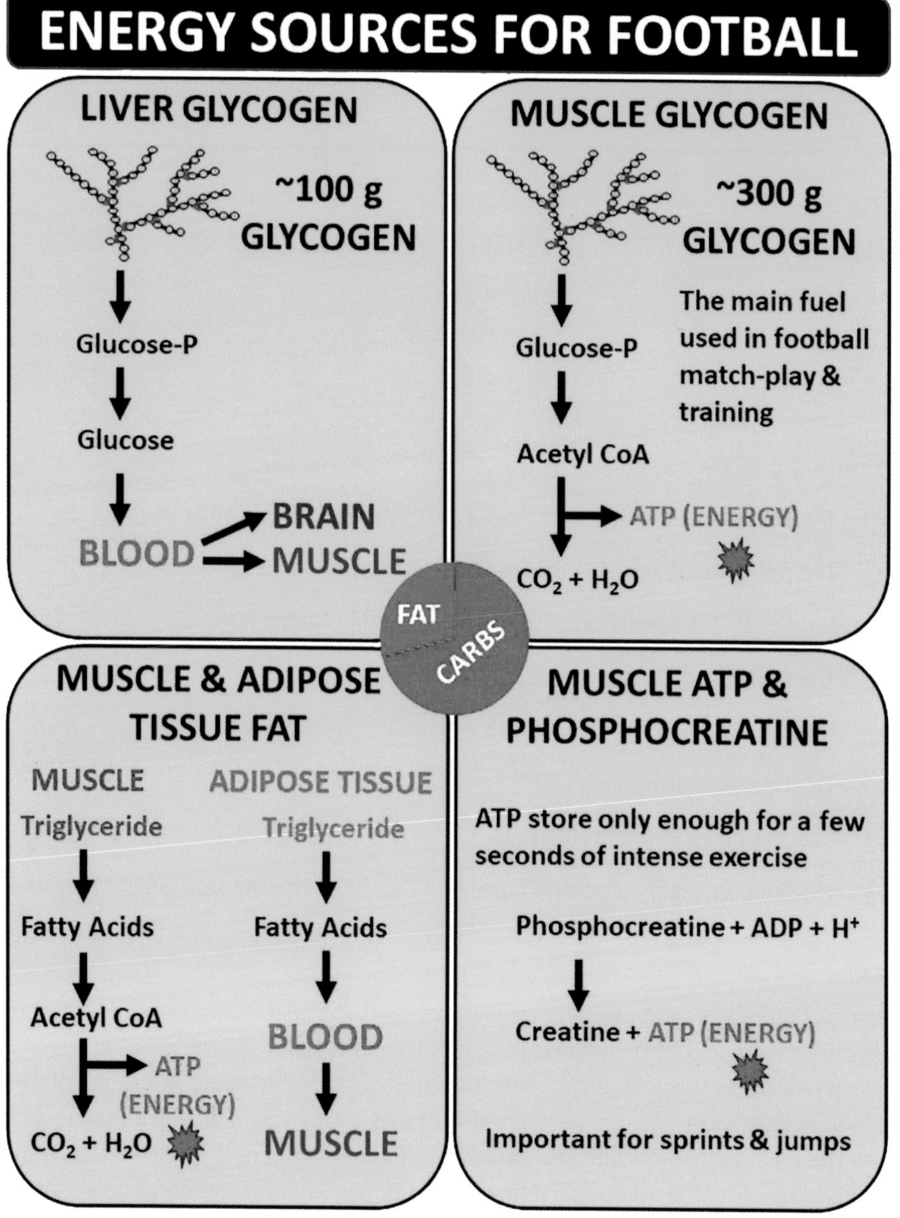

Infographic 3 The major energy sources for playing football.

CHAPTER 4

The Physiological and Nutritional Demands of Football

- The Nature of the Game and How It Has Evolved
- The Influence of Skill and Tactics (Think Barcelona Versus Oldham Athletic)
- Positional Differences in Energy Demand During Match Play
- The Fuels Used During Match Play
- Fatigue Development During Match Play
- The Demands of Training
- Keeping Players Fit and Healthy
- The Support Team Including Those Who Can Influence the Nutrition of Players

The first chapters of this book have largely dealt with the basics of food composition, the role of nutrients and how energy is obtained for exercise. Armed with that knowledge, we can now apply these facts and principles to the particular needs of football players. In this chapter, we will examine the physical and energy demands of football match play, the main fuels used and the causes of fatigue in different phases of the game. We'll also consider the additional demands of training and the various people that can influence the nutrition of a player. I'll begin by describing the characteristic features and consequent energy, metabolic and nutrient demands of playing football.

The various physical activities that footballers engage in during both training and match play constantly change every few seconds and, for this reason, football is classed as an intermittent, high-intensity sport. During a football match, players engage in a variety of activities from walking to sprinting, changing direction, jumping and striking the ball (passing and shooting), as well as tackling and other forms of contact with opposition players. In addition, mental functioning is important for timing of ball strikes and tackles, quick reactions, passing accuracy, decision making and staying concentrated. In outfield players, heart rate is maintained at an average of 85% of maximum and the average relative exercise intensity is at 70% of aerobic capacity (also known as maximal oxygen uptake, which is commonly abbreviated as VO_2max) over the duration of the match. The total amount of energy expended for a player completing the full 90 minutes is typically about 1,600 kcal, and carbohydrates provide about 60–70% of the total energy supply. The remainder comes from fat oxidation and PCr breakdown. The total match-day energy expenditure has been estimated at about 3,500 kcal.

THE NATURE OF THE GAME AND HOW IT HAS EVOLVED

The physical and technical demands of match play for elite outfield male footballers have increased substantially in recent years, mostly as a result of tactical modifications. Recent analyses of professional, high-level matches have revealed that the total distance covered is on average 10.9 km, with 1,150 m of high-intensity running and over 170 high-intensity actions (figure 4.1). The total distance covered by sprinting amounts to 350 m and, on average, players perform 57 sprints per game. In addition, the introduction of new technology has revealed that players make, on average, 35 passes during a game, of which 83% are successful. All these values, apart from total distance covered, which has remained the same, are higher than they were 10–15 years ago. These physically and technically demanding tasks make effective nutritional strategies for bolstering player performance even more important. The ability to sustain high-intensity exercise periods is probably the most crucial aspect of performance in football because it is known that, other than considerations of pure skill and passing accuracy, the amount of high-speed running is the major distinguishing factor between top-class players and those at a lower level. Equivalent data for elite female players is rather limited but suggests that elite, international-level female players cover approximately the same average total distance as their male counterparts, but they run less at high speeds.

At the time of writing this book, no studies have been performed to assess the physiological demands or fatigue responses of goalkeepers specifically. It is common for goalkeepers to perform extended (45–60 minute) pre-match warm-ups and, while they cover less total distance and perform fewer high-intensity activities, they are rarely substituted and need to be prepared for a full 90-minute match. A reasonable estimate is that they expend about 3,000 kcal on a match day – in other words about 500 kcal less than the outfield players.

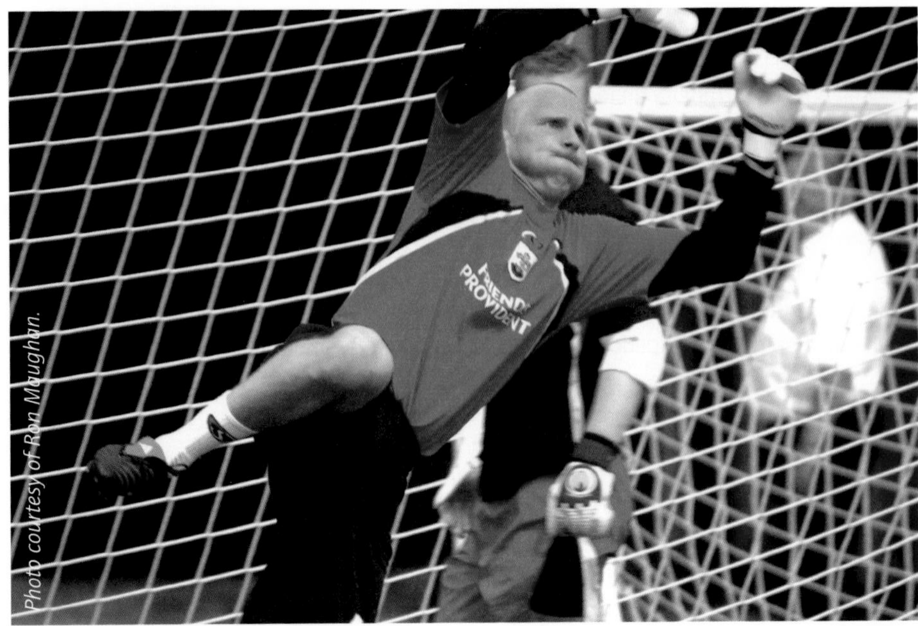

Photo 4.1 Although goalkeepers perform extended pre-match warm-ups, they cover less total distance and perform fewer high-intensity activities than outfield players, so on match days they expend about 500 kcal less than the outfield players.

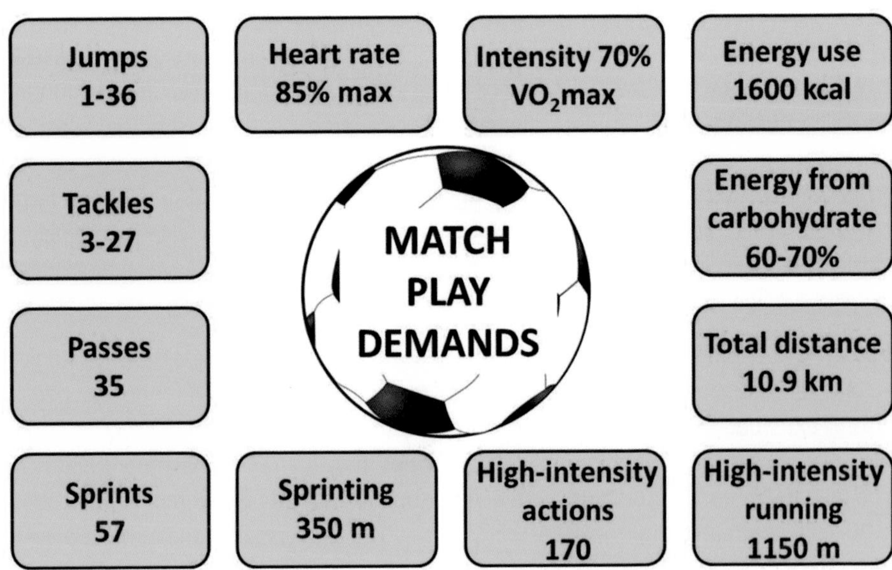

Figure 4.1 The physical and technical demands of match play for the average outfield player.

THE INFLUENCE OF SKILL AND TACTICS (THINK BARCELONA VERSUS OLDHAM ATHLETIC)

Team performance is determined not only by running ability (speed and endurance) but also by match tactics and the amount of ball possession, as well as skilful executions of in-play actions such as jumping, heading the ball, tackling, passing, shooting and dribbling. These actions also require a high level of cognitive functioning (quick reactions, timing of ball strikes and tackles, and effective rapid decision making). Minimising fatigue relative to the opposing team is an important strategy in modern football, since most goals are conceded in the last 15 minutes of each half (figure 1.2) and are attributed, at least in part, to fatigue. Generally, teams with the higher percentage of ball possession run less distance and expend less energy. Having the ability to play this way is one of the main reasons why teams such as Barcelona, Manchester City and Bayern Munich have had so much success in recent years. Lower level, less skilful teams who frequently lose possession of the ball (sadly, I have to include my own beloved Oldham Athletic in this category) are forced to do a lot of chasing of the ball and will always struggle physically against such dominating opposition.

POSITIONAL DIFFERENCES IN ENERGY DEMAND DURING MATCH PLAY

The typical distance covered by a top-class outfield player during a match is 10–13 km, but midfield players cover greater distances than other outfield players. However, most of this distance is covered by walking and low-intensity running, which require only relatively small increases in energy supply compared with being at rest. In terms of energy production, it is the high-intensity exercise periods that are most important. It is well known that the amount of high-intensity exercise separates top-class players from players of a lower standard. Time–motion analysis has revealed that international players perform 28% more high-intensity running and 58% more sprinting than professional players of a lower standard. The number of tackles and jumps depends on the individual playing style and position in the team, and at the highest level, has been shown to vary between 3 and 27 tackles and between 1 and 36 jumps per match. In top-class matches, sprinting speeds of the fastest players reach peak values of around 32 km/hour (20 mph), and we know that when a player sprints more than 30 m, he needs a longer time to recover than from the typical average sprints (10–15 m) during a game.

There are major individual differences in the physical demands of players, in part related to their position in the team. Central defenders cover less overall distance and perform less high-intensity running than players in the other outfield positions, which is probably closely linked to the tactical roles of the central defenders and their lower physical capacity. In contrast, full-backs cover a considerably greater distance at high speeds, but they perform fewer headers and tackles than players in the other playing positions. Generally, the forwards cover a similar distance at a high intensity to the full-backs and midfield players, but perform more sprints than the midfield players and defenders. Midfield players perform as many tackles and headers as defenders and attackers. They cover a total distance, and distance at a high intensity, similar to the full-backs and forwards, but generally sprint less. These positional differences in energy demands have an important influence on what players should be eating. The players who cover a lot of distance – such as full-backs and box-to-box midfielders – expend more energy than centre-backs or goalkeepers, so will need considerably more dietary calories.

Players in all team positions experience a significant decline in high-intensity running towards the end of the match. This indicates that most elite soccer players exhaust much of their physical capacity and become fatigued – to varying degrees – during a game. This can, of course reduce their effectiveness and possible contribution to team success in the latter stages of a game, and is one of the most common reasons that players are substituted from mid-way into the second half of a match. Other reasons may include injury, the risk of a red card, poor form, missing too many chances to score or not following their manager's instructions. Of course, individual differences are not only related to position in the team but to a player's individual role. Some midfielders, for example, may play a holding role and support defenders in breaking up attacks by the opposing team, whereas others may be box-to-box midfielders, meaning that they will cover further distances, as well as greater distance at a high intensity. Individual differences in playing style and physical performance should be taken into account when planning the training and nutritional strategy. Exactly the same principles apply to female and academy players.

THE FUELS USED DURING MATCH PLAY

Aerobic energy production appears to account for more than 90% of total energy consumption during match play. Nevertheless, anaerobic energy production plays an essential role during soccer matches. A top-class soccer player has 150–250 brief intense actions during a game, indicating that the rates of anaerobic PCr utilisation and glycolysis are frequently high during a game, which is supported by findings of reduced muscle PCr levels and several-fold increases in blood and muscle lactate concentrations. During intensive exercise periods of a game, PCr becomes partially depleted but is partly restored during subsequent periods of less-intense activity, such as jogging, walking or standing still. In blood samples taken

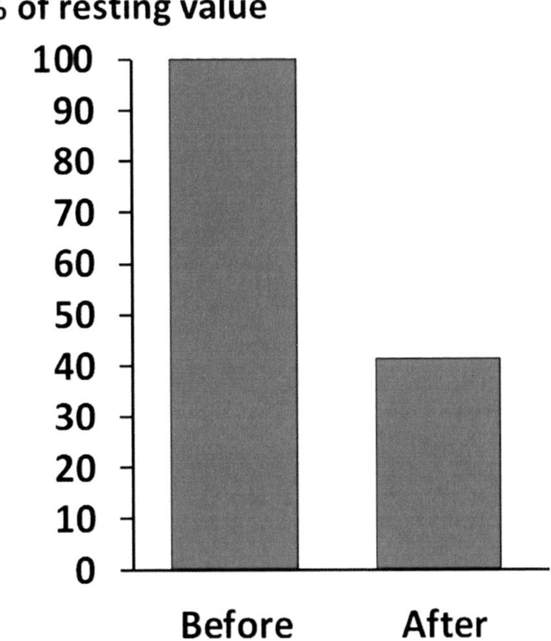

Figure 4.2 The percentage change in total thigh muscle glycogen content after a football match. Data from Bangsbo et al. (2006).

at rest, the lactate concentration is typically about 1 millimole per litre (mmol/L) and after top-class soccer matches, the lactate concentration averages 3–9 mmol/L, and individual values frequently exceed 10 mmol/L during match play. These findings indicate that the anaerobic energy systems are heavily taxed during some periods of match play.

Glycogen in the working muscles seems to be the most important fuel for energy production during games of football and is depleted typically by 60–90% of pre-match values by the end of a match (figure 4.2). However, muscle triglycerides, blood free fatty acids (FFA) and glucose are also used as substrates for oxidative metabolism in the muscles. Blood-glucose concentration, however, tends to be well maintained (or even above normal resting levels) during a game.

FATIGUE DEVELOPMENT DURING MATCH PLAY

At high standards of competitive play, it is noticeable that players suffer from fatigue during the second half and this is reflected in a reduction in work rate (less distance covered and fewer sprints). Studies using Prozone technology to analyse time spent in different activities during English Premier League matches have found that in the last 15 minutes of a game, high-

Table 4.1 Distance covered in soccer matches when players started the game with low or high muscle glycogen stores

Muscle Glycogen (g/kg muscle)			Distance Covered (km)			% Distance Covered	
Before	Half-time	End	1st half	2nd half	Total	Walking	Sprinting
15	4	1	6.1	5.9	12.0	27	24
7	1	0	5.6	4.1	9.7	50	15

Pre-exercise glycogen content was manipulated by feeding a high-carbohydrate or low-carbohydrate diet for the 3 days following the last game. Data from Saltin and Karlsson (1973).

intensity running distance is about 20% less than in the first 15 minutes for outfield players in all positions, with similar deficits for high-intensity running with and without ball possession. There is also a noticeable decline in high-intensity running immediately after the most intense 5-minute period of the game with the greatest deficits (40–50%) in attacking players and central defenders. It is common to see more goals scored in the later stages of games as players become tired and more mistakes are made. The development of fatigue during the game seems to be related to the depletion of the muscle glycogen stores, and it has been shown that players who started a match with low glycogen content in their thigh muscles covered 25% less distance than the others (table 4.1). Furthermore, players with low initial muscle glycogen content covered 50% of the total distance walking and only 15% sprinting, compared with 27% walking and 24% sprinting for the players with normal-to-high muscle glycogen levels. Blood lactate concentration is consistently lower at the end of a game compared with values at half-time, and this ties in with observations that the greatest rate of decline in muscle glycogen occurs in the first half of the match. Players who start matches with low glycogen stores in their leg muscles are likely to be close to complete glycogen depletion by half-time, and these findings have important implications for the training and nutritional preparation of players.

The fatigue that sets in towards the end of a game may be caused by a depletion of glycogen concentrations in a considerable number of individual muscle fibres. Muscle glycogen is typically reduced by 60–90% during a game and is by far the most important fuel for energy production. In two experimental studies in which muscle tissue biopsy samples were taken before and after a game of football, thigh muscle glycogen was found to have decreased to 42% of resting pre-match levels by the end of a football match (figure 4.2), and some 47% of muscle fibres were completely, or almost, empty of glycogen after the game (figure 4.3).

In other words, depletion of individual fast- and slow-twitch muscle fibres has been demonstrated despite muscle glycogen at the whole-muscle level only being moderately lowered. In addition, muscle glycogen is stored in specific compartments within muscle fibres, which have been recently demonstrated to be important for muscle function, and

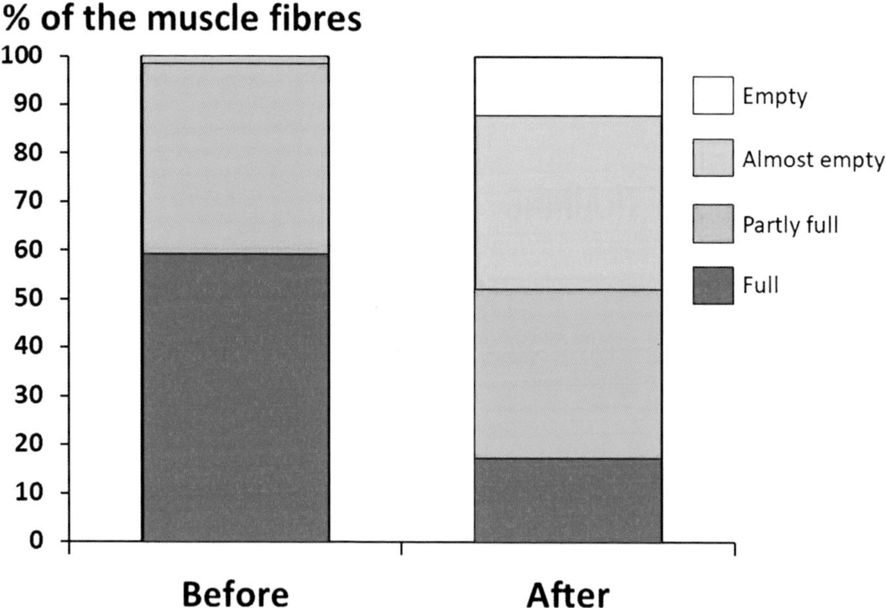

Figure 4.3 Relative glycogen content in muscle fibres before an immediately after a football match. Data from Krustrup et al. (2006).

this should be considered as well as global muscle glycogen availability. Traditionally, the relationship between muscle glycogen depletion and the onset of fatigue has been attributed to a decreased rate of ATP resynthesis due to inadequate carbohydrate fuel substrate availability at the whole-muscle level, but emerging evidence points to a direct coupling between muscle glycogen content and the mechanisms that result in muscle excitation and contraction. This level of detail is beyond the scope of this book, but for the reader who wants to learn more about this, the review papers by Hargreaves and Spriet (2020) and Vigh-Larsen and colleagues (2021) are recommended; details of these can be found in the list of reference sources at the end of the book.

As well as towards the end of a game, fatigue or reduced performance also seems to occur at two other stages in the game: (1) after short-term intense periods in both halves and (2) in the initial phase of the second half. A player's ability to perform maximally appears to be impaired in the initial phase of the second half, which may be due to lower muscle temperatures compared with the end of the first half. Thus, when players perform low-intensity activities in the 15-minute half-time interval between the two halves, both muscle temperature and performance are better preserved compared with just sitting still. On days when the weather is hot and humid, dehydration and an elevated body core temperature approaching 40°C, which results in mental and perceived physical fatigue, may also contribute to the deterioration in performance. In conclusion, fatigue or impaired performance in football (and probably most other sports involving multiple sprints) occurs during various phases in a game, and different physiological mechanisms appear to operate in different periods of a game.

THE DEMANDS OF TRAINING

In addition to playing matches, players have to train regularly to maintain fitness, learn and practice new skills, and try out new tactics and dead ball situations. Training may be either individual to focus on ball skills and a particular player's strengths or weaknesses or team-based such as 5-a-side games, passing, running and dribbling drills. During the season, the average daily training loads of players are somewhat less than those experienced in match play including: total distance (7 km versus 10 km), high-speed running distance (300 m versus 1,150 m), sprint distance (150 m versus 350 m) and average running speed (5 km/hour versus 7 km/hour). Absolute daily training loads depend on many factors. For example, the day after a match is usually a rest/recovery day for the players who had at least 45 minutes of game time; some training sessions on subsequent days will focus on high-intensity work, while others will focus more on tactics and free-kick/corner drills, particularly as the next game approaches. Training on the day before a match will generally be light to avoid glycogen depletion, fatigue or injury.

In the traditional in-season scenario of one match per week, players may complete four or five 'on-field' training sessions where the absolute training load will vary from day-to-day according to the coach's aims and the proximity of the next game. Players may also undertake additional 'off-field' sessions, such as jumping and running performance tests, strength training, cycle ergometer work and other gym-based activities. The aim is to stimulate both aerobic and strength training adaptations while simultaneously rehearsing technical skills and tactics.

In professional clubs, most training sessions will take place in the morning, meaning there is an opportunity for some pre-training nutrition at breakfast and post-training nutrition at lunchtime. For young academy players, and also in the amateur game, most training sessions will take place in the evenings. In all forms of football, nutrition plays an important role in assisting players to be able to carry out regular training while remaining relatively weight stable and healthy.

KEEPING PLAYERS FIT AND HEALTHY

The prevention of illness is a key component in player health management. Illness prevention strategies are not only important to allow uninterrupted training but also to reduce the risk of illness that can prevent participation or contribute to underperformance in matches. The immune system is the body's main line of defence against infection. Several nutritional strategies are effective in helping to maintain robust immunity, although other considerations for illness prevention are also important including good personal, home and training-venue hygiene, managing the training and competition load, getting adequate recovery and sleep, proactive psychological stress management and implementing player monitoring to detect early signs and symptoms of illness, overreaching and overtraining. Good hygiene practice in the storage and preparation of food for use in the training ground restaurant and post-match buffet venue (such as the changing room) is also important to minimise the risk of serious gastrointestinal illness caused by bacterial contamination. The four main things to remember for food good hygiene are: cross-contamination, cleaning, chilling and cooking. These are known as the 4 Cs and further details can be found on this topic in the next chapter and by reference to the UK Food Standards Agency website (https://www.food.gov.uk/business-industry/food-hygiene).

THE SUPPORT TEAM INCLUDING THOSE WHO CAN INFLUENCE THE NUTRITION OF PLAYERS

Most readers will be familiar with the roles of managers, assistant managers and coaches who make decisions on matters relating to team selection, match tactics and player transfers. Some managers and coaches have their own strong views on nutrition based on their previous experience and may influence, in particular, what foods, beverages and snacks are available to players at the training ground and what players should eat and drink on match day and the day before. A good example of this is the changes to his players' diet that Antonio Conte introduced at Chelsea after taking over from José Mourinho in 2016. Although being an Italian, Conte banned pizza, as well as ketchup, brown sauce and vinegar for his new players and told them to use salt, pepper and herbs if they wish to spice up their meals. He also made sugary and fizzy drinks off-limits. Pep Guardiola also banned pizza after joining up with Manchester City, but Conte's rules appeared much stricter as he also had cereals and pasta on his hit-list, replacing them with salads and chicken as lunch options in Chelsea's club canteen. In contrast, another Italian manager, Claudio Ranieri, who was the boss at Leicester City at that time, had previously rewarded his players with a pizza meal at an Italian restaurant when they kept their first clean sheet during their Premier League title-winning season in 2015–16. To be fair, this was a bit of a joke, and a treat for the players who were somewhat surprised to learn that they had to make up their own pizza toppings at the restaurant, which was no doubt a lesson in nutrition in itself!

All top clubs employ a team of sport science staff, which generally includes one or more exercise physiologists, strength and conditioning specialists, and match analysts. Some players may even have their own personal trainer. The physiologist is often the leader of the sport science support team, reporting directly to the manager on issues related to player fitness and well-being, and he or she will frequently liaise with a qualified sport nutritionist or dietitian and performance chef. These members of the team assist players with appropriate food choices to ensure that they have a balanced, varied and healthy diet that is sufficient to meet the energy and nutrient demands of regular training and competition. Some players also employ their own performance chef to prepare and cook their food in their homes, and the chefs usually take advice or instruction from the club nutritionist on the specific macronutrient needs of the players which will vary from day-to-day according to training load and match schedules.

Other members of the support team include physiotherapists, masseurs and the team doctor. The doctor may also be consulted on matters to do with nutrition and, in particular, the potential need for, and use of, supplements if blood tests reveal a deficiency of an essential micronutrient, such as vitamin D or iron. Some clubs may also employ a psychologist, although, in reality, it is the manager who often acts in that capacity to boost player confidence or inspire players to produce good match performances. The size of the multidisciplinary support team of science and medical experts has grown over the years. This mostly reflects the increasing desire of clubs that are paying huge wages to players – and whose value is measured in tens of millions of pounds – to now manage all aspects of player care and performance. It is essential that nutrition is integrated into the performance team. This means being a fundamental part of the team´s performance and/or medical meetings, where the priorities for each individual player are discussed in detail.

It is also important to be aware that some players' nutrition choices may be influenced by what they have seen on TV, Amazon and Netflix programmes or read about on social media platforms and the internet. Often the information available from such sources is biased and blatantly incorrect! Then there is the player's agent and the owners and directors of the club who effectively pay the players' wages. Some owners like to have an influence on team matters (much to the chagrin of many a manager!) and this can include some influence on what the players eat and drink.

Finally, there are the players' family and friends whose influence on the players' nutrition can be good or bad. The player's family might include their spouse and one or more children, and it is usually the spouse who does the food shopping and prepares and cooks the meals taken at home. Players in a team may often socialise with each other, but many will also have friends outside football who can have a potentially damaging effect on a player's choice of food and drink. Some of the older readers of this book may recall that Paul Gascoigne, the hugely talented former Newcastle, Tottenham Hotspur and England player, had a lifelong pal who liked eating fast food and drinking beer. His name was Jimmy 'Five Bellies' Gardner, which tells you all you need to know really!

PLAYER NUTRITION INFLUENCES

Players may make their food choices based on a whole variety of influences and sources of information which can lead to confusion

Manager & Coaches	Nutritionist or Dietitian	Club Doctor
S & C Coaches		Performance Chefs
Personal Trainers		Personal Preferences
Team Mates		Nationality Culture/Religion
Partner & Family		External Gurus
Friends		Internet & Social Media
Club Owners	Agents & Sponsors	TV Programmes Amazon/Netflix

Players should get their nutrition advice mostly from the club nutritionist or dietitian working in concert with the doctor & chefs

Infographic 4 The various people, factors and sources that can influence a player's food choices.

CHAPTER 5

Nutrition for Training Days

- Training Goals: Improving Fitness and Preparing for the Next Match
- Energy and Macronutrient Needs for Training
- Essential Micronutrient Requirements
- Supplements Used to Support Training
- Eating and Drinking on Training Days
- How Nutrition Can Help to Keep Players Healthy Throughout the Season
- Cultural and Religious Influences on a Player's Food Choices
- Food Preferences, Allergies and Tolerance Issues
- Is It Possible to Be a Vegetarian or Vegan Footballer?
- Good Food Hygiene Practices

As explained in the previous chapter, in addition to playing matches, players have to train regularly to maintain fitness, develop team cohesion, work on their strengths and weaknesses, learn or practice new skills and try out new tactics and dead ball situations. Training load often varies considerably on a day-to-day basis: some days may be mostly for recovery and the day before a match usually involves only a light training session, whereas others can be quite intense. That means, of course, that the day-to-day nutritional requirements will also be different. Nutrition to support the players' energy and specific macronutrient needs is the major focus of this chapter, although I will also cover some of the more important micronutrient needs, the potential value of certain

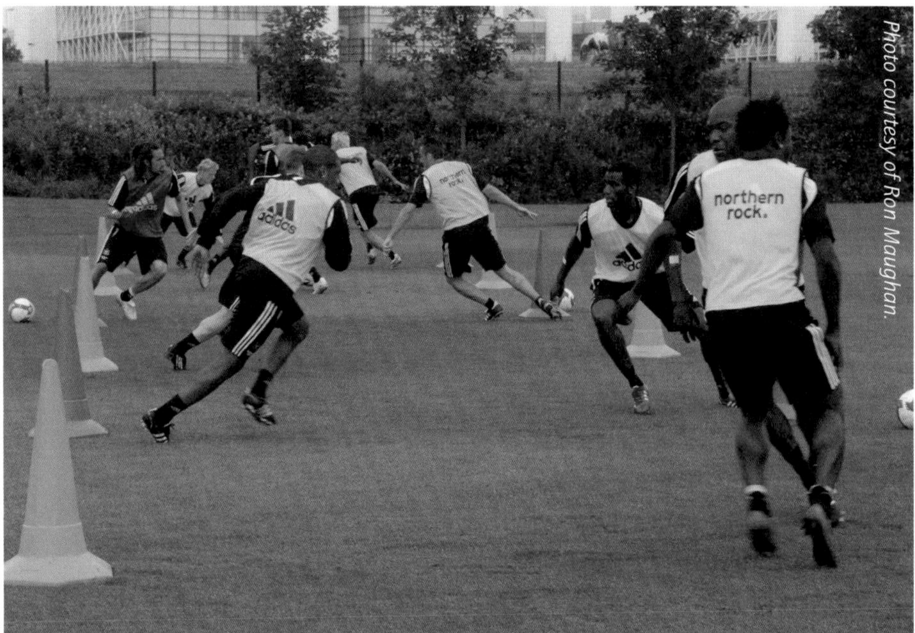

Photo courtesy of Ron Maughan.

Photo 5.1 Football training has an impact on energy and nutrient needs.

dietary supplements to support hard training and explain the importance of nutrition and good food hygiene practices to protect players' health.

When the players return for pre-season training – which has often been preceded by a holiday – the aim is to lose any excess weight and improve fitness through a programme of 5–6 weeks of intensive training, in which training loads may be up to double what they are during the competitive season. Once the new league season begins, usually in August, training will typically take place on 4–5 days per week if there is just one match per week, but may be limited to only 2 days per week during congested fixture periods as recovery, rather than adaptation and fitness building, becomes the more important focus.

TRAINING GOALS: IMPROVING FITNESS AND PREPARING FOR THE NEXT MATCH

During the season, when there is one game every six or seven days, the average daily training loads of players amount to covering about 7 km, running 300 m at high speed and sprinting 150 m (figure 5.1). Absolute daily training loads depend on many factors. For example, the day after a match is usually a rest/recovery day

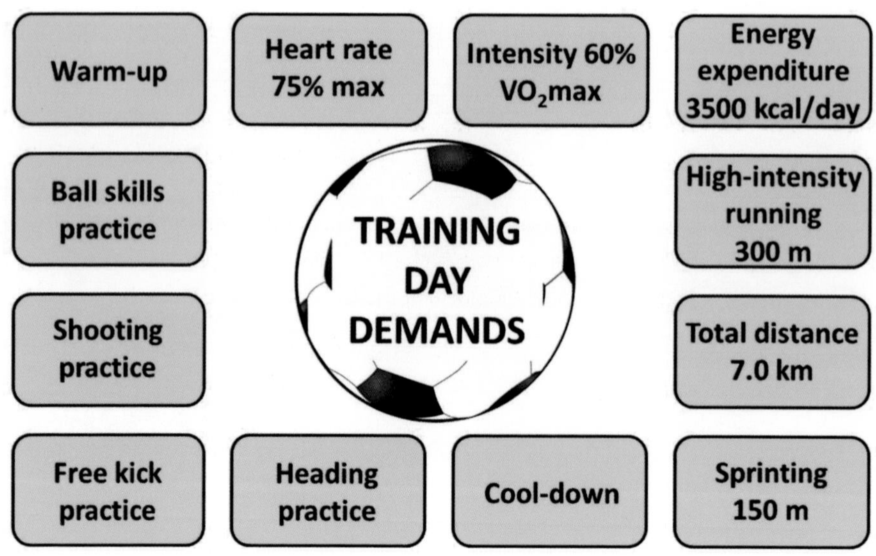

Figure 5.1 The physical and technical demands of a typical training day for the average outfield player.

for the players who had some game time; some training sessions on subsequent days will focus on high-intensity work and practicing team formations and tactics that are planned to be used in the next match. The aim is to stimulate both aerobic and strength training adaptations to improve, or at least maintain, fitness while simultaneously rehearsing technical skills and tactics, particularly as the next game approaches. Training on the day before the match is usually very light and will focus mostly on the specific tactics to be used against the upcoming opposition and free-kick/corner drills and shooting practice. At times during the season, when there are two games per week and there may be only three days from one match to the next, all training sessions will normally be lighter and shorter than in the one-game-per-week scenario, with the focus on recovery and immediate preparations for the next match, at least for those players getting regular game time. The issue of using appropriate nutrition to optimise rapid and effective recovery will be covered in chapter 7. In the remainder of this chapter, I will focus on describing the recommended nutritional strategies that can be employed to facilitate effective training and keep players healthy throughout the season.

ENERGY AND MACRONUTRIENT NEEDS FOR TRAINING

As mentioned at the start of this book, nutrition recommendations for elite football are based on the UEFA expert group consensus paper published in the *British Journal of Sports Medicine* in October 2020. A total of 31 experts, including yours truly, contributed to the writing of this review. The experts included six basic and applied researchers with expertise in sport nutrition, five nutritionists currently working in elite football, 14 who had a background of both research and field-based practice, and six were members of the UEFA Medical Committee.

The energy expenditure of outfield players (during a 7-day in-season micro-cycle consisting of two games and five training days) from the English Premier League was recently quantified as about 3,500 kcal per day (for the average player weighing 75 kg) with goalkeepers' energy expenditure being about 600 kcal per day less. In general, larger, heavier outfield players will have higher total daily energy requirements than this, and for smaller, lighter players, the needs will be a little less than average. For this reason, it is more appropriate to express energy and macronutrient needs as kilocalorie or gram amounts per kilogram body mass (g/kg BM) rather than as absolute amounts. Current recommendations for the intake of macronutrients (i.e. carbohydrate, protein, fat and water) to support training are summarised in table 5.1.

We will begin by examining the macronutrient needs for training starting with carbohydrate which, as previously mentioned, is the main fuel used in both match play and intensive training sessions.

CARBOHYDRATE REQUIREMENTS

The main stores of carbohydrate (CHO) in the body are in the form of glycogen, a large molecule composed of thousands of linked glucose (the same sugar that is in the blood) molecules that can be broken down rapidly when needed as a source of energy. Given the important role of muscle and liver glycogen in supporting energy production and performance in moderate- to high-intensity exercise, as outlined in the previous chapters, meeting daily carbohydrate requirements for football training is a priority. Although players can adjust their daily carbohydrate intake according to the perceived training load, they are generally recommended to consume about 4 g of carbohydrate per kilogram body mass (abbreviated as g CHO/kg BM from now on) on most training days, with 6 g CHO/kg BM on the day before a match and match day itself, and up to 8 g CHO/kg BM on the day after a match to promote recovery. Alternatively, given the lower absolute daily training loads on typical training days (i.e. one session per day in a one-game-per-week micro-cycle), daily intakes ranging from 3–6 g CHO/kg BM may

Table 5.1 Recommendations for macronutrient intake to support football training

Macronutrient	General	Before Training	During Training	After Training
Carbohydrate (CHO)	3–6 g CHO/ kg BM/day for low-moderate intensity training 6–8 g CHO/ kg BM/day for high-intensity training or match preparation	1–2 g CHO/kg BM consumed 2–4 hours before training begins	None for low-moderate-intensity training 30–50 g CHO/ hour as beverage or gel for high-intensity training	1–4 g CHO/kg BM consumed in post-training meals
Protein (PRO)	1.2–1.6 g PRO/ kg BM/day with 0.4 g/kg BM/meal every 3–4 hours	0.4 g PRO/kg BM consumed 2–4 hours before training begins	None	0.4 g PRO/kg BM consumed in each post-training meal
Fat	20–35% of the total daily energy intake (approx. 1.0–1.8 g fat/kg BM/ day for an average energy expenditure of 3,500 kcal/day)	Pre-training meal will likely have a lower fat content than other meals	None	Typically 0.2–0.8 g fat/kg BM in post-training meals though fat content less crucial than for PRO and CHO
Water (H_2O)	1.5–2.0 L H_2O per day as drinks plus additional volumes according to fluid losses during training sessions	5–7 mL H_2O/kg BM consumed 2–4 hours before training begins	Drink fluid in volumes sufficient to limit fall in BM to no more than 2% of pre-training BM Drink regularly (e.g. every 20–30 minutes) in small portions to avoid overfilling stomach	Drink fluid to satisfy thirst or up to 1.5 L for each kilogram of body mass loss Consumption of fluid in post-match meal with carbohydrate and protein will increase fluid absorption and retention

In this and some other subsequent tables of this book, the following abbreviations are used: CHO – carbohydrate; PRO – protein, H_2O – water; BM – body mass.

be sufficient to promote fuelling and recovery. In accordance with the lower absolute loads during training compared with match play, it is unlikely that most players require any carbohydrate intake during the training sessions themselves, and daily needs can be satisfied by the carbohydrate consumed in regular meals. High-carbohydrate foods include potato, rice, pasta, corn, cereals, bread, jam, honey and several fruits including banana, apple and mango. Sports dietitians and performance chefs are trained to turn the theoretical recommendations of macronutrient intake into foods, and advice is often provided in g/kg BM/day or g/hour. For example, you have just read that that the recommended carbohydrate intake for training is typically about 4 g/kg BM/day. Table 5.2 is a handy way to figure out what a football player needs to ingest to hit those targets. This table illustrates the amount of carbohydrate available in various high-carbohydrate foods and it also tells you which of these foods have a high, moderate or low glycaemic index (GI) and glycaemic load (GL). The GI represents how much the blood-glucose level is elevated (figure 5.2) in the first two hours after consuming an amount of the food containing 50 g CHO compared with ingesting 50 g of pure glucose. Foods with a high GI raise blood sugar levels to relatively high levels quite quickly. Low-GI foods are digested

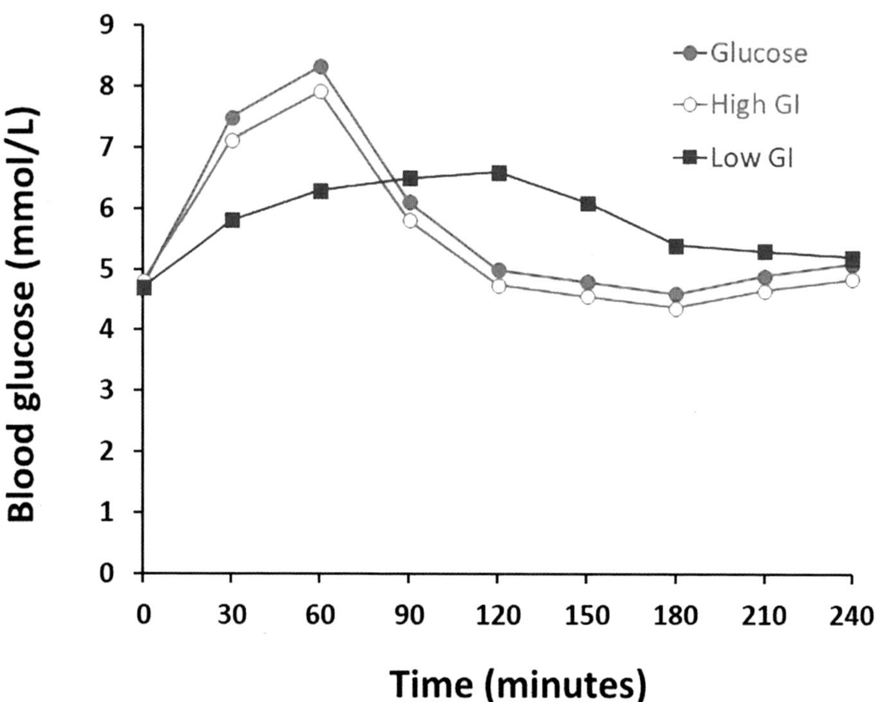

Figure 5.2 The blood-glucose response to consuming a high or low glycaemic index (GI) food containing 50 g CHO compared with 50 g of pure glucose.

Table 5.2 Carbohydrate content of foods that provide at least 10 grams of carbohydrate per normal size serving; also shown are the values for GI and GL in comparison to 50 grams of glucose

High-GI Foods (GI = 70 or more)	GI	Serving size (g)	CHO content (g)	GL per serving
Glucose	100	50	50	50
Pancakes, buckwheat	102	80	23	23
Typical sports drink (e.g. Gatorade)	89	250 (mL)	15	13
Rice bubbles/pops/crispies	88	30	26	23
Baked potato	86	150	27	26
Pretzels	83	30	20	16
Puffed rice cakes	82	25	21	17
Corn flakes	81	30	26	21
Bread, white, wheat flour	75	30	15	11
Weetabix	75	30	22	12
Boiled potato	75	150	28	16
Popcorn	72	20	12	9
Rice, white, boiled	72	150	42	30
Moderate GI Foods (GI = 56–69)	**GI**	**Serving size (g)**	**CHO content (g)**	**GL per serving**
Bagel, white	69	70	35	24
Doughnut	67	47	23	17
Croissant	67	57	26	17
Oreo cookies	64	40	32	20
Coca-Cola	63	250 (mL)	26	16
French baguette with butter and jam	62	70	41	26
Bread, white, toasted	60	30	15	7
Digestives (cookies/biscuits)	59	25	16	10
Ice cream, vanilla	57	50	10	6
Blueberry muffin	57	70	39	22
Long-grain rice, boiled	56	150	41	23

Moderate GI Foods (GI = 56–69)	GI	Serving size (g)	CHO content (g)	GL per serving
Honey	56	25	18	10
Fruit cocktail, canned	56	120	16	9
Low-GI Foods (GI = 55 or less)	**GI**	**Serving size (g)**	**CHO content (g)**	**GL per serving**
Potato crisps/chips	54	50	21	11
Sweet corn	52	150	32	17
Cookies/biscuits, chocolate	52	45	30	16
Banana	52	120	24	12
Porridge (wheat or oats)	51	250	30	15
Orange juice	50	250 (mL)	26	13
Muesli	49	30	20	10
Spaghetti, white, boiled	49	180	48	24
Baked beans	48	150	15	7
Ice cream, low fat, vanilla	46	50	15	7
Grapes	46	120	18	8
All-Bran cereal	44	30	20	9
Custard	43	100	17	7
Orange or peach	42	120	11	5
Rye bread	41	30	12	5
Rice noodles, boiled	40	180	39	15
Apple juice	40	250 (mL)	29	12
Apple	38	120	15	6
Pizza, Super Supreme (Pizza Hut)	36	100	24	9
Smoothie, raspberry	33	250 (mL)	41	14
Skimmed milk	32	250 (mL)	13	4
Milk, full fat	31	250 (mL)	12	4
Crème Fraîche	30	150	17	5
Lentils	30	150	17	5
Kidney beans	28	150	25	7
Low-fat yoghurt	24	200	14	3

Table 5.3 A list of common sports nutrition products that can provide 30 g of high-GI CHO

Product	CHO content (g)	Amount providing 30 g
Sports drink	6–8 g/100 mL	400–500 mL (15–18 fl oz)
Gel (one packet)	24–30	1–1.5
Cereal energy bar	20–40	0.75–1.5
Chews	80 g/100 g	40 g (8 chews)
Jelly beans	94 g/100 g	35 g (15 jelly beans)

and absorbed more slowly, which helps you achieve a lower but more stable level of blood sugar. Foods with a low GI are typically foods that are higher in fibre.

Foods may be classed as high, medium or low GI with the corresponding GI values being 70 or more, 56–69 and 55 or less, respectively. The GL is the GI divided by 100 and multiplied by the number of grams of carbohydrate present in the normal serving size of the food. The GL values of foods are generally classed as 20 or more, 11–19 and 1–10 for high, medium and low GL, respectively. A player's carbohydrate intake can be further supplemented with sports drinks, gels, cereal-based energy bars and jelly beans, or other forms of candy that are all high GI sources of carbohydrate (table 5.3). Studies have shown that medium and high-GI foods are the best types of carbohydrate for muscle glycogen resynthesis, so when recovery is the priority, such as for post-match meals, these would be the preferred choice.

Current recommendations for the intake of carbohydrate to support training are summarised in table 5.1.

FAT REQUIREMENTS

Dietary fat is an important part of a player's training nutrition as an energy source, a source of fat-soluble vitamins (A, D, E and K), omega-3 fatty acids and the two essential fatty acids linoleic acid and alpha-linolenic acid. Players are often advised to adjust fat intake to allow protein and carbohydrate requirements to be met within total energy targets, and to follow general population guidelines regarding a minimal (i.e. as low as possible) intake of harmful *trans*-fatty acids (which are higher in some margarines and processed foods) and a limited intake (up to 20 g/day) of saturated fats (highest in fatty cuts of meat, egg yolk and dairy products). This typically leads to a fat intake that provides 20–35% of total dietary energy. While some players may restrict fat intake to reduce total energy intake, or because they think it is 'healthy', over-restricting fat intake to less than 15–20% of total daily energy intake often requires an unnecessary avoidance of a range of foods with valuable nutrient contents and could lead to an inadequate intake of fat-soluble vitamins A, D, E and K and essential fatty acids. Good food sources of healthy unsaturated fats include avocado, oily fish such as salmon, sardines, trout and mackerel, vegetable oils, nuts and seeds. Foods that contain some saturated fat but are also nutritious include eggs, milk, cheese and yoghurt. Current recommendations for the intake of fat to support training are summarised in table 5.1.

PROTEIN REQUIREMENTS

Daily football training places stress on the muscles and tendons, and there is a need to remodel and repair these protein-containing structures to maintain and improve their integrity and function. Players will almost certainly benefit from provision of higher quantities of protein than are needed by the general population. The recommended daily allowance (RDA) for protein is 0.8 g/kg BM/day, but higher intakes up to 1.6–2.2 g/kg BM per day appear to enhance training adaptations, reduce post-match muscle soreness, improve recovery and are optimal for immune function. Such a level of protein intake can be achieved easily from a mixed diet, provided that the energy intake is sufficient to meet the demands of training. For that reason, special protein supplements in the form of milkshakes, whey protein or specially formulated post-workout recovery drinks are probably not needed for most players, although they provide a convenient and easily digestible alternative to foods immediately following a match or an intensive or gym-based resistance exercise training session, particularly for players whose appetite may be temporarily suppressed for a while following the performance of intense exercise. Where protein supplements are consumed at a dose of 0.3–0.4 g/kg BM, whey protein is definitely considered superior to other protein sources (e.g. casein, soy, collagen etc.), owing to its higher leucine content and digestibility. Leucine is one of the 20 amino acids that are found in protein, but it is considered to be a special amino acid as it is the only one that is known to directly stimulate muscle protein synthesis, which is important for muscle repair, growth and adaptation to the training stimulus.

Ideally, three or four discrete protein-containing meals should be consumed each day, with at least 0.4 g/kg BM per meal. For a player weighing 75 kg that equates to 30 g of protein per meal. This is because research has shown that around 25–30 g of protein has to be consumed in a meal to achieve close to the maximal rate of muscle protein synthesis. Below this amount, the rate of protein synthesis will be considerably lower. Amounts in excess of 30 g per meal produce no further substantive rise in protein synthesis; in other words, the anabolic response to protein ingestion peaks at around 0.4 g/kg BM. Most people do not follow a repeated, but relatively constant, intake of protein over the course of a day. It is more common for people to consume the largest amount of protein in their evening meal, somewhat lower amounts for lunch and the lowest amount in their breakfast. The recommended feeding strategy requires judicious planning of meals to emphasise protein at each main eating occasion (i.e. breakfast, lunch and dinner) to provide a sufficient dose to stimulate body protein remodelling.

Good food sources of protein include lean meat, poultry, eggs, fish, prawns, milk, cheese, beans and pulses. Bread, rice and pasta also supply some protein. Dietary protein quality may be important for players as all nine essential amino acids must be provided. Animal sources of protein are generally superior to plant foods in this respect (table 5.4). At least 2–3 g of the essential amino acid leucine is needed per meal for optimal boosting of muscle protein synthesis, and leucine content is highest in dairy proteins (i.e. whey and casein) and meat (table 5.5). Emerging research on protein consumption before sleep suggests that this may be important for football players. Overnight is a natural regenerative phase and yet is also a time when nutrient intake is usually very low or absent. Preliminary evidence supports pre-sleep protein ingestion at a dose of about

Table 5.4 Examples of foods that will provide 30 g of protein

Food	Typical portion size (g)	Amount needed for 30 g protein (g)	Energy content in the amount needed for 30 g protein (kcal)	EAA in the amount needed for 30 g protein (g)	Leucine in the amount needed for 30 g protein (g)
Bread (white)	75	357	838	97.2	2.2
Spaghetti (boiled)	50	1,000	861	15.2	3.3
Milk (semi-skimmed)	200 (mL)	909 (mL)	418	15.4	3.0
Egg (boiled)	60	240	352	14.4	2.4
Steak, stewing (raw)	175	148	261	13.7	2.4
Chicken (roast)	85	112	159	12.8	2.2
Lentils (boiled)	155	395	395	11.9	2.3
Potato (boiled)	150	2,000	1,500	11.4	1.9

Note the very different amounts of food and the different energy contents for the same amount (30 g) of total protein and for similar amounts of essential amino acids (EAA).

Table 5.5 Leucine content of various protein sources

Protein source	Leucine (g/100 g protein)
Whey protein isolate	14
Milk protein	10
Egg protein	8.5
Muscle (meat) protein	8
Soy protein isolate	8
Wheat protein	7

0.4 g/kg BM an hour or two before bedtime to improve training adaptation during periods of high training volume.

Ingestion of protein just before bedtime may also improve sleep quality, reduce muscle soreness and improve recovery of muscle function after hard training sessions and match play, and this will be discussed in more detail in chapter 7. Current recommendations for the intake of protein to support training are summarised in table 5.1.

WATER REQUIREMENTS

Water is an essential macronutrient, although, of course, it comes with zero calories. Most sedentary people consume about 2 L of water per day with 1.2 L coming from drinks and 0.8 L from solid foods. On resting and recovery days, footballers should aim to drink 1.5–2.0 L (20–27 mL/kg BM) of watery fluids in addition to the water they get from eating food. On training days, more water will be needed to offset fluid lost in sweat and expired air, and fluid needs will be influenced by ambient temperature, humidity, exercise intensity and exercise duration, which can all affect the individual's sweat rate. Maintaining an appropriate hydration status will help support players' health and football performance.

Water is lost from a player's body primarily in the form of sweat, urine and respiratory losses, whilst water is gained by the ingestion of foods and fluid. Sweating is the main mechanism used by the body to dissipate the excess metabolic heat generated as a consequence of football training and match play in both cool and hot environments. Note that most players will wear warm underclothing, as well as tracksuits, hats and gloves, when they train in cold weather conditions so they can still sweat a lot. Evaporation of sweat from the surface of the skin causes a cooling effect that helps to prevent body temperature from rising by more than a degree or two, which can otherwise cause fatigue and the risk of life-threatening heat illness. However, the loss of water in sweat can also lead to dehydration if fluid losses are not replaced. Dehydration reduces both sweat rate and skin blood flow making it even more difficult for the active player to prevent a rise in his core temperature. Starting a training session in a well-hydrated state and drinking regularly during training is therefore important for both the health and performance of the player, especially in warm weather.

Changes in the hydration status of a player can be monitored using daily measurements of body weight, urine colour and urine concentration. Urine colour should be very pale yellow when a player is well hydrated. Dark yellow would suggest that the player may well be somewhat dehydrated. Urine concentration is a more reliable measure of hydration status and can be easily be determined from a hand-held device known as an osmometer, which can almost instantly produce a reading of urine osmolality from a small sample of urine that a player collects mid-stream into a sample bottle. Osmolality is simply a measure of the dissolved particle content of a given volume or mass of urine (1 L of urine weighs about 1 kg) and the units are in milliosmoles per kilogram (mOsmol/kg), so it is directly related to the overall concentration of a sample of urine. A urine osmolality of less than 700 mOsmol/kg is indicative of normal hydration. A value of over 900 mOsmol/kg can be taken to indicate dehydration (or hypohydration, which is the preferred scientific term). To ensure they are well hydrated before starting training, players should drink 5–7 mL/kg BM of fluid in the 2–4 hours before the training session begins. Players are encouraged to drink fluids with their meals (e.g. breakfast) as the sodium present in most foods helps to promote fluid retention in the body. This practice will also allow any excess fluid to be voided, and should result in the desired pale yellow urine colour. Some clubs instigate occasional random checks on the urine osmolality of players when they arrive at the club training venue. Players who arrive in a dehydrated state can be expected to be admonished and possibly fined.

Players will lose some fluid due to sweating during training sessions. Sweat rate is influenced by the intensity of exercise, ambient temperature and humidity, clothing and acclimation status. However, there is a wide variation in sweat rates between individuals, such that sweat rates may vary from 0.5 L/hour to 2.5 L/hour and are generally lower in female players because of lower body mass and absolute work rates compared with their male counterparts. A loss of fluid from the body amounting to more than 2% of body mass (that would be 1.5 kg for a player weighing 75 kg) can increase cardiovascular strain, impair cognitive function, increase the perception of effort and is associated with reduced physical as well as technical football performance. To this end, players should aim to drink fluids to replace sweat losses, sufficient to prevent a deficit of more than 2% of pre-exercise body mass during exercise, but avoiding gains in body mass. This is particularly important when training in high ambient temperatures, which exacerbates the detrimental effects of dehydration. Water is an appropriate beverage to replace sweat losses, although the inclusion of some carbohydrate (20 g/L) and sodium (500–1500 mg/L) as found in most commercial rehydration beverages will improve water absorption and partially replace sodium losses in sweat. Furthermore, providing chilled (8–10°C) beverages with some fruit flavouring will promote voluntary fluid intake.

Variable quantities of electrolytes, particularly sodium, are also lost in sweat. Individual assessment of sweat-electrolyte concentration and sweat rate is recommended as players with high sweat sodium concentrations and high sweat losses will need greater fluid replacement during exercise than others. These measurements can be made by the club sport science support staff. Sweat losses can be calculated as follows to help players understand their personal fluid needs and determine personalised drinking plans for exercise at different intensities and under various environmental conditions:

Sweat rate (L/hour) = Sweat loss (L) / Exercise duration (hours)

Sweat loss (L) = Body mass before exercise (kg) – Body mass after exercise (kg) + Volume of any fluid ingested during exercise (L) – Volume of any urine voided before post-exercise body mass is measured (L).

An observational study published in 2021 reported sweat losses and voluntary (unprescribed) intakes of fluid (water or a commercial sports drink) during both high- and low-intensity training sessions involving 14 players of the men's first team squad of FC Barcelona (Spanish first division; La Liga) in both cool (15°C and 66% humidity) and hot weather conditions (29°C and 52% humidity). Fluid intakes were recorded on four separate training days during the competitive season and each outdoor football-specific training session lasted 60–70 minutes. This was a purely observational study and no advice was given to the players. As expected, on average, the players experienced a reduction in body mass that was relative to the session intensity and level of heat stress, but the individual differences were large. During the high-intensity session in hot conditions, the players' sweat rates averaged 1.4 L/hour but ranged between 1.1 and 1.8 L/hour for the lightest and heaviest sweaters. Even so, none of the players incurred sweat losses greater than 2% of body mass. The exercise intensity seemed a slightly more important factor than the temperature (table 5.6). Therefore, recommendations for fluid and carbohydrate intake should be specific to the individual player and exercise occasion. Assessing players' sweat rates during training sessions should therefore be the first step in personalising players' fluid intake

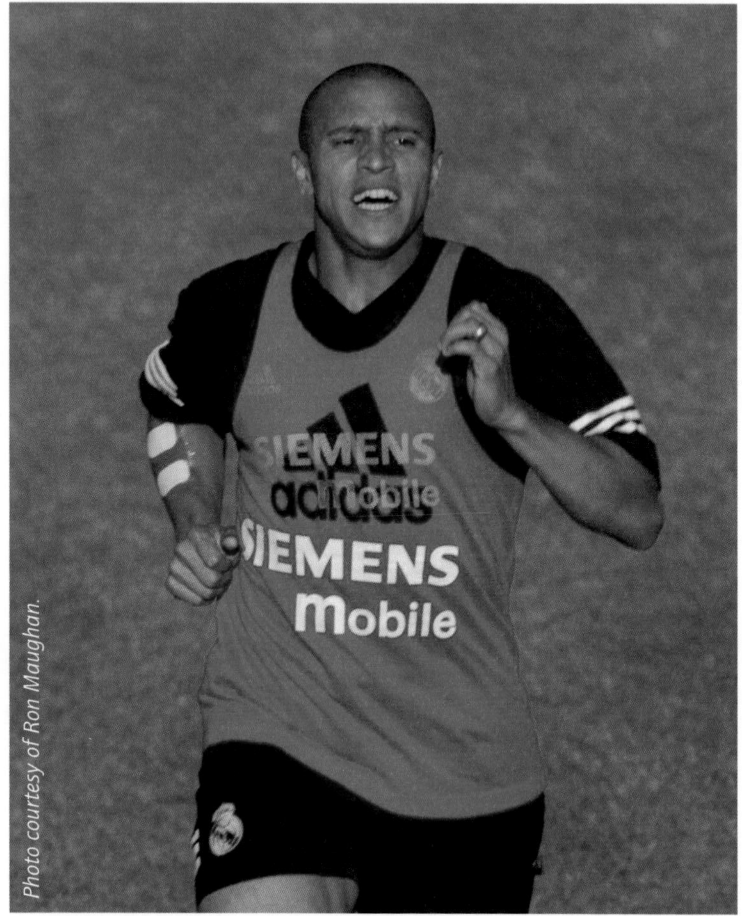

Photo 5.2 Roberto Carlos, the Brazil and Real Madrid player, wearing sweat patches on his forearm (and under his shirt) in training to collect sweat for analysis of its sodium content.

recommendations. In addition, the measurement of sweat sodium concentrations can be used to estimate salt losses.

After exercise, players should aim to replace any fluid and electrolyte deficit. In most situations, there is sufficient time to restore hydration and electrolyte imbalances with normal eating/drinking practices, starting with the post-training meal. Current recommendations for fluid intake to support training are summarised in table 5.1 and a typical training-day nutrition plan is illustrated in table 5.7.

Table 5.6 Average (with range in brackets) sweat losses and fluid intakes during low- and high-intensity football-specific training sessions in cool and hot conditions for players from FC Barcelona

	Condition			
	Cool		Hot	
Intensity	Low	High	Low	High
Sweat rate (L/hour)	0.55 (0.20–0.85)	0.98 (0.67–1.50)	0.81 (0.50–1.20)	1.43 (1.10–1.81)
Salt (NaCl) loss (g/hour)	1.1 (0.4–2.1)	2.2 (1.5–2.8)	1.6 (0.8–3.0)	3.2 (1.9–4.7)
Fluid intake (L/hour)	0.39 (0.18–0.72)	0.51 (0.22–1.06)	0.57 (0.31–0.90)	0.66 (0.27–0.93)

Data from Rollo et al. (2021).

Table 5.7 Typical training-day nutrition recommendations for elite footballers

Timing	Feeding
07:00: Wake up	Individual preparation. Drink 250 mL water
08:00–8:30: Breakfast at home	1 g CHO/kg BM + 0.4 g PRO/kg BM + 5–7 mL H_2O/kg BM
10:30–12:30: Training session	Drink water or CHO-electrolyte beverage according to sweat losses to limit fall in body mass to less than 2%
13:00–14:00: Lunch	1–1.5 g CHO/kg BM + 0.4 g PRO /kg BM + fluid
14:00–15:00: Meetings	
15:00–16:00: Gym or massage	Fluid according to thirst
18:00–19:00: Dinner at home	1–1.5 g CHO/kg BM + 0.4–0.6 g PRO/kg BM + fluid
19:00–21:00	Fluid as required according to thirst
22:00–22:30	0.4 g PRO/kg BM
23:00: Sleep	

ESSENTIAL MICRONUTRIENT REQUIREMENTS

The demands of both training and match play for elite footballers may also increase the requirements for some micronutrients to support metabolic processes within the body. The micronutrients include vitamins, minerals and trace elements essential for growth and development of the body. Their various roles and dietary sources were described in chapter 2. The most frequently reported cases of sub-optimal status are for vitamin D, calcium and iron. Deficiencies of these essential micronutrients can be harmful to both the health and performance of the player, and lack of sufficient vitamin D and/or calcium can make bone fractures more likely. Occasionally, supplements may be required for these micronutrients, at least on a temporary basis. Deficiencies of most other micronutrients are rare but may occur on restricted diets and vegetarian or vegan diets. Vegans avoid all animal products so supplementation with vitamin B12 (needed for normal red and white blood cell production) is essential as this only comes from animal food sources. For any player, a daily multi-vitamin tablet supplying the RDA for all 13 vitamins can be taken for insurance without any risk to health, and can be a useful strategy to avoid deficiencies, particularly if dietary energy intake is being restricted to lose excess weight during pre-season. Let us now look in a little more detail at the three micronutrients whose status is most likely to be of concern even for players who are not vegetarian, vegan or failing to meet their daily energy requirements.

VITAMIN D

Inadequate vitamin D status has been reported to impair muscle function and recovery and to compromise immune health, so it is essential that football players who are deficient are identified and treated accordingly. Vitamin D is a unique vitamin in that it can be synthesised in the skin via sunlight exposure, with less than 20% of daily needs typically coming from the diet. The average daily dietary intake across the world is approximately 100–250 IU (note that 40 IU is equivalent to one microgram (µg) of vitamin D), which is less than the current RDA of 400 IU (10 µg) in the UK. The ability to synthesise vitamin D from sunlight is dependent on geography and meteorology, with the solar UVB radiation being insufficient to convert 7-dehydrocholesterol in the skin to vitamin D in the winter months at high latitudes (i.e. Northern Europe, including the UK, Russia and much of North America). Given that many footballers reside in countries far from the equator, and that many of them use sunscreen during the summer months, it is not surprising that footballers occasionally present with vitamin D deficiencies. Several scientific studies on athletes, including games players, indicate that as many as 55% can have inadequate or severely deficient vitamin D status between the months of November and March, despite much of their training being outdoors. Vitamin D deficiency has been associated with increased risk of respiratory infections (and also longer lasting and more severe illness symptoms), and infection rates in the general population are generally highest in the winter months. If a deficiency is observed (it can be detected using a blood test that measures the serum concentration of 25-hydroxy vitamin D) or anticipated (e.g. in the winter months) then a supplement of 2,000 IU/day of vitamin D3 is recommended. In a number of randomised controlled trials, Vitamin D supplementation has been reported to reduce respiratory infection incidence by one-third. In 2020, over 30 observational studies showed that incidence, symptom severity and death from COVID-19 are inversely correlated with serum 25-hydroxy vitamin D concentrations. Vitamin D supplementation is already familiar to many athletes and sports teams because there is some evidence that it improves athletic performance and muscle repair. Thus, football players should consider vitamin D3 supplementation to serve as an additional means by which to reduce the risk of respiratory infections, including COVID-19 and its consequences.

Doses higher than 4,000 IU/day (the tolerable upper intake level set by the European Food Standards Agency) can be harmful and are not recommended. Good dietary sources of vitamin D include red meat, liver, egg yolk, oily fish, mushrooms and fortified foods – such as most fat spreads, some breakfast cereals and milk (in some countries).

CALCIUM

Calcium is important for the maintenance of bones and teeth and the processes of muscle contraction and nerve conduction (table 2.4). The largest store of calcium in the body is in the skeleton, and this store is mobilised when dietary intake is inadequate, leading to demineralisation and weakening of bone, which increases the risk of fractures and is obviously most undesirable in a sport such as football, which involves physical contact and occasional knocks and falls. Dairy products (e.g. milk, cheese, yoghurt) are the main dietary sources of calcium, but it is also found in green leafy vegetables, nuts and soya beans. The UK RDA for calcium is 700 mg/day for adults and 1,000 mg/day for adolescents. If supplements are to be used, calcium carbonate and calcium citrate are well absorbed. Calcium status cannot be readily established by the measurement of the blood serum calcium concentration, but measurement of the circulating levels of the hormones involved in its deposition and mobilisation from bone (calcitonin and parathyroid hormone) can give some indication, together with an assessment of dietary calcium intake based on a 7-day weighed food intake record.

IRON

Iron is important for oxygen transport in the blood by the haemoglobin present in red blood cells, and for the burning of fuel in the muscles, heart and other tissues of the body (table 2.5) because it is an essential component of myoglobin (an intracellular trapper of oxygen) and the cytochromes present in the electron transport chain within the mitochondria. Iron is also essential for immune function. The current UK RDA for iron is 14.8 mg for females and 8.7 mg for males. Iron deficiencies may present as lethargy and reduced performance and can be identified through blood screening by the measurement of the concentrations of blood haemoglobin and serum ferritin. A diet rich in iron, particularly red meat, liver, tuna, seafood, green leafy vegetables, beans, nuts, seeds and vitamin C (which assists the absorption of iron from plant food sources) is recommended to avoid the development of iron deficiency. Iron supplements are only recommended after consultation with qualified medical and dietetic practitioners as otherwise there is a real danger of harmful iron toxicity.

SUPPLEMENTS USED TO SUPPORT TRAINING

Good nutrition choices can support the health and performance of footballers, whereby the intake, type, quantity and timing of foods, fluids and supplementation can optimise the performance and recovery of players both within and between matches. Several other foods and supplements may help to promote health and reduce illness risk during the season. Some dietary supplements may be effective in improving the performance of footballers, and some may permit higher training loads to be achieved with reduced fatigue, although there is no guarantee that they will work for everyone. It is, of course, important to try these out in training first, before being applied in a match situation in case of adverse side effects such as tummy upsets, diarrhoea or headaches. Here we look at some of the more common supplements used in elite football to boost performance and recovery in training. Other supplements that are commonly used on match day will be discussed in the next chapter.

SPORTS FOODS AND DRINKS

Footballers will have clear nutrition guidelines to follow on training and match days. These guidelines will be provided by the club nutritionist or one of the other sport science support staff. Due to the usual organisation of training sessions in a day (concurrent 'on-pitch' sessions followed by resistance work) with limited breaks in training and match play, it isn't always possible for players to consume foods in the form of meals, particularly if training is somewhere other than the club training ground or if a canteen is not available on site. In this situation, sports foods and drinks providing appropriate amounts of carbohydrate and protein, or both, can provide a convenient alternative to proper food to meet nutrient targets. Products with good evidence for consideration include carbohydrate-electrolyte drinks, carbohydrate gels, sports bars and confectionery, recovery shakes, protein drinks and liquid meal supplements.

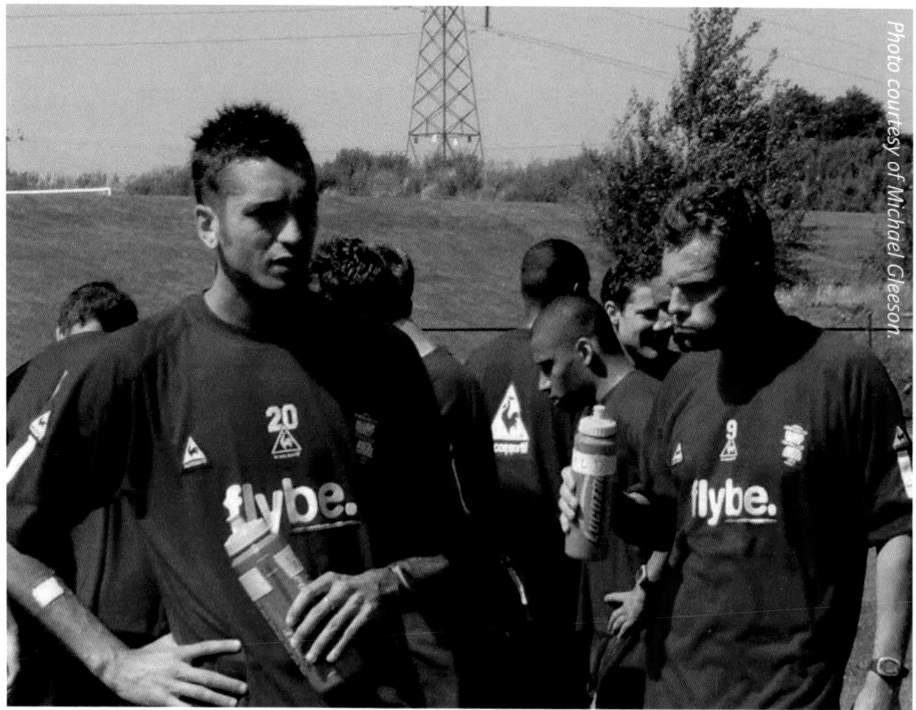

Photo 5.3 Carbohydrate-electrolyte drinks provide some fuel for players, together with some sodium and water to replace sweat loss during hard training sessions, particularly in warm weather as this photo from a pre-season training session at Birmingham City's training ground shows.

CREATINE

Increasing dietary creatine can increase the creatine (and more specifically the PCr) content of the muscles. This provides a greater energy store for rapid use during very high-intensity exercise such as sprinting (you can refer back to chapter 3 for a recap on this topic if necessary). The breakdown of PCr can also help to neutralise the acidity that is produced in this type of exercise. Increasing the free creatine content of the muscles may also permit improved performance of repeated sprints, which are important in both training and match play. Vegetarian and vegan players may experience greater benefits as the vegetarian diet contains very little creatine, and these individuals start from a lower level of creatine in the muscles.

A proven approach to load the muscles with creatine is to take 20 g/day (divided into four equal daily doses), for 5–7 days. This is then followed by a maintenance phase, which means taking a single daily dose of 3–5 g/day for the duration of the supplementation period. One potential disadvantage of creatine loading is that many players can gain

1–2 kg in weight due to an increase in muscle water content. An alternative approach of taking 2–5 g/day for 4 weeks may avoid the associated increase in body weight. It generally takes about 4–6 weeks following chronic creatine supplementation for levels to return to normal. As with all dietary supplements, there is a risk of a doping violation due to contamination with banned substances. Any supplements that are used should be obtained from a reliable source that uses an approved batch testing scheme for its products. In the UK, this scheme is called Informed Sport.

β-ALANINE

β-alanine (pronounced beta-alanine) is a nonessential amino acid, but not one that is found in proteins. It combines with another amino acid called histidine (one of the nine essential amino acids) to form a compound called carnosine (which is naturally present in muscle), which acts to mop up acidity in the muscles during high-intensity efforts, thereby delaying fatigue and increasing performance. Taking β-alanine supplements daily (about 6 g/day given as 1.5 g every 3–4 hours) over a few weeks increases the muscle content of carnosine by up to 80%. As with creatine, this could be beneficial for the performance of some players (attacking full-backs and speedy forwards in particular) in both training and match play.

CAFFEINE

Caffeine is a stimulant that is found in coffee, chocolate, cola and energy drinks; it can also be taken as a powder or pill or be a constituent of a specially formulated sports drink, cereal bar or a chewing gum. Caffeine can improve performance in a variety of exercise tasks, probably via direct effects on muscle and on the brain. There may be improvements in the performance of tasks that require sustained alertness and concentration, and there is some evidence that caffeine use may improve skill and fine motor control. Early studies on caffeine and exercise performance in the 1970s and 80s established that an effective dose was about 3 mg/kg BM (so that's a little over 200 mg for a player weighing 75 kg) and that higher doses than this were not any more effective but more likely to induce unwanted side effects, which can commonly include anxiety, nausea, tremor and reduced sleep quality. More recent research has suggested that the effective dose is probably much smaller than previously thought and benefits have been reported with doses as small as 100–200 mg, allowing players to gain benefits without some of the potential adverse effects of higher caffeine doses. The usual protocol is to take about 2 or 3 mg/kg BM in the form of anhydrous caffeine (i.e. pill or powder form), consumed one hour prior to exercise. A strong cup of coffee provides about 100 mg of caffeine and is just as effective as pills or powder as a performance and cognitive function enhancer. Match-day protocols for caffeine supplementation will be described in the following chapter. Great care should always be taken if caffeine supplements are to be used. Doses higher than 3 mg/kg BM will not produce greater improvements in performance and are strongly discouraged, as more serious side effects can occur, including high heart rate and arrhythmias, muscle tremor and headache. If training takes place in the evening it is best to avoid caffeine as it is likely to impair a player's ability to sleep well.

RISKS OF TAKING SUPPLEMENTS

Care must always be taken in the use of supplements and a benefit/risk analysis should be carried out (figure 5.3). The main risk of taking supplements for the professional player is the risk of a positive doping test because the supplement is contaminated (accidentally or otherwise) with a substance that is on the World Anti-Doping Agency's banned list. Perhaps the safest approach is to use only pre-tested batches, but the only

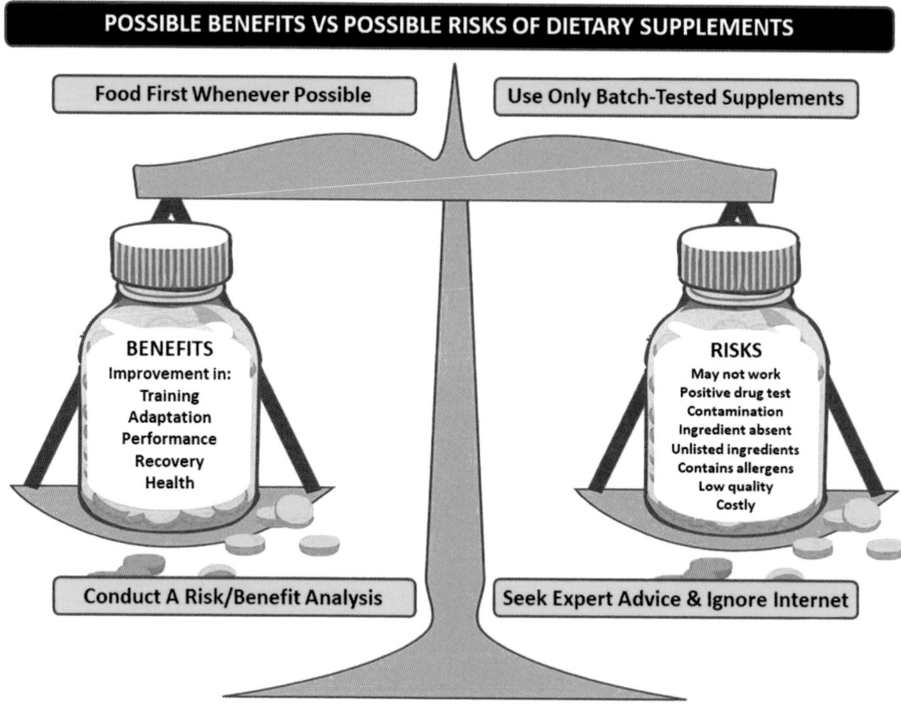

Figure 5.3 Supplements may have some benefits for some players but there are risks in taking them. A benefit/risk analysis should always be conducted before making a decision to take a supplement.

truly safe approach is not to take any supplements at all. Regulation of supplements is not as strict as for medicines. Other than the possibility of being contaminated with banned or toxic substances, some supplements may not actually contain what it says on the tin/bottle/sachet or may only contain a much smaller amount than is advertised. It is worth mentioning a quote about dietary ergogenic supplements by one of my most respected colleagues, Professor Ron Maughan: '(1) If it works, it's probably banned. (2) If it's not banned then it probably doesn't work. (3) There may be some exceptions.' These have become known in the sport nutrition world as 'The Rules of Maughan' and Ron is right, there are relatively few exceptions: the three supplements discussed (i.e. creatine, β-alanine and caffeine) can be included in this rather limited exclusive list. A couple of others that could also be included (nitrate and bicarbonate) are mentioned in the next chapter. It is also worth knowing that some supplements may be effective for some people in some sport or exercise situations, but what seems to work for one particular sport or activity (e.g. cycling, marathon running, sprinting, weight lifting) may not necessarily work for another such as football, rugby or tennis, so be very wary of broad (and often unrealistic) claims about performance enhancement by companies that manufacture or sell supplements. I, for one, am always wary of anyone trying to sell me something! Always 'check the evidence first – for efficacy, side effects and safety' is my motto.

EATING AND DRINKING ON TRAINING DAYS

So far, we have covered the energy and nutrient requirements for training but in reality, of course, players eat food not isolated nutrients. In professional clubs, most training sessions take place in the morning, typically starting around 10:00–10:30am and will last a couple of hours. Players therefore have the opportunity to fuel up and rehydrate after a night's sleep at breakfast time, usually eaten at home, before travelling to the club training venue. Most players will live less than an hour's drive away and they should be aiming to finish their breakfast at least two hours before the start of the training session. This allows sufficient time for the stomach to be emptied and for the digestion, absorption and assimilation of the nutrients in the meal to take place. It also allows the player to be well hydrated by the start of training. A suitable breakfast is half a pink grapefruit or large orange, 40 g of cereal (e.g. Weetabix, Shredded Wheat or muesli) with added fruit (e.g. 20 blueberries, 10 cherries or 5 strawberries) and 125 mL of whole milk, followed by scrambled or poached eggs on toast or a mixed vegetable and olive omelette with a slice of wholemeal bread. A mug of tea or coffee (with milk if preferred), 150 mL fruit juice and a 250 mL glass of water are good beverages to have with breakfast. Such a meal will provide approximately 600 kcal, 75 g of CHO, 30 g of protein, 18 g of fat and 700 mL of water. The latter includes the water content of the food as well as the beverages consumed. Additional examples of suitable breakfast meals are provided in chapter 12.

After training, the players will normally take lunch in the training ground canteen, which in many cases is akin to a high-end restaurant buffet and usually prepared by an excellent chef. The menu will mostly feature good quality lean meats and fish with freshly cooked vegetables, fresh salad, or both, and a suitable selection of high-carbohydrate foods such as boiled potato, boiled rice or pasta (e.g. egg noodles, spaghetti, linguine, penne) and bread. Fresh mixed fruits, nuts, yoghurt and/or reduced fat ice cream make suitable desserts. In case you were wondering, there is nothing wrong with players eating a dessert following their main meal. A good choice of dessert will provide additional carbohydrate and have a high micronutrient content. Sensible beverages include cold water, mineral water, or low-calorie soft drinks (e.g. tonic, ginger ale, cola) or fresh fruit juices (e.g. orange, tomato, cranberry) with no added sugar. Green tea is a good choice if a hot drink is preferred.

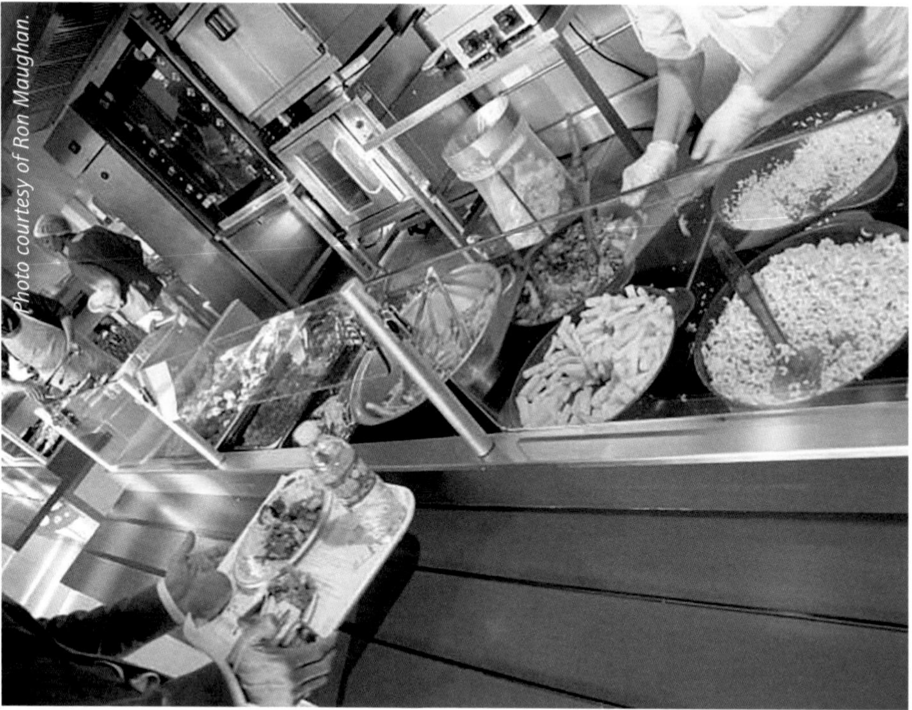

Photo 5.4 A typical professional football training ground canteen has plenty of appropriate foods to refuel the player after a morning training session.

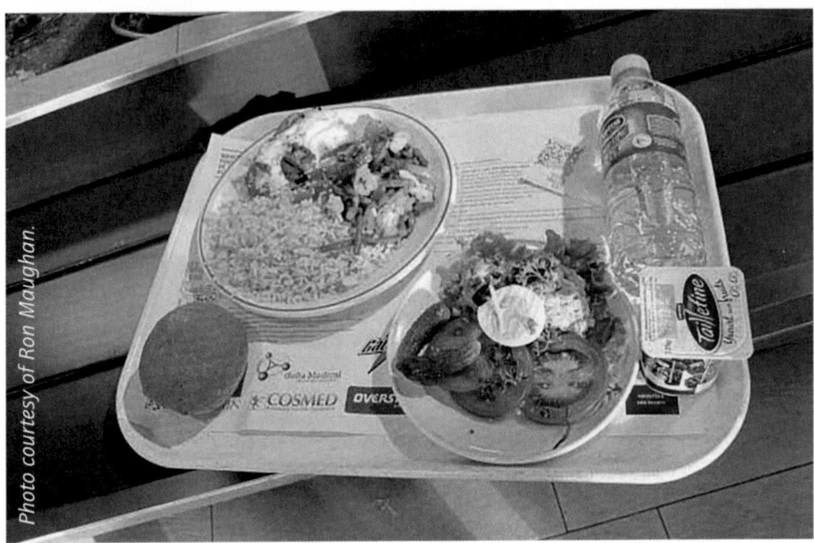

Photo 5.5 A typical training-day lunch for a professional player following a morning training session.

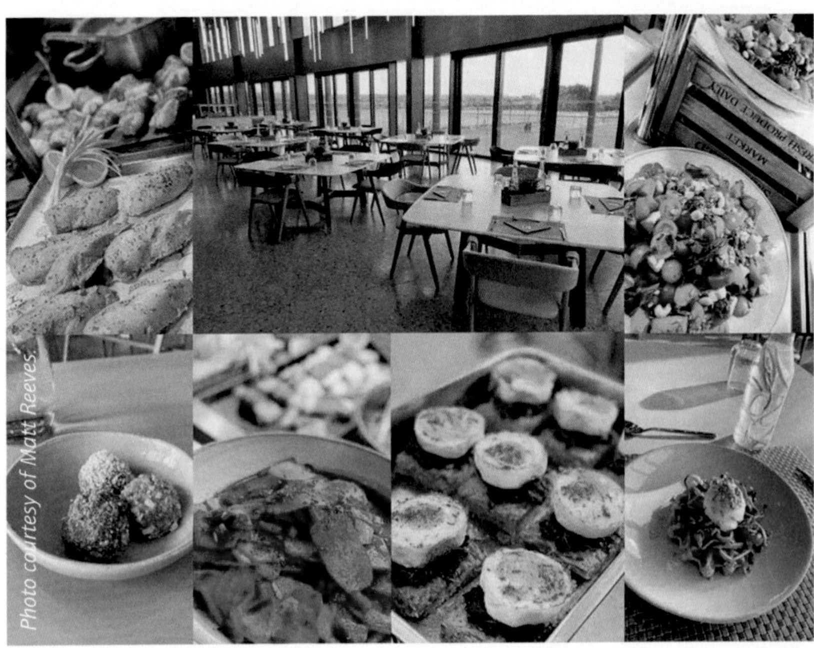

Photo 5.6 The training ground canteen used by the players and support staff at Leicester City FC and a selection of the foods on offer.

Alcoholic drinks are usually absent for health reasons and also because many players will be driving home in the afternoon. Dinner will normally be taken in the evening back at the player's house and usually prepared by the player's partner or by a bought-in performance chef who will have been briefed by the club nutritionist on what nourishment is needed. Examples of some suitable meals for breakfast, lunches and dinners are provided in the final chapter of this book including several recipes by top performance chefs Rachel Muse and Bruno Cirillo who regularly prepare meals for elite footballers.

For young academy players, and also in the amateur game, most training sessions will take place in the evenings. This provides a different set of potential problems and solutions and the needs of these players will be discussed in detail in chapters 10 and 11.

HOW NUTRITION CAN HELP TO KEEP PLAYERS HEALTHY THROUGHOUT THE SEASON

Prolonged strenuous exercise, hard training and psychological stress are known to depress immunity. Hence, the high physical and psychological demands of participation in elite football can increase the risk of illness. The most common illnesses in elite footballers are the common cold, influenza, chest infections and gastrointestinal illness. Since early 2020, the COVID-19 pandemic has also become a serious concern for everyone, including professional footballers. Several factors are associated with depressed immunity or increased risk of illness, or both (figure 5.4), including: higher than normal training loads, fixture congestion, nutritional deficiencies or low energy intake (particularly when attempting to lose excess body weight), environmental extremes, including the winter months when most viral infections are more prevalent, long-haul travel, poor sleep, psychological stress and depression. Perhaps surprisingly, poor oral health has also been reported in elite players, which can affect their ability to train, match-day performance and recovery from pain, psychosocial impacts and effects on eating and sleeping. Players should take responsibility for their oral health and have regular check-ups by a dentist.

Preventing or at least minimising the risk of illness is a key component in player health management. Illness prevention strategies are important to achieve uninterrupted training and to reduce the risk of illness that can prevent participation, or contribute to underperformance in both training and matches. In the 2018–19 English Premier League season, there were 66 absences due to illness and 62 in the previous season with an average duration of 11 days. The COVID-19 pandemic in 2020–21 has, of course, provided an impetus to focus even more on these issues.

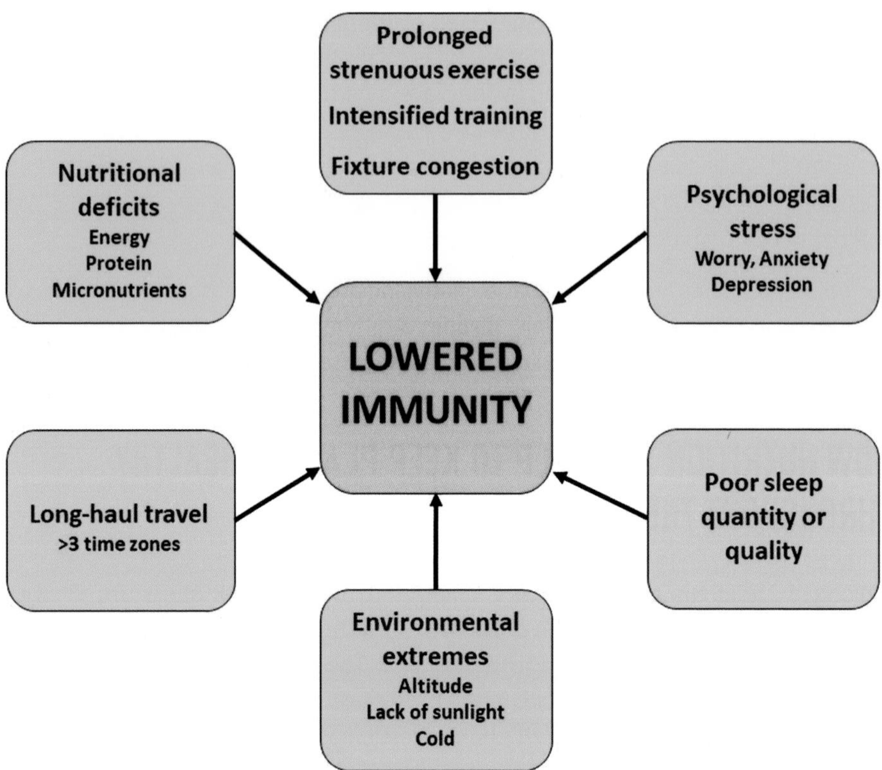

Figure 5.4 Factors that can lower immunity and increase the risk of infection in footballers and other athletes.

Several nutritional strategies may be effective in helping to maintain robust immunity, although other considerations are also just as important in reducing infection risk, including good personal, home and training-venue hygiene, managing the training and competition load, ensuring adequate recovery and sleep, psychological stress management and monitoring of players to detect early signs and symptoms of illness, overreaching and overtraining.

Several nutritional measures can be employed to maintain robust immunity and reduce infection risk in players (table 5.8). For most players, and particularly for those who are illness-prone, these should be implemented throughout the season or, at least, during the autumn and winter months and during periods of fixture congestion when infection risk is highest.

Good hygiene practice in the storage and preparation of food for use in the training ground restaurant and post-match buffet venue (such as the changing room or team bus) is important to minimise the risk of serious gastrointestinal illness caused by bacterial contamination. A description of good food hygiene practices can be found at the end of this chapter.

Table 5.8 Nutritional measures to maintain robust immunity in football players

Nutritional measure	Dosage	Reason
Avoid deficiencies of essential micronutrients	Meet RDA for essential micronutrients	Deficiencies of iron, copper, selenium, zinc, folate, vitamins B12, C, D and E can all impair immunity
Avoid total energy and carbohydrate deficits	Meet daily energy and CHO requirements	Low energy availability is associated with illness and restricting carbohydrate (e.g. 'training low' or Atkins-style diets) may increase immunosuppressive stress hormone responses
Ensure adequate protein intake	At least 1.2 g/kg BM/ day	Required for optimal immune function. There is also some evidence that ingesting up to 3 g protein/kg BM/ day can reduce respiratory tract infection incidence in overreaching athletes
Measure and monitor the vitamin D status of players and supplement with Vitamin D3 if inadequate or deficient	2,000 IU/day	Required to correct a deficiency or to avoid the possibility of a deficiency during the winter months
Ingest probiotics containing *Lactobacillus* and/or *Bifidobacterium* species	Minimum dose of 10^{10} live bacteria (known as colony forming units or CFU) per day	Probiotics stimulate some aspects of immunity and may reduce infection incidence in athletes. Help to maintain a healthy gut microbiota
Regularly consume fruits and plants, supplements or beverages with high polyphenol content (e.g. fruit juices, non-alcoholic beer and green tea)	At least five portions of fruit and vegetables per day on at least 5 days per week	High plant polyphenol intake is associated with reduced incidence of respiratory illness in physically active people
At the onset of a cold take zinc acetate lozenges	75 mg/day until illness symptoms disappear	Reduces duration of cold symptoms by a day or two
Avoid binge drinking of alcohol	Limit alcohol intake to no more than 2 units per day	Known to impair the functioning of immune cells

Finally, a cautionary note about drinking alcohol. Although drinking large volumes of alcohol is no longer common in professional football compared with 20 years ago, players may still occasionally drink alcohol in social settings with teammates, friends and family, or as a means to relieve stress, anxiety or depression, and this more likely to occur after a match. Occasional intake of small amounts of alcohol is not harmful, but players should be aware that imbibing alcohol can interfere with recovery by impairing the ability to (a) restore liver and glycogen reserves, (b) repair damaged muscle and (c) achieve rehydration. Drinking large doses of alcohol in a single session (binge drinking) can also directly suppress immunity and players should therefore minimise, or avoid, alcohol intake during key blocks of training and following match play when recovery is a priority.

CULTURAL AND RELIGIOUS INFLUENCES ON A PLAYER'S FOOD CHOICES

In the English Premier League, 66% of all players are non-UK nationals and this picture of increased globalisation with its variety of cultural and religious beliefs, some of which have an influence on a player's nutrition, is mirrored in other major European leagues (48%) and in the MLS (49%), with lower proportions in Asia (18%) and Latin America (14%). In addition, there are many international club and national team tournaments, pre-season camps, pre-season tours, friendly games and commercial obligations meaning that travel to foreign countries is now a common occurrence for top clubs and their players. This poses several related challenges for performance and nutrition support staff. Practitioners need to be aware of the cultural considerations for all players, and should collaborate with the club chefs to ensure all foods are culturally acceptable within the catering provision for training and match days.

Many players from Africa, Eastern Europe, the Middle East and Asia are practicing Muslims. Ramadan is an important time for Muslim players when they are required to fast from dawn until sunset for one month. Many Muslim players will continue to train and compete during Ramadan, although each must decide on how to best approach this situation to maintain their performance and overall health. The available evidence indicates that elite players can maintain performance over Ramadan if their training, sleep, food and fluid intake are appropriate and well controlled. Where possible, training for Muslim players should be scheduled to allow for the most appropriate nutrition support. When training is scheduled after sunset, players can benefit from food and fluid consumption before, during and after training. Players should make the most of the important meals: Suhour (the pre-dawn meal) should be eaten as close as possible to sunrise, high in carbohydrate, as well-being used to contribute to daily protein and fluid targets. Iftar (the first meal after sunset) is important to support recovery and to meet the overall nutrition needs for the day. Players should still fuel according to the demands of training or match day (maintaining the overall intakes outlined in the earlier parts of this chapter). Making use of fluids and sports foods may reduce gastrointestinal discomfort. Sufficient fluid and electrolyte intake should be spread in small amounts over waking hours after sunset, to fully replace sweat losses.

FOOD PREFERENCES, ALLERGIES AND TOLERANCE ISSUES

When it comes to likes and dislikes with regard to food items, elite footballers are no different to anyone else, so the nutritionist and chef must provide a selection of foods to meet the desired nutrient requirements and not just assume that all players will be willing to eat the same things on any particular day. This is especially important for the food on offer at the training ground where a suitably varied menu should be available so that, for example, a player can choose to have hot or cold food, salad or cooked vegetables and can select from a variety of protein-rich food sources such as lean meats, poultry, fish, eggs, dairy, beans and legumes and a variety of high-CHO foods such as potato, pasta, corn, rice and bread.

Although very rare, some players may suffer from a food allergy, which is an adverse response to a particular food item or ingredient that is mediated by the immune system. It occurs each time a person consumes a given food and is absent when the food is avoided. Reactions can range in severity from minor abdominal discomfort through to a life-threatening inflammatory reaction known as anaphylaxis, with reactions generally developing within minutes of exposure. Anaphylaxis is indicated by more than one of the following: an itchy rash, throat or tongue swelling, shortness of breath, vomiting, lightheadedness, low blood pressure, fainting and temporary blindness. The most common food items that can cause allergic reactions in susceptible individuals include fish, shellfish, peanuts and tree nuts. Food allergy is determined by a thorough medical and nutrition history to guide validated diagnostic methods, such as skin prick measurement of food-specific immunoglobulin E (a type of antibody associated with allergy and inflammation) levels or carefully controlled food challenges.

Food intolerances are reactions that are not immune-mediated (e.g. lactose, gluten intolerance). Intolerances to certain foods are much more common than allergies. The symptoms (e.g. abdominal bloating or pain, loose stools, fatigue or headache) can occur from hours to days after exposure, meaning that the problem cannot easily be attributed to a particular food item. At the present time, aside from lactose intolerance, there are no validated diagnostic methods for establishing food intolerance. Other common conditions include coeliac disease (autoimmune disease), for which validated medical testing exists. It is important that validated diagnostic testing is firstly conducted, under the guidance of a medical doctor, before undertaking an exclusion diet in response to allergy or intolerance-related symptoms.

IS IT POSSIBLE TO BE A VEGETARIAN OR VEGAN FOOTBALLER?

Some people who prefer a plant-based diet may wonder if it is possible to be a vegetarian or vegan footballer. The answer is, yes, it is possible to be a vegetarian or vegan and still play at the elite level in football. There are, in fact, many different types of vegetarian diet. Vegetarian diets generally exclude meat, fish and poultry, but allow consumption of eggs, cheese and other dairy products. Stricter vegan diets exclude all animal products including dairy, eggs and honey. Other varieties include lacto-vegetarian (permits dairy but not eggs), ovo-vegetarian (permits eggs but not dairy) and flexitarian (includes meat, poultry, fish, eggs, or dairy but only occasionally or in small quantities). The recent popularity of vegetarian diets among elite footballers appears to reflect current public trends. The impact of a vegetarian diet on athletic or football-specific performance has not been established, although such diets are considered to be healthy provided that they are diverse and well-balanced. However, compared with a mixed omnivorous diet, there is an increased risk of lower calcium, iodine, iron, zinc, vitamin B12 and omega 3 fatty acid and creatine intakes, although protein needs are commonly met in athletes as long as daily energy requirements are met and a variety of plant-based protein-rich foods are eaten.

GOOD FOOD HYGIENE PRACTICES

Good hygiene practice in the storage and preparation of food for use in the training ground restaurant and post-match buffet venue (such as the changing room or team bus) is important to minimise the risk of serious gastrointestinal illness caused by bacterial contamination. This is all in the control of the club's support staff, including the nutritionists and the chefs. There are also some situations, like eating in hotels, where some degree of control can be lost. One example of this is described by Sir Alex Ferguson in his autobiography published in 2013. He recalls the events on the night before the Champions League final in Rome in 2009 when his Manchester United side, which at the time included the likes of Ronaldo, Giggs, Scholes and Ferdinand, played Barcelona, which included Messi, Henry, Busquets and Eto'o in their ranks. The United team stayed in a hotel in the Eternal City and had their meals in the hotel restaurant, which was a room with very dim lighting; the food came late and it was cold. Sir Alex states that he took a chef there but he was dismissed by the hotel staff who totally blanked him. The next day, several players were feeling unwell. The game that night was lost, with several of United's players underperforming according to their manager's and their own expectations. All of this was, very possibly, due to a lack of good hygiene practice in the hotel restaurant. Hopefully, this particular anecdote will help you appreciate that a good understanding of food hygiene can be important in football and many other sports!

The four main things to remember for food good hygiene are: cross-contamination, cleaning, chilling and cooking. These are known as the four Cs (figure 5.5) and further details, including useful guidance documents and hygiene training videos can be found on the UK Food Standards Agency website (https://www.food.gov.uk/business-industry/food-hygiene). A summary of the more important guidelines is provided here:

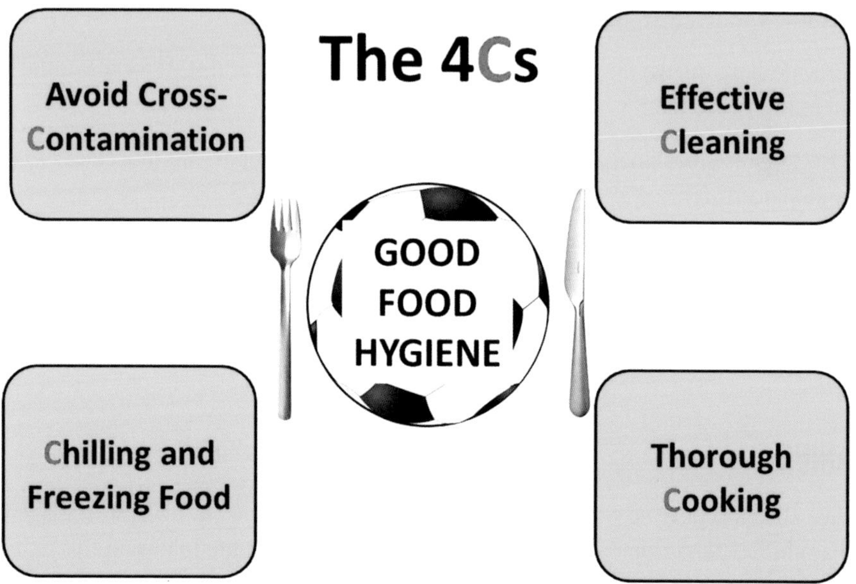

Figure 5.5 The four major considerations to ensure good hygiene for the preparation, storage and cooking of food.

CROSS-CONTAMINATION

Cross-contamination is when bacteria are spread between food, surfaces or equipment. It is most likely to happen when raw food touches (or drips onto) ready-to-eat food, equipment or surfaces. Cross-contamination is one of the most common causes of food poisoning. Here is what needs to be done to avoid it:

- Clean and disinfect work surfaces, chopping boards and equipment thoroughly before you start preparing food and after you have used them to prepare raw food.
- Use different equipment (including chopping boards and knives) for raw meat/poultry and ready-to-eat food unless they can be heat disinfected in, for example, a commercial dishwasher.
- Wash your hands before preparing food.
- Wash your hands thoroughly after touching raw food.
- Keep raw and ready-to-eat food apart at all times, including packaging material for ready-to-eat food.
- Store raw food below ready-to-eat food in the fridge. If possible, use separate fridges for raw and ready-to-eat food.
- Provide separate working areas, storage facilities, clothing and staff for the handling of ready-to-eat food.
- Use separate machinery and equipment, such as vacuum packing machines, slicers and mincers, for raw and ready-to-eat food.
- Separate cleaning materials, including cloths, sponges and mops, should be used in areas where ready-to-eat foods are stored, handled and prepared.
- Make sure that all relevant staff know how to avoid cross-contamination.

CLEANING

Effective cleaning gets rid of bacteria on hands, equipment and surfaces, so it helps to stop harmful bacteria from spreading onto food. You should do the following things:

- Make sure that all staff involved in food handling, preparation and cooking wash and dry their hands thoroughly before handling food.
- Clean and disinfect food areas and equipment between different tasks, especially after handling raw food.

- Clear and clean as you go. Clear away used equipment, spilt food etc. as you work and clean work surfaces thoroughly.
- Use cleaning and disinfection products that are suitable for the job, and follow the manufacturer's instructions.
- Disinfection products should meet BS EN standards. Check product labels for either of these codes: BS EN 1276 or BS EN 13697.
- Do not let food waste build up.

CHILLING

Chilling food properly helps to stop harmful bacteria from growing. Some food needs to remain chilled to keep it safe, for example, food with a 'use by' date, cooked dishes and other ready-to-eat food, such as prepared salads and desserts. It is very important not to leave these types of food standing around at room temperature. So, make sure you do the following things:

- Check chilled food on delivery to make sure it is cold enough.
- Put food that needs to be kept chilled in the fridge straight away.
- Cool cooked food as quickly as possible and then put it in the fridge.
- Keep chilled food out of the fridge for the shortest time possible during preparation.
- Regularly check that your fridge and display units are cold enough (<8°C).
- For freezing food, ensure that food packages are stored at <18°C and ensure food is completely defrosted before cooking.

COOKING

Thorough cooking kills harmful bacteria in food. So, it is extremely important to make sure that food is cooked properly by following these guidelines:

- Cooking food at a temperature of 75°C or more will kill virtually all bacteria.
- When cooking or reheating food, always check that it is steaming hot all the way through. It is especially important to make sure that you thoroughly cook poultry, pork, rolled joints and products made from minced meat, such as burgers and sausages. This is because there could be bacteria in the middle of these types of

products. They should not be served pink or rare and should be steaming hot all the way through.

- Whole cuts of beef and lamb, such as steaks, cutlets and whole joints, can be served pink/rare as long as they are fully sealed on the outside.
- Hot food that is not served immediately should be kept at a minimum of 63°C.

The previous information is adapted from *Food Hygiene: A Guide For Businesses*, Food Standards Agency. Available at https://www.food.gov.uk/business-industry/food-hygiene. This information is licensed under the Open Government Licence v3.0. To view this licence, visit http://www.nationalarchives.gov.uk/doc/open-government-licence/OGL.

TRAINING DAY NUTRITION

MACRONUTRIENTS
Carbs 45-65%
Protein 15-20%
Fat 20-35%
Water

ENERGY
Typically consume
2500-3500 kcal/day
to match energy needs
Important to eat a well-balanced & diverse diet

ESSENTIAL MICRONUTRIENTS
Vitamins/Minerals
Any deficiency can cause ill health & impair performance

DAILY CARBS
3-8 g/kg BM
Depending on the specific training scenario & individual player training goals

VITAMIN D
Aim for serum
25(OH)D >75 nmol/L
Spring/Summer: sunlight
Autumn/Winter: supplement 2000 IU vitamin D3/day

DAILY PROTEIN
1.6-2.2 g/kg BM

0.3-0.4 g/kg BM high quality protein per meal

IRON
>8 (♂) - >18 mg/day (♀)
Test serum ferritin & blood haemoglobin
Eat meat, seafood, green leafy vegetables
Avoid tea & coffee at main meals

DAILY FAT
1.0-2.0 g/kg BM
with <0.5 g/kg BM from saturated fats

WATER
>2 L/day
Arrive at training well-hydrated & avoid body mass deficit of >2% during training sessions

CALCIUM
>700 mg/day (♂)
>1000 mg/day (♀)
Eat dairy products, green leafy vegetables, nuts, soya beans

Infographic 5 Training-day nutrition.

CHAPTER 6

Nutrition for Match Days

- Pre-Match Nutrition
- In-Play Nutrition
- Half-Time Nutrition
- Supplements to Boost Match-Day Performance
- Extra-Time Nutrition
- Post-Match Nutrition
- Influence of Different Match Timings
- Nutrition for Travel

The most important day of the week for any footballer is match day. Poor nutrition choices in the lead up to a match may result in substandard performances on the pitch that could well influence the outcome of the game. Careful consideration of the composition, amount and timing of food and fluid intake is therefore vital to ensure that players are prepared as well as possible when they walk out onto the pitch, and that is the main focus of this chapter. Appropriate food selection, according to the preferences and tolerances of individual players, is also important, as is good hygiene practice in the use of drink bottles and preparation of foods to be consumed in the lead up to the game to avoid gastrointestinal upsets before or during a match.

PRE-MATCH NUTRITION

Nutritional preparation for a match essentially begins the day before the match (MD-1). Training on MD-1 will have been light, and a high-carbohydrate intake of 6–8 g/kg BM over the day should ensure optimal muscle and liver glycogen content is achieved. Nutrition on MD-1 is the most important day for fuelling carbohydrate requirements, and, despite what many people might assume, what is eaten on the day before a match actually has a bigger impact on match performance that what is eaten in the pre-match meal on match day itself. Many top professional players believe in always preparing themselves for the toughest game possible and that means making sure you're fuelled sufficiently enough – particularly getting your muscle glycogen stores fully stocked up. Leaving that to the morning of match day is way too late.

A classic meal that many players enjoy for evening dinner on MD-1 is spaghetti bolognese made with high-quality lean minced beef steak which is relatively easy to digest compared with other red meat dishes. Others like Manchester United's captain Harry Maguire prefer a lasagne which has a fairly similar macronutrient composition to spaghetti bolognese. Some players may prefer chicken or fish with their pasta and sauce, but the main focus is on boosting the body's glycogen stores by eating plenty of carbohydrate while also consuming some high-quality protein.

On match day itself, it is generally recommended that players consume a carbohydrate-rich meal 3–4 hours before warm-up so play can begin with adequate carbohydrate (in the form of glycogen) stores in the liver and muscles. This may be particularly important for matches with a lunchtime kick-off, as liver glycogen levels will be at least 50% depleted after a night's sleep (figure 6.1). You may recall from chapter 3, that the liver supplies most of the blood sugar (glucose) that will be used by the brain, heart and the working muscles during exercise. In fact, glucose is normally the only fuel used by the brain and it needs about 6 g glucose per hour, even when we are asleep.

Some suitable meal plans for pre-match meals are described in chapter 12. The meal should supply some carbohydrate (1–2 g/kg BM) that has a low fibre content, some protein (about 0.2–0.4 g/kg BM; the actual amounts are not so important for this particular meal) and be relatively low in fat, which tends to delay the emptying of the stomach. Ideally, when the player steps onto the pitch, all the food he or she has eaten should have been emptied from the stomach, digested and absorbed. Running on a full, or even half-empty, stomach is not a good idea as it can result in a 'side stitch', also known as exercise-related transient abdominal pain, which is felt on either side of your abdomen, although more commonly on the right side. Symptoms may range from

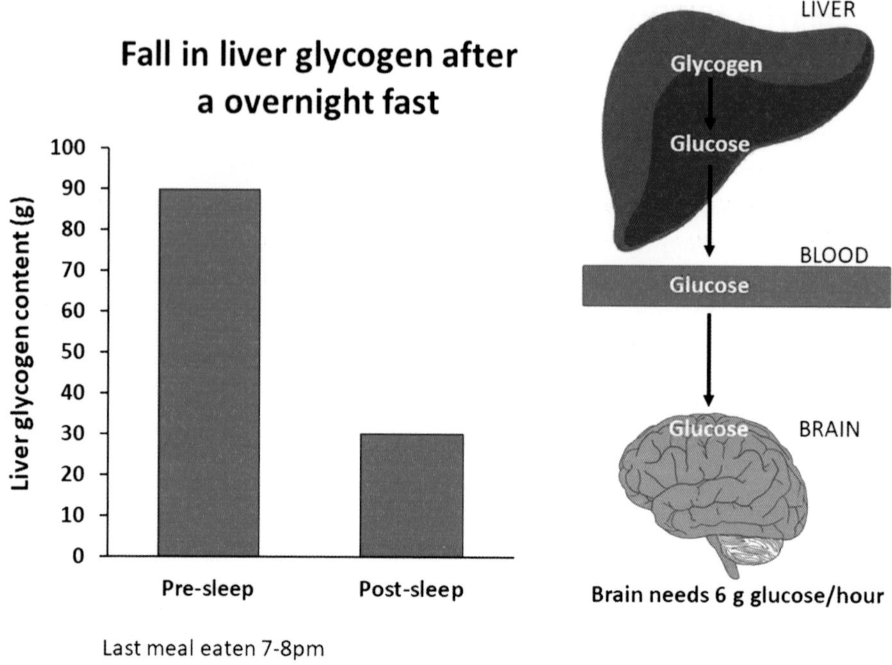

Figure 6.1 The effect of an overnight fast on the liver glycogen content. Liver glycogen breakdown helps to maintain the blood-glucose concentration and, even when we are sleeping and our muscles are relaxed, the brain uses about 6 g of blood-borne glucose per hour.

cramping or a dull ache to a pulling sensation or a sharp, stabbing pain. Side stiches can affect anyone but younger players may be more likely to get a side stitch than senior players. The pre-match meal should also make players feel good so an individual's food preferences and comfort should be considered, rather than rigid strategies focused solely on meeting carbohydrate-intake guidelines. Often players will get to learn what foods suit them best before a match and will stick with this as a normal routine ahead of most matches. It is usual for professional players to eat their pre-match meal together at the training ground canteen (for home games) or at a hotel or on the team bus (for most away games).

Tom Parry, head nutritionist at Manchester City FC, says that 'generally, we won't serve red meat the night before the game.' Fish, chicken and beans are usually the preferred alternative sources of protein. He also says, 'We definitely won't serve red meat for the pre-match meal because it's just too hard to break down. It's a waste and there is no point because it's just going to be sat in the stomach.' Clearly, when it is close to kick-off, issues of food's digestibility take preference over nutrient content, and the emphasis is very much on achieving good hydration and appropriate carbohydrate intake. Hence, pre-match meals are generally simpler and less exotic than some of the meals that players may enjoy on training days. Chicken, pasta and tomato sauce remains a staple favourite of many players.

Because of concerns over possible gastrointestinal discomfort, some players prefer to eat very little in the hours before a game. For example, Ilkay Gundogan, the Manchester City attacking midfielder, has said that 'personally, I like to feel light before a game. So if we play in the afternoon I have a good breakfast but for the pre-match meal I just have my coffee and maybe a piece of banana bread and that's it.' At the end of the day, it is the individual player's personal preference that has to win out, albeit if in terms of scientific considerations it might not be quite the ideal nutritional strategy.

Several scientific studies have shown that high-carbohydrate intakes before (and during a match when possible) can delay fatigue and enhance the players' capacity for intermittent, high-intensity exercise. Some studies also indicate that this can also help to improve or sustain players' technical performance. For example, carbohydrate ingestion seems to improve passing, dribbling speed and shooting performance, but the effects on sprinting, jumping and mental function are less consistent. In one study, increased dribbling speed was observed when professional youth footballers consumed a 500 kcal breakfast containing 75 g CHO compared with a meal containing half this amount 2–3 hours before a before a match. Players should also aim to start the match well hydrated. In addition to fluid consumed as part of the pre-match meal, this can usually be achieved by drinking 5–7 mL/kg BM of water (that's 375–525 mL for a player weighing 75 kg) 1.5–2 hours before kick-off, which allows time for any excess fluid to be emptied from the bladder before the warm-up begins.

Some clubs encourage players to ingest a pre-match ergogenic supplement. One strategy is to drink a 70 mL concentrated beetroot juice (containing 300 mg of nitrate) shot 2–3 hours before kick-off and a second shot that contains 100–200 mg of added caffeine 1 hour before kick-off. Both nitrate (the active ingredient in beetroot juice) and caffeine are known to improve endurance by different mechanisms, so combining the two could have additive effects and there is some, albeit limited evidence, that this is the case. Caffeine may also improve mental function, as mentioned previously. This particular pre-match nutritional strategy was suggested by yours truly to Matt Reeves, and subsequently used by Leicester City's first team squad during their English Premier League title-winning season in 2015–16. I have been asked on numerous occasions if I think that made a real difference or, indeed, did it help them to that title win. The honest answer is I don't know. There were many other factors involved in that unexpected success, not least the acquisition of the midfield dynamo N'Golo Kante, the form of Jamie Vardy (who scored in a record-breaking 11 consecutive Premier League games) and the mercurial Riyad Mahrez, plus the outstanding man-management of the newly appointed manager

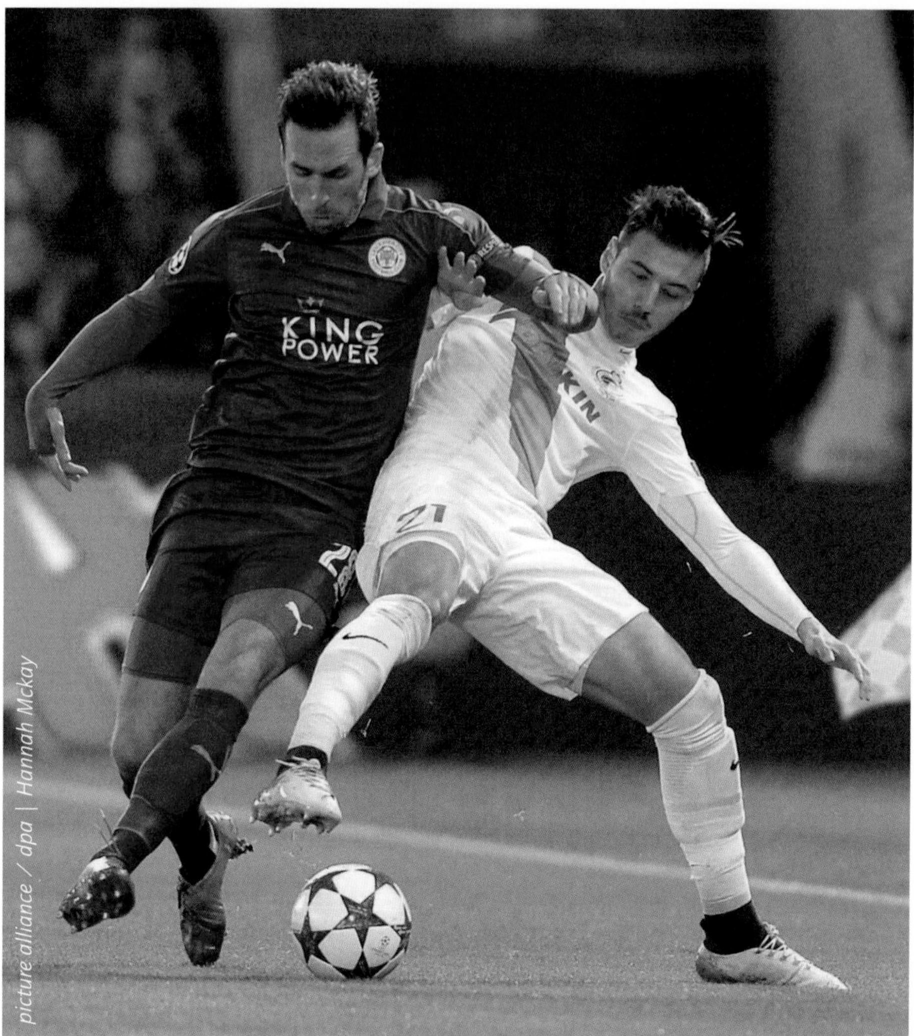

Photo 6.1 Nutrition has a role to play in helping players to perform well in a match and recover quickly afterwards.

Claudio Ranieri. And essentially that will always be the case for the nutritionist who comes up with a novel idea that might potentially improve player performance. Your new idea, preferably based on evidence from scientific studies, perhaps in other situations relevant to football, could be viable, but as with other nutritional strategies, should first be tested in training. And even if it appears to work in that scenario, there is no guarantee that it will translate to the ultimate goal of regularly winning competitive matches as there are always so many other factors involved. Ultimately, it is the sport nutritionist's job in a football club to recommend what they think is the best way, in a nutritional sense, to improve player performance and/or recovery. The rest, you might say, is in the hand of the gods.

It is also common to see players consuming a carbohydrate gel, a sports drink, or both, in the players' tunnel just before kick-off. This provides some additional carbohydrate fuel that can be used during match play. The timing of any carbohydrate intake in the hour before kick-off is important as illustrated in figure 6.2. If some rapidly absorbed carbohydrate is consumed 45–60 minutes before kick-off, there is a large rapid rise in blood glucose that stimulates a substantial release of the hormone insulin, which promotes glucose uptake by the liver, muscles and adipose tissue. However, when exercise begins, the sudden rise in muscle glucose uptake in the presence of high insulin levels can cause the blood-glucose concentration to drop precipitously below normal levels (figure 6.2) in some individuals. Although this transient hypoglycaemia does not usually affect exercise performance, there is a risk it could, for a short time, detrimentally affect mental function as the brain relies on glucose as its source of fuel. The last thing a manager wants is to see his players 'switch off' and concede a goal in the early stages of the game. It seems sensible to avoid this potentially undesirable 'rebound hypoglycaemia' effect, and this can be achieved by delaying the final pre-match intake of carbohydrate until about 5 minutes before exercise is due to begin (i.e. while the players are in the tunnel before coming on to the pitch, just before the start of a match). In this situation, the glucose enters the circulation more gradually (as stomach emptying is slowed down during exercise) and can help to supply the muscle with an additional source of energy while the blood-glucose concentration remains stable, or just slightly increased above normal (as indicated by the blue and dashed lines in figure 6.2). Exercise itself inhibits the secretion of insulin while stimulating the muscles' uptake of glucose from the blood via a mechanism that is independent of insulin.

Manchester City's Tom Parry says, 'If I can get the players to ingest 30-40 grams of carbohydrate just before kick-off then I am happy.' If taken in a sports drink that would mean consuming around 500 mL which many players find to be too much fluid sitting in their stomach to comfortably start match play with, and most players prefer carbohydrate gels which can supply around 30 g of glucose polymer in a volume of less than 100 mL.

IN-PLAY NUTRITION

Scientific studies using protocols that simulate soccer matches have reported performance benefits when carbohydrate is consumed during exercise at rates of about 30–60 g/hour. It seems that most elite players are consuming amounts that are at the low end of this

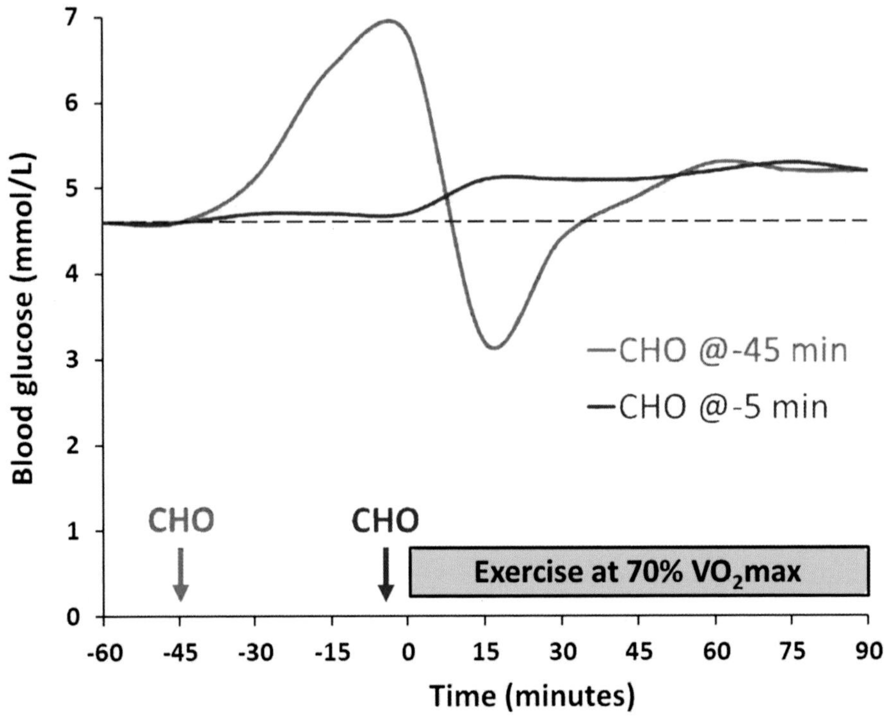

Figure 6.2 The timing of the ingestion of a bolus dose (e.g. 50 g) of carbohydrate before exercise has an important influence on the blood-glucose response. See text for details. The dashed line indicates the normal blood-glucose concentration in the fasted (post-absorptive) state.

scale. For example, players in the English Premier League reportedly ingest, on average, 32 g CHO/hour, just before and during a match. This may be attributed to the rules of the game, which largely limit food and fluid intake, or both, to warm-up and half-time, and the fear or actual experience of gastrointestinal upsets during match play. However, players should use the occasional opportunities for fluid intake, such as unscheduled breaks in play, typically when injured players are receiving on-pitch medical assistance following strong tackles, bad falls or accidental collisions. In recent years, the introduction of the video assistant referee (VAR) in the professional game has provided another opportunity for a drink break while play is stopped to allow a referee to review a VAR decision on the pitch-side monitor.

Dehydration is commonly reported after a soccer match because sweat losses (governed by the intensity and duration of play and environmental conditions) exceed fluid intake (governed by hydration opportunities and individual drinking practices). In cool conditions, net fluid losses are quite small, typically 1–2% of body weight,

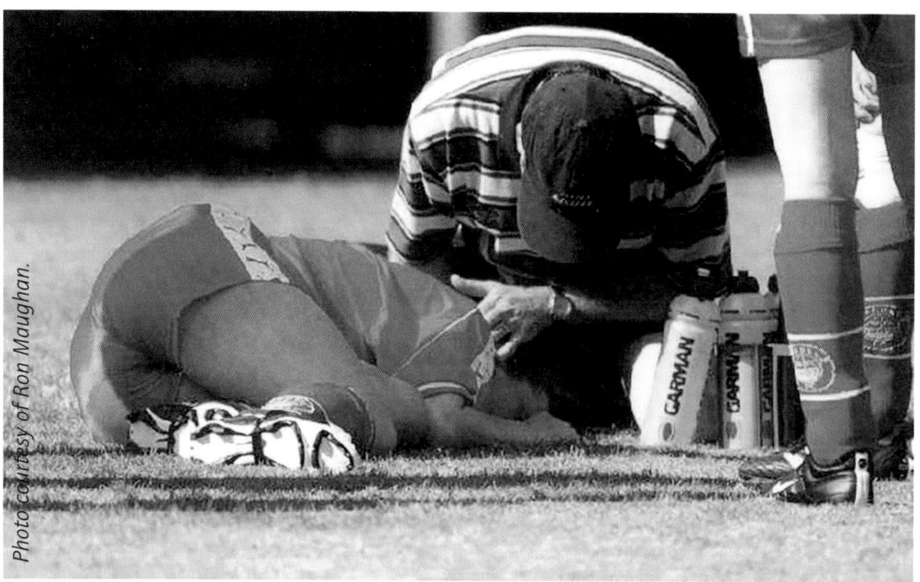

Photo 6.2 When a player is injured and requires treatment on the pitch it provides an opportunity for drinks to be brought on, which can be helpful for players on warm days.

which has little, if any, effect on endurance and mental performance. As long as dehydration is limited to moderate levels (i.e. no more than 2.5% of body weight), it seems that current drinking practices are not a major concern for performance in temperate (13–22°C) conditions. However, in hot conditions, greater fluid losses in match play will occur due to losing sweat at rates of up to 2–3 L/hour, which is likely to impair players' performances. For example, in elite soccer matches played in hot environments (over 28°C), players have been observed to exhibit reduced performance of repeated sprint and jump activities and substantially reduced amounts of high-intensity running in the final 20–30 minutes of the match; this has been mostly attributed to increased body core temperature and dehydration. It is possible that drinking larger volumes than usual, and more frequently, could prevent some of the larger effects on performance in hot environments. Some players will sweat much more than others, so hydration strategies require an individualised approach to prevent excessive dehydration in heavy sweaters, particularly in warm weather conditions. I described in the previous chapter how the individual sweat rates of players can be estimated.

In the winter months, some matches may be played in very cold conditions, including some UEFA Champions League and Europa League matches, or in other leagues around the world that take place in countries located at high northern latitudes (e.g, Canada, Iceland, Finland, Norway, Russia, Sweden). Most players can cope with match play in cold environments by wearing appropriate clothing, such as undergarments and gloves. If the air temperature is not too extreme (note that UEFA regulations specify that when the temperature is -15ºC [5ºF] or colder, the match is postponed unless both teams agree to play) and the work rate is maintained at a high level, cold should not be a problem if appropriate clothing is worn. In cold environments, the body's carbohydrate requirements are increased, whilst dehydration is less likely to develop and may be less detrimental to performance.

HALF-TIME NUTRITION

Because of the in-game limitations to feeding and/or drinking in football, the opportunities to take on fluid and nutrition before the match and during half-time are more important than in many other team sports. Players can rehydrate according to thirst or their anticipated body weight loss at half-time and should be encouraged to drink at least 250 mL of water or a suitable sports drink. A carbohydrate-electrolyte sports drink containing 4–8 g CHO/100 mL is probably the most appropriate choice. Taking a caffeine supplement at half-time can also be considered, particularly if caffeine was not ingested before the match. On cold days, a hot mug of strong coffee may be the most suitable option. Chewing gum containing 100–200 mg of caffeine is readily available and is a suitable choice because it allows for more rapid absorption of caffeine (directly through the lining of the mouth) compared with caffeine in capsules or tablets (figure 6.3). Peak plasma levels of caffeine occur after only 30 minutes with the gum compared with about 60–90 minutes in capsule or tablet form, so if chewed during the half-time interval, the caffeine boost kicks in just when it is needed most: in the final 15–20 minutes of the second half. The gum should be spat out before players return to the pitch to avoid the risk of swallowing it or, worse still, accidentally inhaling it (i.e. what most people might call 'going down the wrong way') during match play, which could be life-threatening.

All match nutrition strategies, including the use of supplements, should be practiced in training and during minor matches to allow individualised protocols to be developed. In training sessions, individual player sweat rates can be determined under different environmental conditions (i.e. cool, temperate and warm weather) so fluid-replacement needs during match play can be predicted with a reasonable degree of accuracy. Weighing players during competitive matches or half-time is obviously unrealistic.

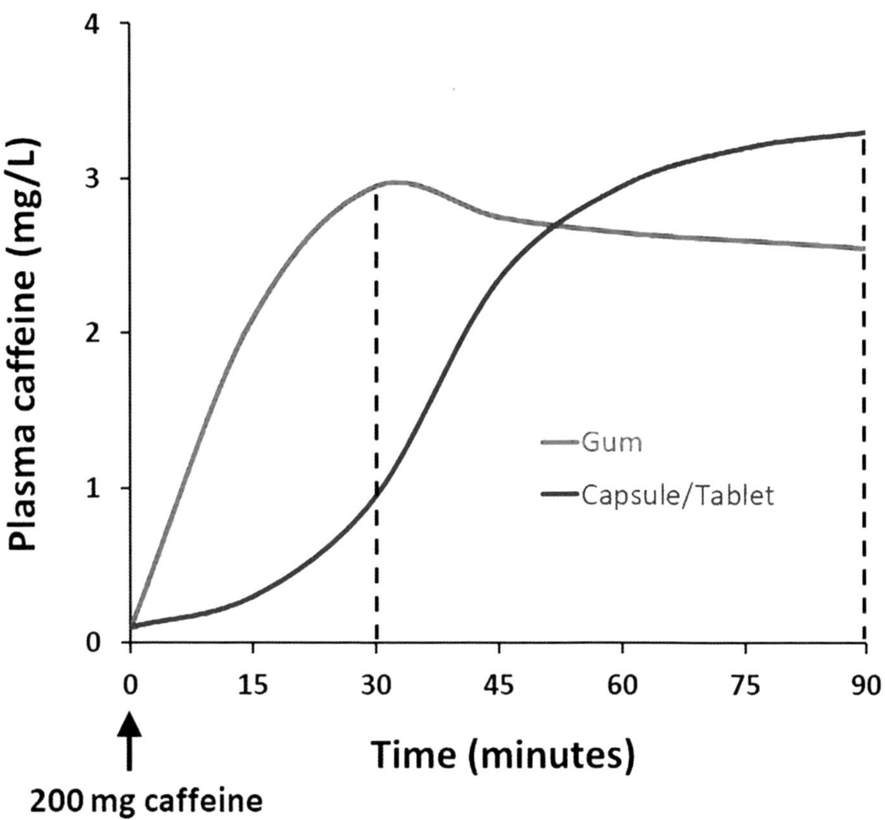

Figure 6.3 Caffeine in a chewing gum is absorbed faster than from a capsule or tablet because some absorption takes place through the lining of the mouth directly into the blood. Peak plasma levels of caffeine occur after only 30 minutes with the gum compared with about 60–90 minutes in capsule form. Data from Kamimori et al. (2002).

SUPPLEMENTS TO BOOST MATCH-DAY PERFORMANCE

I mentioned some of the sport foods and supplements that are commonly used to support training in the previous chapter. Some players also use supplements to boost their performance on match day (figure 6.4). On match day, in addition to caffeine and carbohydrate-containing sports drinks and gels, which I have already discussed in both this chapter and the previous one, there is also evidence that concentrated beetroot juice can improve endurance, so let me explain how: Beetroot is a good dietary source of nitrate (NO_3), which has been shown to reduce the oxygen cost of exercise and improve endurance performance. In the body, the nitrate absorbed from the ingested beetroot juice is converted to nitrite (NO_2) and nitric oxide (NO), which are responsible for the performance-enhancing effect. About 500 mL of beetroot juice is needed to get an effective dose of nitrate (about 300–600 mg) and should be consumed 2–3 hours before kick-off. Beetroot juice is not to everyone's taste and an alternative is to take two 70 mL shots of concentrated beetroot juice, which can be downed in a couple of gulps. Two shots will provide about 600 mg of nitrate. One side effect of drinking beetroot juice (although not harmful) is that it turns the urine pink. There are now also some alternative dietary supplements that contain 250–600 mg of nitrate from rhubarb juice and amaranthus extract and come in a variety of flavours such as apple, grapefruit and orange for those who really can't stomach beetroot. As with any other supplement, it is important to try it out in training first before being applied in a match situation in case of adverse side effects like tummy upsets or an intense dislike of the taste. More prolonged periods of dietary nitrate intake (e.g. 600 mg taken daily over the 3 days before a match) may also be beneficial to performance. High nitrate-containing foods including leafy greens (e.g. spinach, rocket salad, celery), rhubarb and root vegetables including beetroot, can provide a food first solution for longer-term use as an alternative to beetroot juice or rhubarb juice and powder supplements.

Dietary nitrate is absorbed in the gut, enters the blood circulation, and is taken up and concentrated in the salivary glands. When saliva is secreted into the mouth some of the nitrate is converted to nitrite by the oral commensal bacteria. When the saliva is subsequently swallowed the nitrite is absorbed and enters the blood circulation where it is bioactive as nitrite or is further reduced to nitric oxide. Players should note that the use of an antibacterial mouthwash for purposes of oral hygiene kills many of the commensal bacteria in the mouth which means that dietary nitrate will not be effective as a performance enhancer. If you want to take beetroot juice or other forms of dietary nitrate to improve your endurance then use a toothbrush and toothpaste instead.

One other potential supplement that is worth mentioning is sodium bicarbonate ($NaHCO_3$), commonly known as baking soda. Bicarbonate is present in the blood plasma and it acts to mop up acidity (i.e. hydrogen ions, H^+), which contribute to muscle fatigue in high-intensity exercise:

$$H^+ + HCO_3^- \rightarrow H_2CO_3 \rightarrow H_2O + CO_2$$

In theory, this could be beneficial in high-intensity exercise where the production of large amounts of lactic acid causes an increase in levels of acidity in the muscle to the point where they can contribute to fatigue. High doses of sodium bicarbonate (0.3 g/kg BM, which is 22.5 g for a 75 kg player) taken in gelatine capsules (to mask the taste) and washed down with plenty of water with some added citrus fruit cordial, 1–2 hours before all-out efforts lasting from about 1–10 minutes are known to enhance performance, and there may be benefits in longer events including football matches with frequent high-intensity efforts. The main disadvantage is that bicarbonate can cause gut discomfort

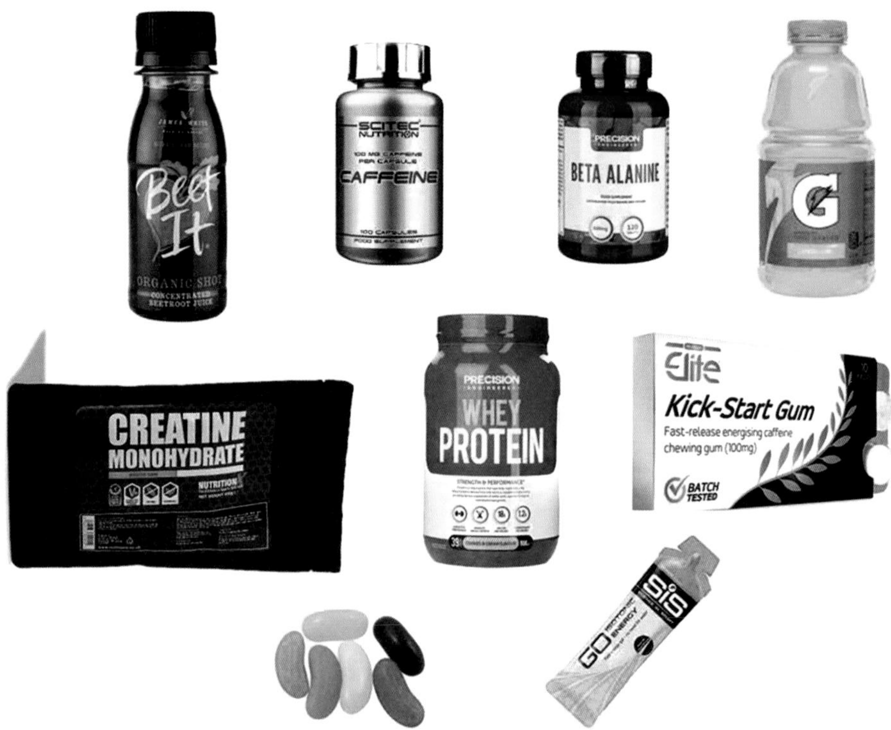

Figure 6.4 Some common supplements that are used by professional footballers to boost their match-day performance.

in some people because when the bicarbonate hits the stomach acid it reacts with it to produce carbon dioxide (CO_2) gas, which can cause bloating and abdominal discomfort, so it is particularly important to try it out in training first. To my own personal knowledge, bicarbonate is only rarely used in football because of the concerns about gastrointestinal upset, but concentrated beetroot juice has become increasingly popular in recent years.

Finally, in this subsection, let's revisit the phenomenon of carbohydrate mouth rinsing that I mentioned in chapter 1. The central nervous system is known to be able to sense the presence of carbohydrate in the mouth via receptors in the oral cavity and, presumably in anticipation of some usable fuel soon becoming available via digestion and absorption, this promotes a sense of well-being, reduces perception of effort during exercise and may have a small (1–3%) benefit for endurance performance, and likely benefits in repeated sprint performance during intermittent exercise. The implications for football are still unclear, but the use of CHO mouth rinsing during breaks in match play (e.g. when an injured player is being treated on the pitch, or when play is stopped to review a VAR decision, or when extra-time is about to begin) could potentially enhance performance in situations where there is limited time to swallow significant volumes of fluid. In scientific studies, only mouth rinsing with a carbohydrate beverage was used (followed by spitting it out) in order to determine if this effect was independent of carbohydrate ingestion, gut absorption and muscle fuel supply, but ideally, players should be encouraged to mouth rinse for 5–10 seconds and then swallow the fluid, not spit it out. Some observations made in recent football tournaments suggest that some players appear to misunderstand the mouth-rinsing strategy and spit out the carbohydrate beverage even when there is time to swallow it! Rinsing and swallowing would allow both the oral receptor and the muscle fuel supply mechanisms to occur simultaneously to improve performance. Let's not forget that some cup matches can extend to extra-time and penalty shoot-outs where both the muscles and brain may benefit from additional fuel support and activation, respectively.

EXTRA-TIME NUTRITION

Soccer match play is typically contested over a period of 90 minutes with a few minutes added at the end of each half (known as 'added time') to account for playing time lost due to halts in play for treatment of injuries, pitch-side monitor VAR reviews by the referee, substitutions and perceived time-wasting (usually by the team that is winning in the later stages of a game). However, in some cup and tournament scenarios, when matches are tied after 90 minutes (plus added time), they proceed to an additional 30 minutes of play, which is called 'extra-time'. In recent years, extra-time has increasingly become a deciding factor in determining the outcome of cup competitions and international tournaments. Since the 1986 FIFA World Cup competition, 33% of matches in the knock-out stages have required extra-time. At the 2014 World Cup finals, 50% of knock-out matches required extra-time compared with 25% of matches at the 2002 and 2010 World Cup competitions, and 38% of matches at the 2006 World Cup tournament. More recently, 31% of knock-out matches played at the 2018 FIFA World Cup proceeded to extra-time, with just one of the match outcomes decided during this period. Of course, when the scores are tied after extra-time, the match result is decided by a penalty shoot-out, which depends on nerve, skill and luck with nothing much nutrition can do to influence the outcome.

Video and GPS analysis of competitive high-level matches that go to extra-time has revealed that outfield players cover an average total distance of 3.2 km with 153 m of high-speed running and 12 sprints. During extra-time, players cover 5–12% less distance relative to match duration (i.e. metres per minute) compared with the preceding 90 minutes. As well as reductions in physical performance due to fatigue, players also exhibit reductions in technical performance (i.e. shot speed, number of passes and dribbles) during extra-time. The rules of the game only allow a limited opportunity for nutritional intervention, so the most effective strategy is likely to be carbohydrate mouth rinsing followed by swallowing the fluid (as described in the previous section). The limited amount of research on nutrition in the short (5-minute) break between the end of the normal game duration and the start of extra-time, suggests that carbohydrate provision may improve dribbling performance during extra-time. Administering nutrition that has ergogenic properties and is rapidly absorbed, such as caffeinated chewing gum, could also be considered in the break before extra-time begins. It can also be expected that players will need longer to recover after matches that go to extra-time, and careful attention to effective post-match nutrition should be a priority.

POST-MATCH NUTRITION

After a match, when it is important for players to start refuelling and rehydration as soon as possible to promote recovery, sports drinks will be handed to players as they leave the pitch at the end of a match and some finger food (e.g. baked sweet potato wedges, chicken, ham or tuna Paninis, tortilla wraps or sandwiches) and sports foods will often be provided in the changing room and during travel after away games. In this situation, sports foods providing appropriate amounts of carbohydrate and protein can provide a convenient alternative to proper food to meet the desired nutrient targets. Products with good evidence for consideration include carbohydrate-electrolyte drinks, carbohydrate gels, sports bars and confectionery, recovery carbohydrate/protein shakes and other liquid meal supplements. The aim is to begin the resynthesis of muscle glycogen at the time when the rate of resynthesis is at its highest, which is in the first few hours post-exercise. Ingestion of about 30 g protein at the same time can speed up the process of muscle repair and adaptation. A recent study showed that dietary protein–derived amino acid incorporation into both contractile and mitochondrial proteins in muscle responds to increasing protein intake in a dose-dependent manner, but that ingesting 30 g protein is sufficient to maximise contractile protein synthesis rates during recovery from a single bout of endurance exercise. Protein ingestion following exercise may also, albeit to a small degree, reduce muscle soreness over the next 24–48 hours (further details about this can be found in the next chapter).

For the main meal after a match, many players like to eat some sort of comfort food. A good chef can create some foods that they call 'fakeaways' because they are intentionally made to resemble takeaway-style foods such as pizza, beef burger, chicken nuggets, chicken chow mein etc., which if made well, and with appropriate ingredients, is a good

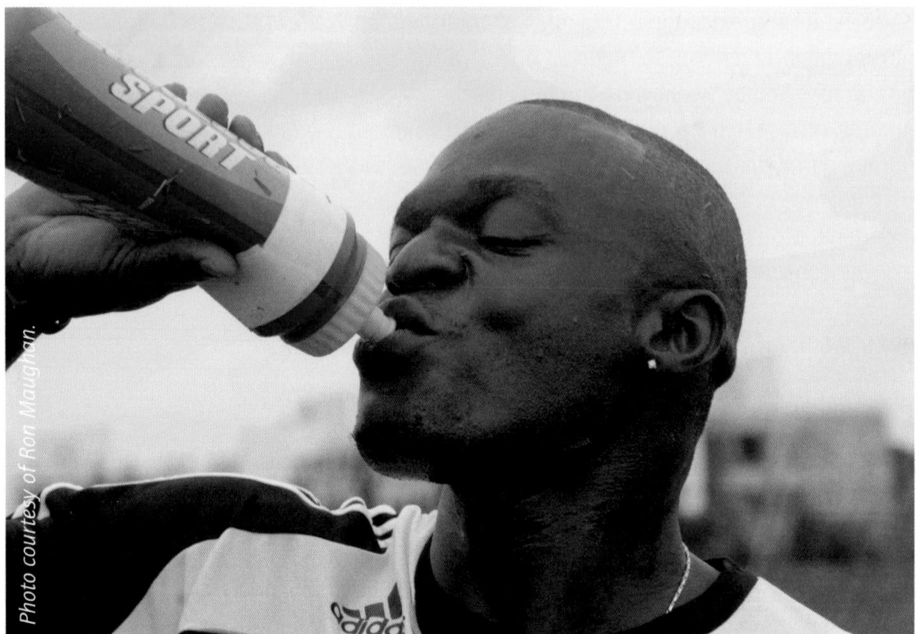

Photo 6.3 After a match it is important for players to start refuelling and rehydrating as soon as possible to promote recovery and it is common to see players drinking a sport beverage as they leave the pitch after the final whistle.

solution to satisfy the players' desire. You will find some examples of these popular meals in chapter 12. These, and other nutritional issues related to recovery, will be covered in more detail in the next chapter. Table 6.1 summarises a typical match-day nutrition strategy for elite footballers for matches that kick-off at 3:00pm.

INFLUENCE OF DIFFERENT MATCH TIMINGS

Only 30 years ago, almost all football league matches in countries such as England, kicked-off at 3:00pm on a Saturday afternoon with the occasional mid-week evening match starting at 7:30pm. Nowadays, television rights provide a huge amount of income to clubs but, in part, the price to pay for that is that games can be scheduled on almost any day of the week at any time between 12:00 noon and 8:00pm. This, obviously, has an impact on the planning of nutrition of the players. Tables 6.2 and 6.3 summarise typical match-day nutrition strategies for matches that kick-off at 1:00pm and 7:45pm, respectively.

Table 6.1 Match-day nutrition recommendations for a 3:00pm kick-off

Timing	Feeding
08:00: Wake up	Individual preparation. Drink 250 mL water
09:00–10:00: Breakfast	50–70 g CHO + 10–20 g PRO
10:00–11:30	Drink fluid according to thirst
11:30–12:30: Pre-match meal	70–150 g CHO + 20–30 g PRO (see chapter 12 for example meals). Beetroot juice?
14:00: Optional ergogenic supplements	Beetroot juice? Caffeine?
14:50: After the warm-up	30 g CHO (e.g., 1 gel = 250 mL sports drink)
15:00: Kick-off	
15:45–16:00: Half-time	30–60 g CHO + 250–500 mL fluid. Caffeine?
16:45: Full time: As players leave pitch and return to dressing room	Sports drink (30–40 g CHO; 500 mL fluid)
17:15–17:45: After a shower and dressing	Finger food snacks containing 50 g CHO Carbohydrate/protein shake (50 g CHO + 40 g protein; 500 mL fluid)
19:00–20:00: Meal (main course and dessert)	100–150 g CHO + 30 g PRO (see chapter 12 for example meals)
	Fluid according to thirst
22:00–22:30: Pre-bed protein and fruit	30–40 g PRO (slow-release casein) + 30 g CHO (e.g. cottage cheese with crackers followed by kiwi fruit or milk-based protein/CHO shake blended with fruit and oats)
23:00: Bedtime (sleep)	

Note the use of ergogenic supplements such as beetroot juice and/or caffeine is a suggestion and not a recommendation. The decision to take supplements is down to the individual and the sport science support staff.

Table 6.2 Match-day nutrition recommendations for a 1:00pm kick-off

Timing	Feeding
08:00: Wake up	Individual preparation. Drink 250 mL water
09:00–10:00: Pre-match meal	70–150 g CHO + 20–30 g PRO + fluid (see chapter 12 for example meals)
10:00–12:00	Drink 500 mL water. Beetroot juice?
12:00: Optional ergogenic supplements	Beetroot juice? Caffeine?
12:50: After the warm-up	30 g CHO (e.g., 1 gel = 250 mL sports drink)
13:00: Kick-off	
13:45–14:00: Half-time	30–60 g CHO + 250–500 mL fluid. Caffeine?
14:45: Full time: As players leave pitch and return to dressing room	Sports drink (30–40 g CHO; 500 mL fluid)
15:15–15:45: After a shower and dressing	Finger food snacks containing 50 g CHO CHO/protein shake (50 g CHO + 40 g protein; 500 mL fluid)
16:30–17:30: Light meal (or larger meal instead of the dinner below if travelling back from an away game)	50–100 g CHO + 20–30 g PRO Fluid according to thirst
19:00–20:00: Dinner (main course and dessert)	100–150 g CHO + 30 g PRO (see chapter 12 for example meals) Fluid according to thirst
22:00–22:30: Pre-bed protein and fruit	30–40 g PRO (slow-release casein) + 30 g CHO (e.g. cottage cheese with crackers followed by kiwi fruit or milk-based protein/CHO shake blended with fruit and oats)
23:00: Bedtime (sleep)	

Note the use of ergogenic supplements such as beetroot juice and/or caffeine is a suggestion and not a recommendation. The decision to take supplements is down to the individual and the sport science support staff.

A particular problem for Muslim players during Ramadan can be playing in matches with an evening kick-off. Some games may not start until 8:00pm when it is still daylight in the spring and summer months in many countries. This means that a player may start a match without having had any food or drink during the day. Of course, the manager

Table 6.3 Match-day nutrition recommendations for a 7:45pm kick-off

Timing	Feeding
08:00: Wake up	Individual preparation. Drink 250 mL water
09:00–10:00: Breakfast	50–70 g CHO + 20–30 g PRO
10:00–12:00	Drink fluid according to thirst
12:00: Light lunch	50–70 g CHO + 20–30 g PRO
16:00: Pre-match meal	70–100 g CHO + 20–30 g PRO
17:00–18:00	Drink 500 mL water. Beetroot juice?
18:45: Optional ergogenic supplements	Beetroot juice? Caffeine?
19:35: After the warm-up	30 g CHO (e.g. 1 gel = 250 mL sports drink)
19:45: Kick-off	
20:30–20:45: Half-time	30-60 g CHO + 250–500 mL fluid. Caffeine?
21:30: Full time: As players leave pitch and return to dressing room	Sports drink (30–40 g CHO; 500 mL fluid)
22:00: After a shower and dressing	CHO/protein shake (50 g CHO + 40 g protein; 500 mL fluid)
22:30–23:30: Dinner (main course and dessert)	100–150 g CHO + 30 g PRO (see chapter 12 for example meals) Fluid according to thirst
24:00: Bedtime (sleep)	

Note the use of ergogenic supplements such as beetroot juice and/or caffeine is a suggestion and not a recommendation. The decision to take supplements is down to the individual and the sport science support staff.

has the option to rest players, but that could be unpopular with the Muslim players in the squad, and besides the player might be very important to the team. However, the manager might consider substituting the player in the second half if the game result is going well. One good example of this took place on April 23, 2021, in the English Premier League when Leicester City were 3-0 up against West Bromwich Albion by half-time. The manager Brendan Rodgers substituted his talented 20-year-old defender Wesley Fofana in the 61st minute and after the match said, 'He's a young player in the middle of Ramadan [which began on April 13 that year] so he's obviously not eaten during the day.' In fact, he had not eaten or drunk anything in the previous 15 hours. Rodgers continued with 'It was just one where I thought I could get him off and he could get some food into him on the bench and just protect him a little bit. I work with lots of players who have similar devotion to their faith, and I think, for a lot of the guys, it gives them strength. He [Fofana] has found incredible strength to play continuously and to train while in Ramadan.' A nice illustration, I think, of good management and sport nutrition in tandem and in practice when cultural or religious issues can impinge on what and when a player can eat and drink. Four days later Leicester had another home, this time against Crystal Palace which the Foxes won 2-1, and Fofana played the full 90 minutes. Both teams contained Muslim players who were adhering to the rules of Ramadan, and a pre-match agreement between the club captains allowed players on both sides to break their fast after 30 minutes of play when the ball had gone out of play for a goal kick. In my humble opinion, in the near future, it would be good to see some official rules put in place to allow this practice in all games involving Muslim players during the holy month of Ramadan.

NUTRITION FOR TRAVEL

For away games that are not against local arrivals, there is obviously a need for travel. Occasionally, particularly for evening kick-offs in the national league and European competitions (e.g. Champions League, UEFA League), teams may stay in a hotel near the location of where the match was played and travel home the next morning. In that situation, a late evening post-match meal can be consumed in the hotel restaurant. However, for the majority of away games, teams will travel home immediately after departing from the match stadium. In that situation, food and drink will be made available on the move via coach, train or aircraft. Often it will be more prudent to have prepared suitable high-quality ready meals and other foods in advance (with careful attention to hygiene, packaging and cooling) that can be reheated on the team coach or consumed cold (e.g. tortilla wraps, filled pitta bread, sandwiches, cereal bars) if travelling by rail or air, rather than relying on what the mode of transport provider has available.

MATCH DAY NUTRITION

CARBOHYDRATE
6-8 g/kg BM/day
On day prior to match & match day to elevate muscle glycogen stores

ENERGY
Typically consume 3500 kcal to match total energy needs on match days

RECOVERY
Begins immediately post-match with fluid, carbs, protein in sports foods & protein shakes

PRE-MATCH MEAL
High in low-fibre carbohydrate 1-2 g/kg BM to replenish liver glycogen stores

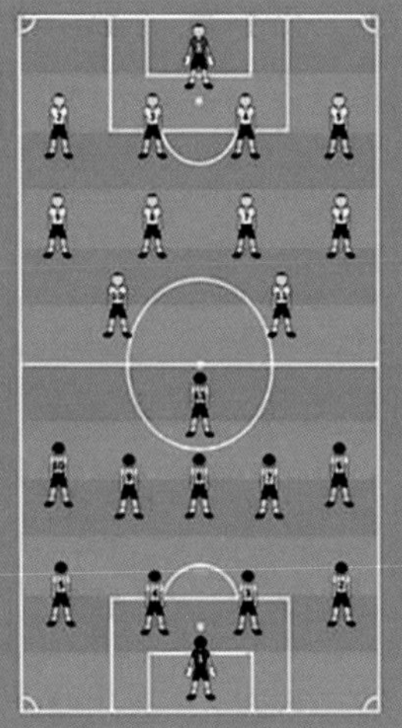

POST-MATCH MEAL
Begin restoration of muscle glycogen & repair by providing 2 g/kg BM carbohydrate plus 40 g high quality protein at 3-4 h intervals

HYDRATION
Start match well-hydrated by drinking 5-7 ml/kg BM fluid 2-4 h before kick-off

BREAKS IN PLAY
Drink water to avoid dehydration on warm days.
Mouth rinse then swallow sport drink

PRE-MATCH ERGOGENIC AIDS
Beetroot shots with pre-match meal
Caffeine 1-3 mg/kg BM 1 h before KO

WARM-UP JUST BEFORE KICK-OFF
Ingest 30 g carbohydrate as gels or sport drinks

HALF-TIME
Ingest 30-60 g carbohydrate as gels or sport drinks.
Caffeine chewing gum (spit out before returning to pitch)

Infographic 6 Match-day nutrition.

CHAPTER 7

Recovery Nutrition

- Post-Match Nutrition: Rehydration, Refuelling and Repair
- Nutrition and Sleep

After a match or a hard training session, players need some time to rest and recover, and good nutrition is an important – some would say essential – part of the recovery process. In this chapter, we will examine nutritional strategies that can help to assist and speed recovery. During congested fixture periods with two or even sometimes three games in one week speedy and effective recovery becomes even more important. This is especially relevant if the manager wants the same players to play in successive matches, which for some clubs can be especially important, particularly some of the less well-off ones that lack the same depth of quality among their squads beyond their manager's first-choice eleven.

The immediate post-match or post-training period should be a time for rest (i.e. relaxation and later a good night's sleep) as well as a time for rehydration (to restore fluid and electrolyte losses), refuelling (to restore glycogen) and repair (i.e. muscle tissue repair and remodelling to alleviate soreness and allow adaptation to the training stimulus); these are known as the 4Rs (figure 7.1). The appropriate amounts of fluid, electrolytes, carbohydrate and protein should be ingested during recovery to accomplish the goals defined by the 4Rs. Eating just before bedtime has also been suggested as a good time to provide additional dietary protein that can be directed toward remodelling muscle proteins while the player is sleeping.

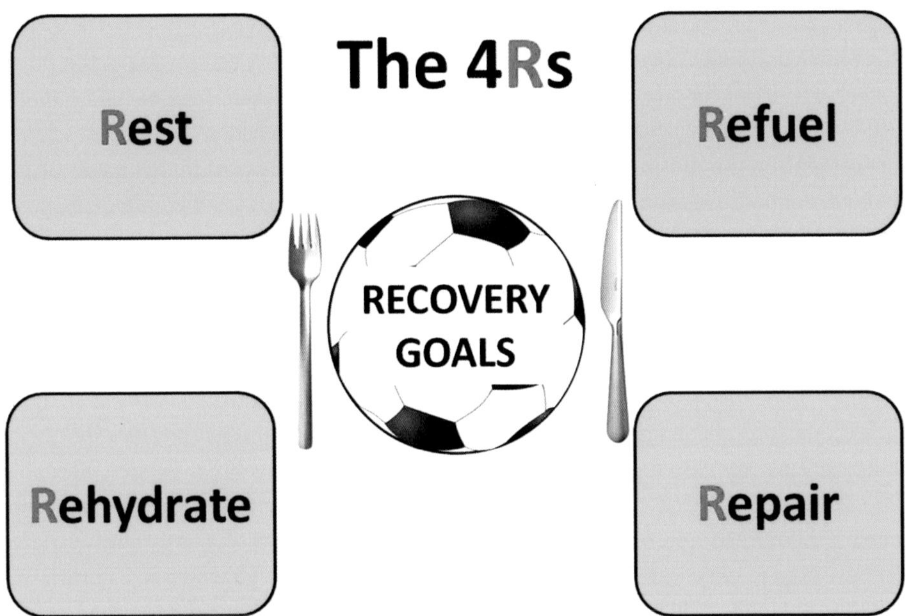

Figure 7.1 The 4Rs that define the goals of recovery: (1) Rest (i.e. relaxation, recuperation and sleep), (2) Refuel (i.e. restoration of muscle and liver glycogen stores), (3) Rehydrate (i.e. restore losses of water and electrolytes), and (4) Repair (i.e. alleviate muscle damage and muscle soreness and allow muscle remodelling and adaptation).

POST-MATCH NUTRITION: REHYDRATION, REFUELLING AND REPAIR

It is important to appreciate that recovery begins straight after a match is finished. Appropriate nutrition can reduce the time that it takes the player to recover. During congested fixture periods, when matches take place 2–3 times per week with some away games requiring long-distance travel, the appropriate timing, quality and quantity of post-match meals can play critical roles in recovery. To optimise muscle protein synthesis for repair and recovery, meals and snacks should be scheduled to target intakes of 20 to 30 g of high-quality protein in 3–4 hour intervals. Furthermore, consuming a high-protein shake that contains 30 to 50 g of protein an hour or so before bedtime can enhance overnight protein synthesis. There is also a need to restore liver and muscle glycogen with carbohydrate intake and to begin this at an early stage of recovery (within 2 hours post-exercise) when the rate of muscle glycogen resynthesis is at its highest.

Players can begin to rehydrate and refuel immediately by drinking a 6–8 g/CHO/100 mL carbohydrate-electrolyte beverage (i.e. a typical sport drink) as they leave the pitch. Convenient finger food (e.g. baked sweet potato wedges, chicken, ham or tuna Paninis, tortilla wraps or sandwiches) and sports foods will usually be provided by the sport science support staff in the dressing room, and this will be followed by post-match meals at the stadium, during travel and/or at home. Some sports foods (e.g. carbohydrate gels, sports bars and confectionery, recovery carbohydrate/protein shakes and sports drinks) may be the preferred option to supply macronutrients, especially to achieve carbohydrate-intake guidelines when appetite may be reduced (even more likely when the team has been beaten in the match) or when sourcing food when playing away from home.

Professor James Morton is a top applied sport nutritionist who has worked in both professional football and cycling at the elite level. He has strong views on the importance of recovery in sports like football. He says, 'Having your best players consistently available is a critical performance challenge. Nonetheless, whilst player availability is one thing, keeping them fresh and firing on all cylinders is another. Winning consistently requires the best players playing to their best at the right time. That is why recovery nutrition is so important in football where in many professional leagues two games in a three or four day period is the norm. From a recovery perspective, those first few hours immediately after each game are often the most challenging to get right, but also a time that could return the biggest performance impact.'

He continues, 'Replenishing muscle glycogen stores, rehydrating, promoting muscle repair and aiding sleep are, of course, the main physiological priorities. Nevertheless, losing to a last-minute goal, dealing with the logistical challenges of home versus away games (potentially affecting the quality of food provision) and coping with late evening kick-off times and travel schedules can all affect the willingness of the players to engage with recovery protocols.' This is despite the obvious rationale and the strong advice being given by the nutritionists and other support staff.

The science on the effectiveness of appropriate recovery strategies is there to back up the recommendations of what and when to eat and drink, but according to James, 'bringing it to life practically is by far the greatest challenge.' Many club support staff will probably have witnessed half-empty bottles of recovery shakes in the dressing room after match, despite the instructions given to the players to consume all the contents. James's recommendations are as follows: 'Recovery needs to be placed at the heart of performance delivery, so that each member of the management and performance support team is crystal clear on what best practice actually looks like. Equally, players themselves must also understand the role that recovery can play in winning consistently and reducing the risk of injury and illness. Their recovery protocol should be personalised to their individual needs in accordance with their physiological requirements and personal dietary preferences. For some, the traditional plate of pasta and a chocolate protein shake may not cut it. Rather, all taste preferences and cultures should be considered when formulating and delivering a detailed and personalised recovery plan.' In other words, it is important to ensure that the correct quantity and type of food is consumed at the correct time. If the players opt to not eat and drink what they have been asked, it is a problem that needs to be addressed. James concludes that 'tracking calories should perhaps be considered just as routine as putting on your heart rate monitor before training each day. More often than not, what gets measured gets done.'

Players should also aim to restore their fluid and electrolyte balance soon after the match (or at least within 24 hours), but this is not a major priority as, in most situations, there is plenty of time and opportunity to recover from any dehydration that may have developed during the second half of a match (or when extra-time is played in cup competitions). Any disturbance in electrolyte balance (particularly falls in body sodium content due to sweating) will be resolved easily with normal eating/drinking practices, as most foods and some drinks (e.g. milk, sports drinks) contain sodium and some other electrolytes, such as chloride and potassium. Often, in various sports, athletes are advised to drink according to how thirsty they feel. However, this may not always be appropriate in many team sports, including football training and match play, as the availability of fluids and the sensation of thirst may not coincide. This requires some forward planning (e.g. understanding individual sweat losses, developing individualised hydration plans, alongside player education) in order to ensure that each player's hydration needs are met. You can refer back to the section on water requirements in chapter 5 for further details about these issues.

RESTORING MUSCLE GLYCOGEN

In addition to energy expended and fluid loss through sweat, players will use around 50–80% of their muscle glycogen stores during a match. The energy, fluid and carbohydrate lost can be easily replaced in post-match meals, but it takes considerably longer to restore muscle glycogen, even when players consume a high-carbohydrate diet for several days post-match (figure 7.2). Glycogen resynthesis is generally slower in games players than in cyclists, runners and swimmers, which is thought to be due to a reduction in glucose uptake by the muscles when some muscle damage has been incurred due to the nature of the physical activity. In-play collisions, tackles, twisting and turning movements, landing from jumps and decelerating from sprints can all cause some damage to muscle fibres, which results in muscle soreness (which is usually most severe 12–48 hours post-exercise). Muscle soreness in the first few days following a football (soccer) or rugby match (a game in which there is more physical contact and soft-tissue injuries than in soccer) can be an indication that some muscle damage is present. In non-damaging sports such as cycling and swimming, complete restoration of muscle glycogen usually only takes 24–48 hours when a high-carbohydrate diet is consumed.

These losses of glycogen during a football match, and their subsequent slow recovery afterwards, are not a major issue when the next match takes place at least 6 or 7 days later. However, failure to quickly restore muscle glycogen levels back to normal may impair training quality and match performance when the next training session or match is only 2–3 days away. Therefore, players are recommended to ingest a high-carbohydrate diet (6–8 g/kg BM/day with 70% of dietary energy from carbohydrate) for the first few days after a match, and players can also take advantage of a relatively new research finding that supplementing with creatine after a game, and for the next 24 hours, can substantially boost muscle glycogen resynthesis. Using this optimal nutritional strategy, muscle glycogen can be fully restored to its pre-match level within 72 hours (figure 7.3).

To rapidly replenish glycogen stores, post-match snacks and meals should target a carbohydrate intake of about 1 g/kg BM per hour for 4 hours (equivalent to a total of 300 g CHO for a 75 kg player). High-GI foods are preferred, as these have been shown to result in greater muscle glycogen resynthesis in the first few hours after exercise compared with equal amounts of carbohydrate from low-GI foods. Following the consumption of snack foods and a protein shake in the dressing room, a main meal with a dessert should be eaten within the next couple of hours. This meal should contain 100–150 g of high-GI carbohydrate and at least 30 g protein. Popular dishes for the post-match meal are those that most of us would call 'comfort foods' and are often similar to takeaway-style meals or 'fast food'. Dishes that these resemble these types of food, but are made with reduced fat content, healthier ingredients and supply the intended dose of carbohydrate and protein can be created, and some examples devised by expert performance chefs are provided in chapter 12.

In addition, when the goal is to restore muscle glycogen stores as quickly as possible, daily carbohydrate intake should be increased from 4–5 g/kg BM (the typical intake of a professional footballer) to about 6–8 g/kg BM for 48–72 hours after the match. This is especially important during congested fixture schedules and after evening games when players can be more tired and may find it difficult to achieve carbohydrate-intake targets following the match, as they will probably only have a few hours remaining before it is time for bed. Failure to achieve nutrition recommendations when recovery time is limited runs the risk of not fully restoring various physiological parameters affected by match play, such as muscle glycogen content, endurance and muscle strength. This will ultimately limit the players' ability to sprint, jump and perform repeated sequences of intense intermittent

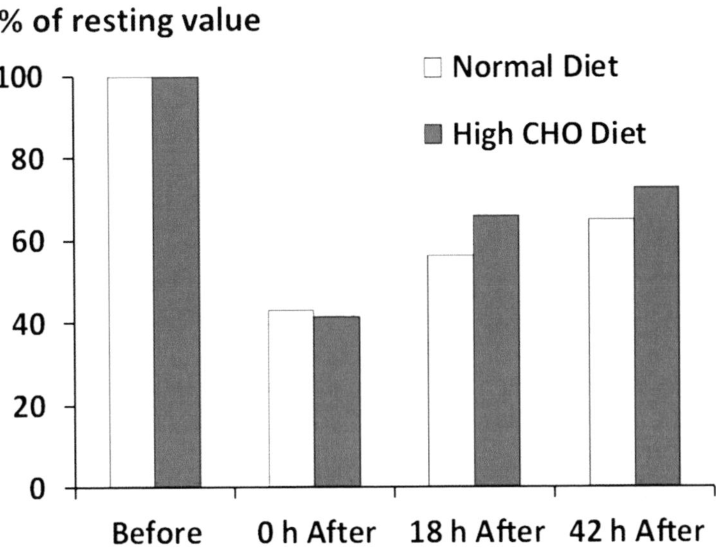

Figure 7.2 Restoration of muscle glycogen after a football match is rather slow, even on a relatively high-carbohydrate diet because muscle damage impairs muscle glucose uptake and glycogen resynthesis. Data from Bangsbo et al. (2006).

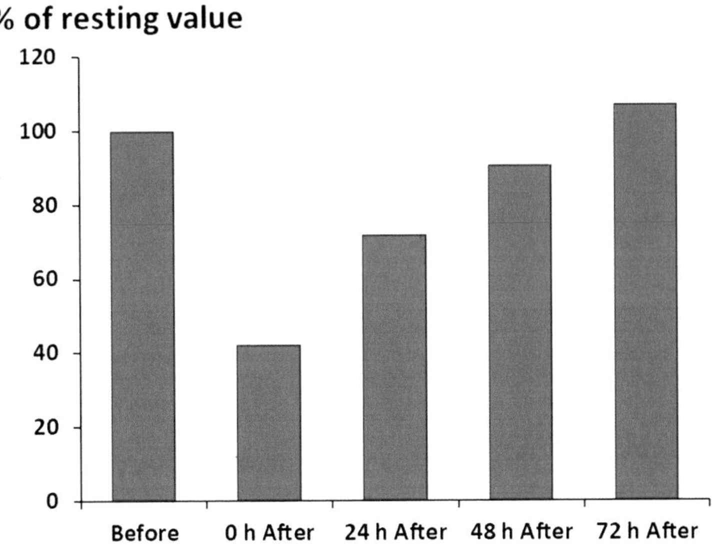

Figure 7.3 Restoration of muscle glycogen content after a football match typically takes about 72 hours if players are put on a carbohydrate-rich diet and supplemented with creatine to optimise muscle glycogen restoration nutrition. See text for details. Data from Krustrup et al. (2011). In this study, muscle glycogen levels were depleted, on average, by 57% immediately after the game. Muscle glycogen levels were still depleted by 27% and 8% at 24 and 48 hours after the game, respectively. At 72 hours after the game, muscle glycogen levels were 7% higher compared with pre-match values.

exercise and so compromise the next match-day performance if it is only a few days away – as it often is during mid-season, with a mixture of domestic and international (e.g. Champions League, Europa League and national team) fixtures. Top players may play 50–60 games per season with most weeks involving two games per week and many miles of travelling.

As previously mentioned, one means of speeding up muscle glycogen resynthesis after a football match, which may be of particular value when the next game is only 2–3 days away, is to ingest creatine (20 g in four separate 5 g doses) together with a high-carbohydrate intake (6–8 g/kg BM) in the first 24 hours after the match. A study has shown that muscle glycogen restoration in the first 24 hours after glycogen-depleting exercise was increased by 82% with co-ingestion of creatine and carbohydrate (compared with placebo and the same amount of carbohydrate), but that no further benefits were evident by continuing this practice for a further 2–5 days (figure 7.4). There are some commercially available recovery shakes that contain around 50 g CHO, 40 g protein and 5 g creatine, and so are ideal to consume straight after a match. On subsequent feeding/drinking occasions, the creatine can be added as a powder to sports drinks consumed with normal foods. Pre-weighed sachets containing 5 g

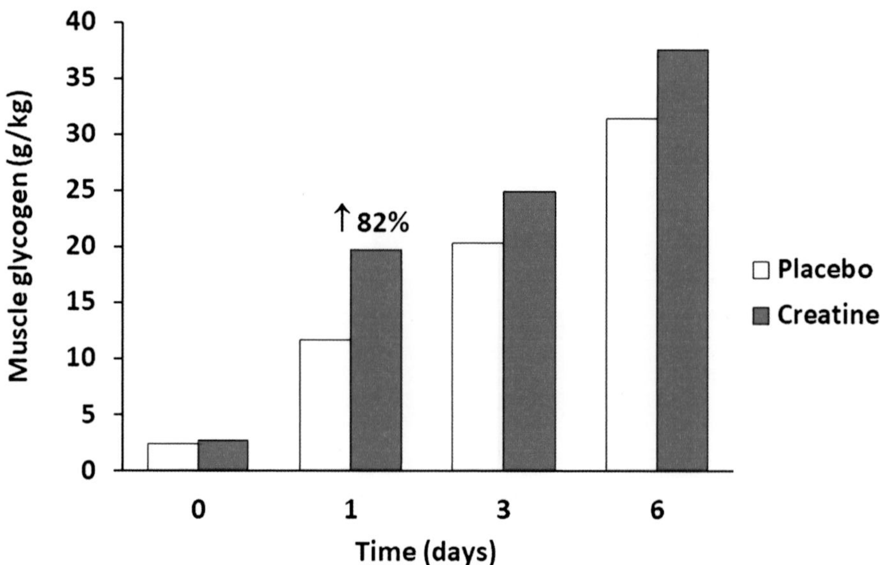

Figure 7.4 Restoration of muscle glycogen content after glycogen-depleting exercise was increased by 82% in the first 24 hours when creatine was co-ingested with carbohydrate. Data from Roberts et al. (2016).

creatine can be given to players for consumption at home the day after a match (most clubs give players a day off to recover at home after match day unless they need treatment for an injury). Although the exact mechanism of action of this glycogen-boosting creatine effect has not been established, there are a number of possibilities and the interested reader is directed to read the Roberts et al. (2016) paper (details can be found in the list of reference sources at the end of the book) to find out what they are. As already mentioned, when this creatine and carbohydrate co-ingestion strategy was used following a 90-minute game of football, muscle glycogen was fully restored within 72 hours (figure 7.3).

REDUCING MUSCLE SORENESS

Players often suffer from some muscle soreness for a day or two after a match due to some exercise-induced muscle damage and soft-tissue injuries from collisions and tackles during match play. I have occasionally heard some managers attribute this delayed-onset muscle soreness to a 'build-up of lactic acid', but that is incorrect. For example, in December 2020 Neil Warnock, the highly experienced manager of Middlesbrough FC, was asked by a television reporter to explain why he had given his players a day off at home the day after a Wednesday night match when they had another match to play on Saturday afternoon (i.e. in less than 3 days' time). Mr Warnock said 'They need to get their lactic acid out, so I ask them to go and have a walk – take the dogs out or something like that – but rest is just as important the day after. They put a big shift in on Wednesday night.' His team had just beaten promotion rivals Swansea City. He continued 'I think sometimes people do things for the sake of it, really. Whereas I don't give a damn, me. I don't mind telling you they played golf yesterday. If I get stick, I get stick. But I think rest is so important.' Mr Warnock is absolutely correct about the need for rest and there is really no point in asking players to come to the training ground the day after a hard game if the intention is to do only a light training session. Some players may have to drive for an hour or more to get there and the same again to go home. Their time would be better spent at home and just doing some light activity like walking or playing nine holes of golf. But Mr Warnock is wrong about the lactic acid, which will be cleared from the muscles within an hour or two of finishing the match. The soreness that players feel the day after a game is due to damage incurred to the microstructure of some muscle fibres in their legs, which causes temporary inflammation and a little swelling of the affected muscles.

This exercise-induced structural muscle damage is difficult to prevent altogether, but muscle soreness and the associated drops in strength and power that occur in the following days might be reduced, to some extent, by nutritional strategies during the post-exercise period. These strategies include the intake of protein (meat, fish, poultry, beans and milk are all good food sources of protein) and foods rich in anti-inflammatory and antioxidant phytochemicals such as berries, cherries, cherry juice, dark chocolate and green tea, which can reduce muscle damage and soreness, albeit to only a small degree. Drinking polyphenol-rich tart cherry juice has become a popular intervention to accelerate muscle recovery in a variety of different sports, but some recent studies of the efficacy of this nutritional intervention in football have not shown improved recovery of markers of muscle function or soreness ratings, so the evidence currently available does not support its use in football.

Several studies have shown that ingestion of two omega-3 fatty acids (called eicosapentaenoic acid, EPA, and docosahexaenoic acid, DHA) derived from fish oil can decrease muscle soreness following damaging eccentric exercise. Several other studies also suggest that improvements in cognitive function, reaction time and attention span result from supplementation with omega-3 fatty acids, and these effects could be important for team games like football. A good dietary source of these anti-inflammatory omega-3 fatty acids is oily fish such as mackerel, salmon, sardines and tuna and oils derived from fish (e.g. cod liver oil) and krill. There are currently no established recommendations for EPA and DHA intake, but the ingestion of about 1 g/day of these fatty acids seems appropriate to obtain the benefits described. A 170 g portion of salmon contains about 2 g of EPA and DHA and about 35 g of protein and is a popular choice with many professional players.

Although ingesting large doses of individual antioxidant vitamins C and E may reduce exercise-induced muscle inflammation and free radical production to some extent, it may also interfere with muscle adaptation and is therefore discouraged, at least during the competitive season. Taking oral non-steroidal anti-inflammatory drugs (e.g. ibuprofen) to provide pain relief is also discouraged, as these can be harmful if consumed regularly.

In professional rugby which, like football, is an intermittent high-intensity team sport in which there are frequent high-intensity collisions, oral cannabidiol (CBD) is increasing in popularity among players to reduce muscle soreness and improve recovery and sleep, despite anti-doping risks. A recent study in professional rugby (both union and league clubs), indicated that 26% of players had either used it (18%) or were still using it (8%). CBD is derived from hemp, a type of cannabis plant which contains over 100 cannabinoids, but has a low content (0.2–0.3% dry weight) of the psychotropic drug tetrahydrocannabinol (THC) found in marijuana (which may contain up to 30% dry weight THC). In the UK, CBD can be legally sold, providing that it does not contain more than 1 mg of the controlled drug in the final 'container' – that is, in the bottle or packet that it is sold in (according to the UK Government Home Office, 2020). In the UK, almost all other cannabinoids, except CBD, remain subject to the Misuse of Drugs Act 1971. There are a variety of forms of CBD that are commercially available for sale, including oils, capsules, sprays, tinctures and gums. Most clubs would probably discourage players from taking CBD due to the risk of a positive doping test. Further research is needed to establish if the claimed effects on soreness, recovery and sleep can be achieved with CBD in athletes and games players, and that its regular use does not produce spikes in other cannabinoids that could result in an anti-doping violation, given that all cannabinoids, except CBD, are currently prohibited substances by the World Anti-Doping Agency (WADA). Many sporting bodies currently advise against CBD use; however, it is clear that some athletes are ignoring this advice and using it to enhance recovery.

Some players like to drink alcohol after a match to help them relax, celebrate an important win or drown their sorrows after a bad defeat. However, it is also important for players to realise that drinking alcohol can interfere with recovery by impairing liver and glycogen resynthesis, muscle protein synthesis and rehydration. Drinking large doses of alcohol has been shown to reduce sleep quality, impair next-day counter-movement jump performance and also directly suppress immune function. Regular drinking of alcohol can also impair wound healing and recovery from injury. Players should therefore minimise, or avoid, alcohol intake altogether when recovery is a priority.

NUTRITION AND SLEEP

The composition of the diet influences sleep duration and quality. For example, deficiencies of total energy, protein and carbohydrate have been shown to be associated with shorter sleep duration. In contrast, one study reported that consuming high-GI carbohydrate meals (that is meals that cause a rapid spike in the blood sugar concentration) about 4 hours before bedtime decreased the time it took to fall asleep after going to bed. This effect was attributed to a decreased plasma fatty acid concentration and a consequent increase in circulating free tryptophan after carbohydrate consumption. Tryptophan is an essential amino acid that is the precursor of the sleep-regulating hormone serotonin and is thought to be important in the proposed relationships between diet and sleep. Increases in tryptophan intake via protein ingestion in the evening have been shown to improve sleep in adults with sleep disturbances and result in enhanced alertness in the morning, most likely as a result of improved sleep quality.

Research on sleep in professional footballers has revealed that they generally have longer than average sleep latency (i.e. it takes them longer to fall asleep after switching off the light) and lower-than-average sleep quality (i.e. they have more frequent awakenings during the night) compared with the general population. This has been attributed to mental anxieties about an upcoming match, coming down from the excitement of competitive match play, caffeine intake before or during matches (especially when it is an evening kick-off), night-time cramps and muscle soreness. Poor sleep could affect both mental and physical performance detrimentally, depress immune function and increase susceptibility to developing respiratory illness symptoms when exposed to a common cold virus. Chronic sleep loss is known to have profound effects on metabolism, but even just one night without any sleep in healthy young adults has been shown to reduce overnight muscle protein synthesis after a standard 600 kcal (14% protein) pre-sleep meal, and also increased plasma cortisol and decreased plasma testosterone. Therefore, improving sleep quality through appropriate nutrition and other behaviours is definitely desirable.

Deficiencies of certain micronutrients have been suggested to affect sleep duration and quality. For example, deficiencies of the vitamins folate and thiamin, as well as the minerals iron, magnesium, phosphorus, selenium and zinc, are associated with shorter sleep duration. Furthermore, lack of selenium and calcium make it harder to fall asleep, and low intakes of vitamin D and lycopene (an antioxidant phytonutrient found in fruits and vegetables) impair the ability to stay soundly asleep. In contrast, the ingestion of certain micronutrients in non-deficient individuals appears to improve sleep quality. For, example, nightly intake of a magnesium or zinc supplement improved sleep quality in long-term care facility residents with insomnia, and in healthy subjects, zinc-rich foods improved sleep onset latency (i.e. shortened the time it took to fall asleep after going to bed and turning off the lights) and increased sleep efficiency compared with placebo. Some other supplements including *Lactobacillus* probiotics and CBD have also been reported to improve sleep quality, but currently, nutritional and supplement intervention studies in elite football players are lacking. Therefore, any interventions of this nature for footballers are largely based on research on athletes in other sports who also experience low sleep quality compared with the general population.

Probiotics are food supplements that contain live microorganisms which, when administered in adequate amounts, can confer benefits to the health and functioning of the digestive system, as well as having a positive influence on immune function. In the general population, studies have shown that probiotic intake can improve rates of recovery from diarrhoea, increase resistance to gut and respiratory infections, and alleviate some allergic and respiratory disorders. Several studies in athletes also indicate that some strains of probiotic – *Lactobacillus* and *Bifidobacterium* species in particular – can be effective in reducing the incidence of the common cold, as was mentioned in chapter 5. However, the benefits of probiotics may extend beyond immunity and reduction of illness risk, according to new research that indicates the gut microbiota can communicate in a bidirectional manner with the brain via the production of neurochemicals by commensal bacteria resident in the large intestine (colon). Probiotics may modify this production of neurochemicals and thus influence mood, stress responses and sleep quality. Microbes and their metabolism can also be influenced in turn by neurochemicals, including catecholamines (e.g. adrenaline and noradrenaline) produced by the human body in response to stress. These interactions likely explain what we like to call our 'gut feelings'!

The body's stress response system maintains homeostasis (i.e. a relatively constant internal environment) against various external stimuli that can disturb it and generate stress. However, an excessive response to stress can trigger both mental and physical health problems. Studies in animals have shown that probiotics and gut microbiota reduce stress reactivity by influencing the neuroendocrine system, and can have positive effects on behaviour and cognitive function (e.g. reduced anxiety, depression and defeatism) under stressful conditions. In humans, recent investigations of the effects of probiotics on both stress-related physical symptoms and stress biomarkers have shown beneficial effects and that the daily ingestion of *Lactobacillus* probiotics can also improve sleep quality (earlier onset of sleep and longer sleep duration with probiotic compared with placebo) in medical students preparing for their academic exams. These findings raise the possibility that probiotics could be of benefit for athletes and football players recovering from intensive training and competition. Recovery involves both physical and psychological issues, and a supplement that could reduce physical symptoms of stress and improve both mood and sleep quality would almost certainly be good for a professional footballer. The importance of mental as well as physical recovery after intense competition is often underestimated, but a quote from someone who has a lot of experience of these issues, Dr Sam Erith, Head of Sports Science at Manchester City FC, is illuminating: 'The longer I do this job the more you see that mood and mind state are such powerful drivers for recovery.' Although further research is required to confirm these effects in the sporting population, it seems likely that probiotic supplements may provide multiple benefits for athletes and games players.

A number of other dietary factors can influence sleep quality (figure 7.5). Players are advised not to consume beverages or foods containing chemical stimulants like caffeine, as this has negative effects on sleep quality. Caffeine (in coffee, cocoa and some soft drinks like Coca-Cola, Pepsi, Red Bull and Monster Energy) and theobromine (in tea) interfere with the actions of adenosine, a metabolite that also serves a signalling function and regulates sleep-wake cycles. The ingestion of caffeine or theobromine before bedtime alters sleep patterns for many hours, including making it harder to go to sleep, reducing total sleep time and worsening perceived sleep quality. So, ideally players should avoid caffeinated beverages, supplements and foods (e.g. dark chocolate, some ice creams and frozen yoghurts) after about 6:00pm. One exception to this general rule could be ingesting caffeine to enhance performance (see chapters 5 and 6 for details) before or during an evening football match. In addition, as already mentioned, drinking alcohol can interfere with recovery processes as well as impairing sleep quality, and is therefore discouraged.

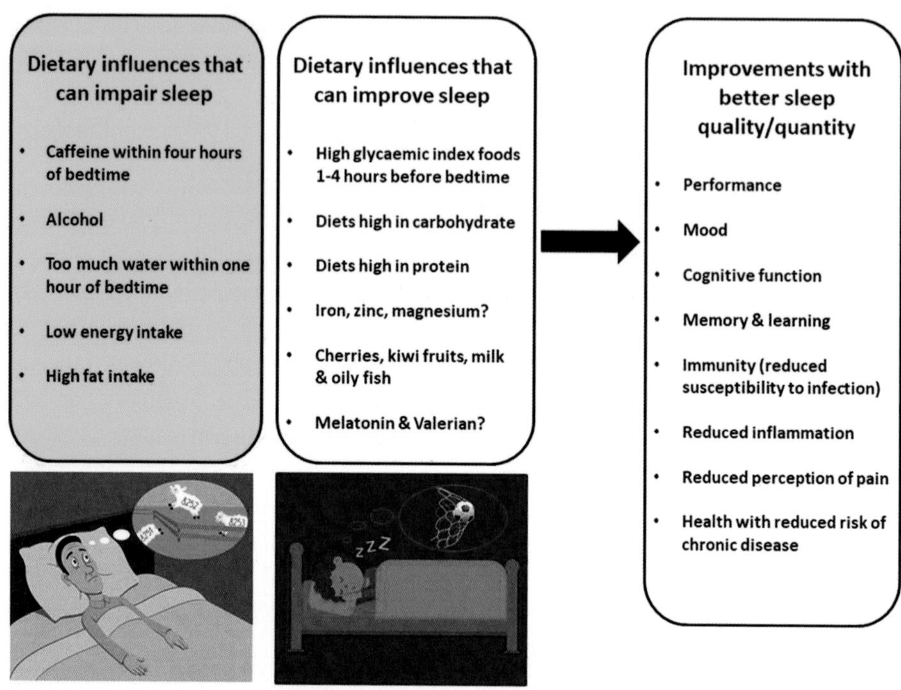

Figure 7.5 Nutrition can have an impact on sleep quality, which has implications for performance, mood and various aspects of health.

Sleep is an integral part of the recovery process, and for that reason some players may choose to limit their caffeine intake for evening matches to just a 100 mg in the form of a caffeinated chewing gum at half-time or avoid caffeine altogether. Some club doctors may advocate taking a melatonin supplement before bedtime. Melatonin is a hormone that your brain produces in response to darkness. It helps with the timing of your circadian rhythms (24-hour internal clock) and with sleep. Melatonin supplements (5 mg slow-release formulation) taken about one hour before bedtime have been shown to improve sleep quality in some healthy active people and are used in the treatment of some sleep disorders. In the UK and several other countries, melatonin is only available as a prescription drug. Other supplements designed to help sleep that are available for over-the-counter purchase include extracts of the root of the herb valerian, but evidence of their efficacy is equivocal. In some people undesirable side effects have been reported such as headaches, dizziness, or stomach problems.

It should be fairly obvious that players should avoid drinking large volumes of any fluid (including plain water) in the hour before bedtime, otherwise it they will feel the need to urinate during the night, which will interrupt their sleep. Urine production is usually at its highest about one hour after consuming a large volume of water so it is best to have your last drink a few hours before bedtime and visit the toilet just before going to bed. A cup (containing no more than 300 mL) of water, milk or a protein shake just before bedtime should be OK, but larger volumes than this should be avoided. In addition, as already mentioned, drinking alcohol can interfere with recovery processes as well as impairing sleep quality and is therefore discouraged.

The consumption of certain whole foods in the hours before bedtime can also affect sleep quantity and quality. For example, consumption of cherries, kiwi fruits, milk and oily fish have each been associated with beneficial effects on sleep quality. Some of these foods have a relatively high content of tryptophan and this may be responsible for their sleep-promoting effects. The intake of bread, pulses and fish has also been shown to extend sleep duration.

The ingestion of protein before bedtime to promote muscle training adaptation, and to repair and reduce muscle soreness, has already been mentioned. One study investigated the effect of ingesting 40 g of milk protein (casein) versus placebo (40 g CHO) before sleep on exercise performance recovery after professional soccer players played a match in the evening. When additional protein was ingested before sleep, the players' average counter-movement jump performance returned to its baseline pre-match value within 36 hours after the match. In contrast, counter-movement jump performance was still below baseline at 60 hours after the match when the carbohydrate placebo was ingested before sleep (figure 7.6). In addition, pre-sleep protein also reduced muscle soreness, which is a common feature of football match play due to the large number of high velocity eccentric contractions (e.g. decelerating after a sprint, bending and turning, and landing from jumps when heading the ball), which results in quite a bit of muscle damage. These results are quite impressive, considering that these players were already ingesting some post-match protein (0.5 g/kg BM) and had a high habitual daily protein intake of about 1.9 g/kg BM. Protein ingested prior to sleep is effectively digested and absorbed during sleep, thereby increasing the plasma amino acid concentration for several hours and stimulating muscle protein synthesis during overnight sleep. When pre-sleep protein intake is combined with exercise performed the same evening (e.g. following an evening match or training session), muscle protein synthesis rates during overnight sleep will be increased further. For players who are looking to increase their muscle mass and strength, protein ingestion before sleep can also be applied in combination with resistance-type exercise training, to further augment the gains in muscle mass and strength when compared with no protein supplementation. Therefore, a high daily protein intake and some protein (about 40 g, or 0.5 g/kg BM) before sleep may be required to optimise recovery and training adaptation in soccer players.

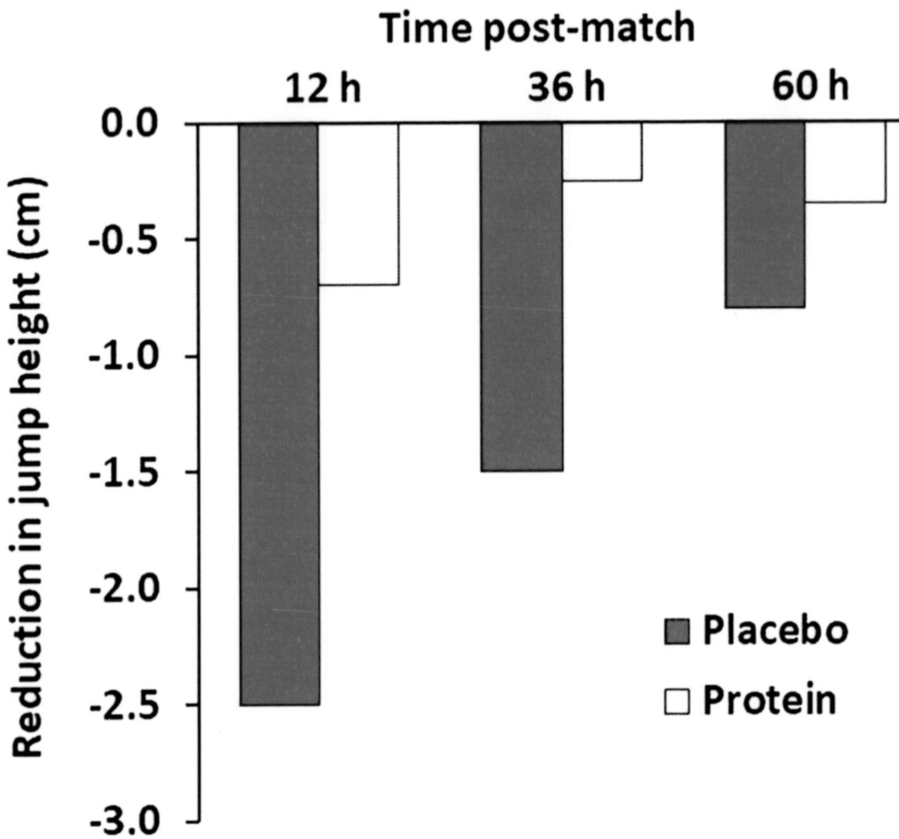

Figure 7.6 Improved recovery of counter-movement jump performance after an evening football match with pre-sleep protein ingestion. Data from Abbot et al. (2018).

Based on the information described in this chapter, it seems that the best nutritional strategy for football players to adopt before sleep to boost their recovery and sleep quality is to consume 30–40 g protein, together with some carbohydrate and a little fruit. For example, cottage cheese with crackers followed by kiwi fruit, or up to 300 mL of a concentrated milk-based protein/carbohydrate shake blended with fruit and oats, ingested around 30–60 minutes before bedtime. By the way, if you were wondering if this pre-sleep food intake might affect your appetite for breakfast in the morning, the research suggests it won't. At the time of writing this book, it is not known whether casein or whey protein is better for pre-sleep protein ingestion to boost overnight muscle protein synthesis. Published studies to date have used slow-release casein, so that is the current recommendation, but look out for new published studies that shed light on this issue. Table 7.1 provides a summary of the match-day nutrition recommendations for post-match recovery after completing a 90-minute match with a 3:00pm kick-off.

Table 7.1 Post-match nutrition recommendations for a 3:00pm kick-off up until bedtime

Timing	Feeding
16:45: Full time: As players leave pitch and return to dressing room	Sports drink (30–40 g CHO; 500 mL fluid)
17:15–17:45: After a shower and dressing	Finger food snacks containing 50 g CHO Carbohydrate/protein shake (50 g CHO + 40 g protein; 500 mL fluid; 5 g creatine)
19:00–20:00: Meal (Main course and dessert)	100–150 g CHO + 30 g PRO (see chapter 12 for example meals) Fluid according to thirst
22:00–22:30: Pre-bed protein and fruit	30–40 g PRO (slow-release casein) + 30 g CHO (e.g., cottage cheese with crackers followed by kiwi fruit or up to 300 mL of a concentrated milk-based protein/CHO shake blended with fruit and oats)
23:00: Bedtime (sleep)	

RECOVERY NUTRITION

IMMEDIATELY POST-MATCH

Sport drink
Gels
Finger-food in dressing room
Recovery protein shake

To begin process of muscle glycogen restoration, rehydration & muscle repair ASAP

MATCH-DAY +1

Consume 6-8 g/kg BM/day CARBOHYDRATE

Consume 20-25 g high-quality PROTEIN at 3-4 hour intervals amounting to a total of 1.6-2.2 g/kg BM/day

Drink FLUIDS according to thirst

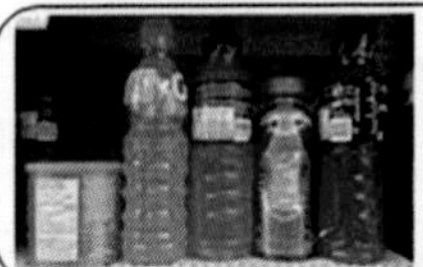
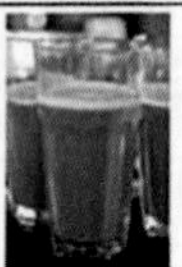
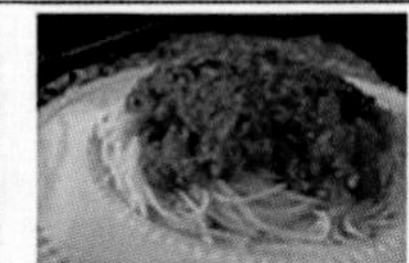
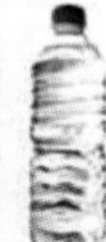
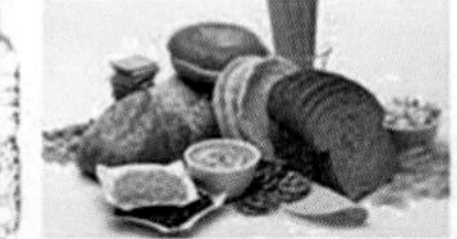
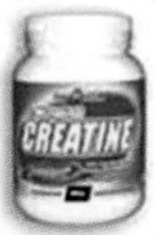

POST-MATCH MEALS

Consume 4 g/kg BM CARBOHYDRATE within the first 4 hours post-match

Consume 20-25 g high-quality PROTEIN at 3-4 hour intervals

Drink FLUIDS (about 1.5 times the volume (mass) of sweat losses) to fully rehydrate

WHEN NEXT MATCH IS ONLY 3 DAYS AWAY

Consume 5 g CREATINE with high carbohydrate post-match & MATCH-DAY +1 meals to provide 20 g CREATINE within 24 hours post-match

Can increase muscle glycogen resynthesis by 80% in first 24 hours after exercise

Infographic 7 Nutrition for recovery.

CHAPTER 8

Body Weight and Composition

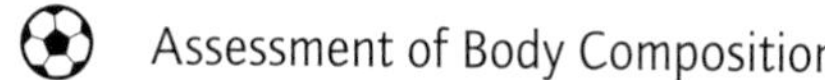

- Assessment of Body Composition

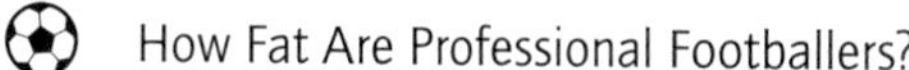

- How Fat Are Professional Footballers?
- Is There an Ideal Body Composition for a Professional Footballer?
- Changing a Player's Body Composition

In this chapter, I will attempt to explain the importance of body composition in football and how it can be manipulated, at least temporarily, by changing the nutrition and the exercise training, or both, of the player. One of the very best applied nutritionists in football I have ever met was a guy called Nick Broad who worked for Blackburn Rovers, Birmingham City and then Chelsea when José Mourinho (2004–2007) and Carlo Ancelotti (2009–2011) and three others (with considerably shorter reigns) managed the club. Tragically, Nick died at the age of only 38 in January 2013, in a road traffic accident, shortly after he joined Ancelotti at Paris Saint-Germain. Nick once let me know that one of the managers he worked with (who shall remain unnamed) had told him 'Your role is to make sure that there are no fat bastards in my team.' That may not be the most scientifically precise instruction a person in his position could receive, but it is a familiar refrain in many football clubs. Arsène Wenger has stated that one of the nutritionist's main roles is 'To ensure that players are in the best physical condition for the match: with an optimal level of body fat and muscle mass' – which is a nicer way of putting it while emphasising the importance of body composition in the mind of the manager or coach.

Nick also revealed to me that part of his job involved going shopping with players and teaching younger footballers how to cook, but most of his work was cutting-edge science, measuring biomarkers in saliva and blood to find out how well players were responding to training, or recovering from matches. He sent samples to me via courier and I analysed them in my lab at Loughborough University and sent him back the results within 24 hours. Nick's forward thinking and attention to detail were a credit to his profession, and one of the reasons Chelsea have had so much success in the past two decades; the other two reasons being lots of money to spend on the best players, courtesy of the billionaire owner Roman Abramovich, and the appointment of Mr Mourinho (at least according to Mr Mourinho). Nick's abiding motto was 'feed the players quality food', so under his tutelage, the lucky Chelsea players enjoyed the very best meats, fish, poultry, fish, fruits and vegetables that money could buy.

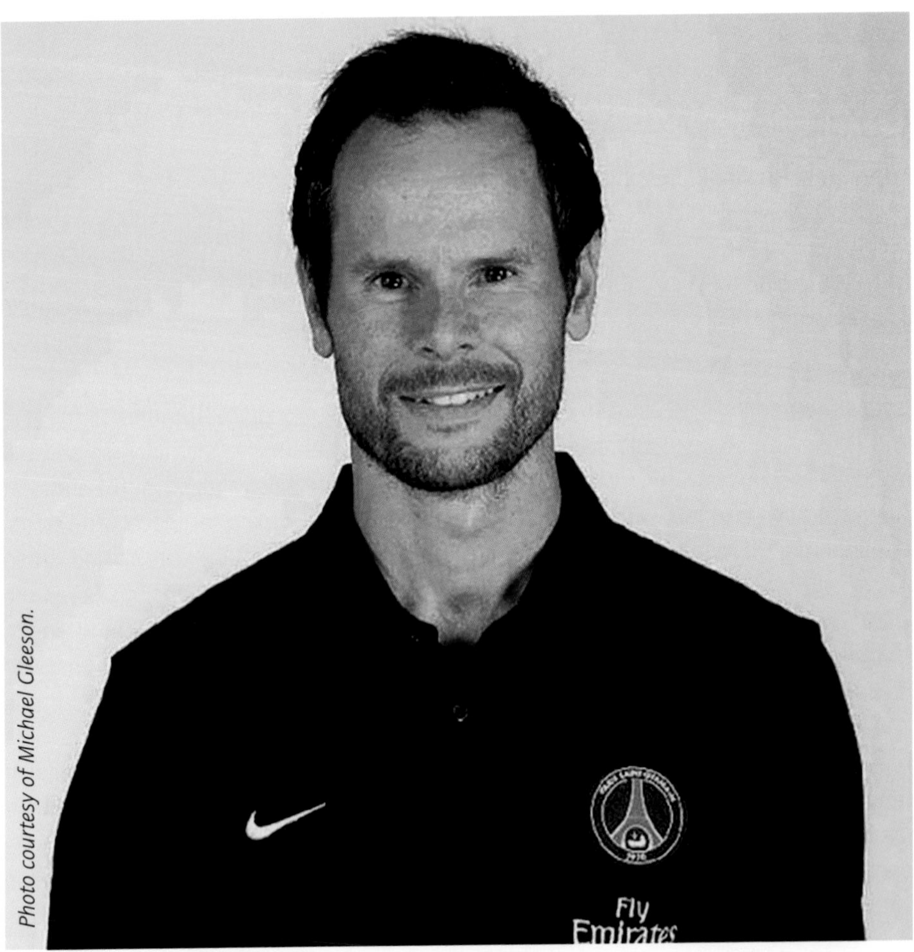

Photo 8.1 The late Nick Broad (1974–2013) who was a brilliant applied sport nutritionist who worked with players at Blackburn Rovers, Birmingham City, Chelsea and Paris Saint-Germain.

Nick and I were once at a scientists-only conference together, and at the end of the day, the organisers arranged a type of 'pub quiz' (with a little alcoholic lubrication, I must admit) along the lines of BBC's 'Mastermind' with people asked to arrange themselves into teams of four for a quiz about their specialist subject (obviously sport nutrition in this case) and general knowledge. Nick happened to be in my team, and when asked for suggestions for the name of the four-person (all-male) team we had, he immediately came up with 'Quality Meat'. His early demise was a great loss to the whole sport nutrition community. RIP Nick!

ASSESSMENT OF BODY COMPOSITION

Assessment of body composition plays an important role in nutritional evaluation, particularly in a sport obsessed with body image. Along with body mass, an estimation of body-fat percentage has traditionally been the requisite regular test demanded by football managers. The evaluation of skeletal muscle mass and body-fat mass can contribute important information to the assessment of nutritional status, and reflects the physical attributes of the player. However, it is not easy to measure and is usually estimated from anthropometric prediction models – validated against the 'gold standard' method of magnetic resonance imaging (MRI) – using measurements of skinfold thickness at three or more sites on the body (e.g. upper arm, beneath the shoulder blade and just above the hip) and limb circumferences (e.g. upper arm, mid-thigh and calf). In addition, a number of other techniques are also being utilised in the modern game, although these require expensive equipment and technical expertise, which would normally be out of the reach of lower-league and amateur clubs.

Dual-energy X-ray absorptiometry (DEXA) is one such technique that is excellent for the body composition assessment of footballers. DEXA can accurately identify fat and lean tissue, and can be used both for whole-body measurements of body composition and for providing estimates of the composition of specific sub-regions (e.g. trunk or legs). The DEXA instruments differentiate body weight into the components of lean soft tissue, fat soft tissue and bone (known as the three-compartment model) based on the differential attenuation by tissues of two levels of X-rays. DEXA can also be used to measure bone density. The X-ray radiation used in DEXA is a low dose, but even so, it should not be used more than just a few times each year. Many clubs will pay for the use of hospital or university facilities to get DEXA or MRI measurements made on their players, especially those who are recovering from long-term injury lay-offs, or when the players return for the start of pre-season training. Players can no longer hide that extra fat that may have accumulated during periods of off-season overindulgence!

Other methods that are used in football to assess body-fat percentage include underwater weighing and air displacement plethysmography (commonly known as BOD POD). These methods both provide a measure of body density that is related to percentage body fat. For clubs that do not have the necessary facilities or equipment and cannot afford MRI or DEXA, anthropometry (i.e. the manual measurement of skinfolds and limb and waist circumferences) provides an acceptable, cost-effective, practical assessment of body composition, when conducted by someone with appropriate technical training (e.g. a sport science graduate). Specialist calipers with a millimetre scale are used to assess skinfold thicknesses, but it requires some technical expertise to do this in a reliable and reproducible way.

The simplest way to measure body fat for most people who do not have access to a science lab or technical expertise, is to use an electronic scale that incorporates a bioelectrical impedance device. Bioelectrical impedance analysis (BIA) is based on the principle that different tissues and substances have different impedance (resistance) to an electrical current. For example, impedance or conductivity is quite different for fat tissue and water. Adipose tissue – of which only about 10% is water – has high resistance, or impedance, whereas muscle – of which up to 77% is water – has low resistance. A BIA device sends a small, safe electrical current through the body to measure impedance and so can be used to estimate percentage body fat (although it is not as accurate or reliable as the other

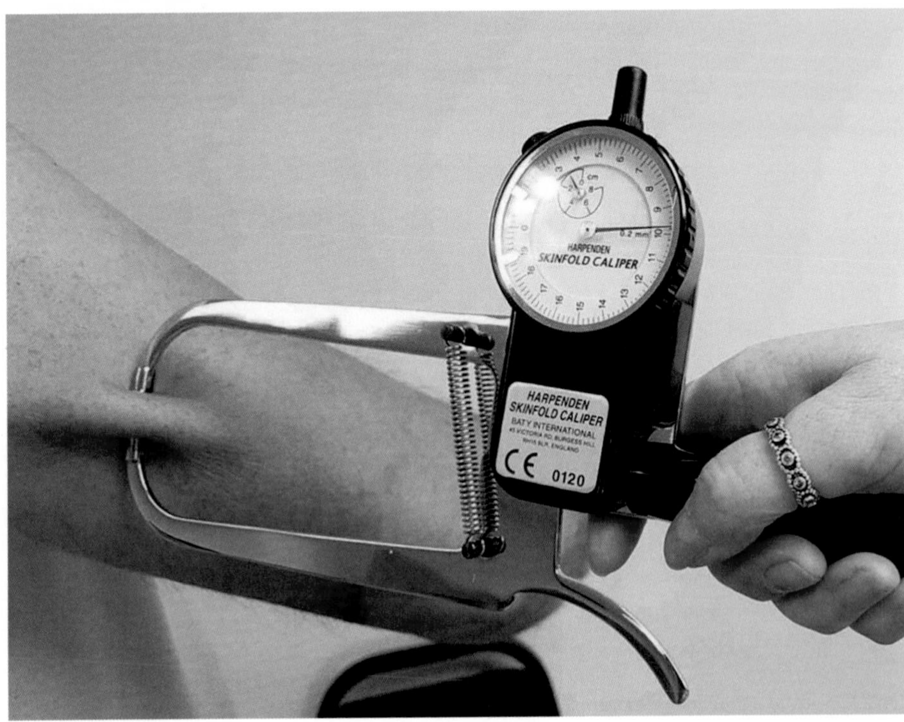

Photo 8.2 Measurement of skinfold thickness using skinfold calipers.

methods I have already described). For consistency, it is best to make BIA measurements in the morning before breakfast and after having gone to the toilet.

HOW FAT ARE PROFESSIONAL FOOTBALLERS?

In football, carrying excess weight in the form of body fat can be detrimental to performance in activities that require movement of the whole body. This is because the energy and oxygen cost of movement is related to body weight, so the heavier the player, the more energy and oxygen needed to cover a given distance. You never see any overweight cyclists competing in the Tour de France, where the male riders are very lean and generally only have about 4–6% body fat. Similarly, elite male and female marathon runners only have 5–11% and 10–15% body fat, respectively. In football, the male outfield players are quite lean, with a body-fat percentage of about 7–15%; for elite female players the usual range is 13–20%. These levels of body fat are all somewhat lower than that of the average person (see table 8.1).

Body fat consists of essential body fat and storage fat. Essential body fat is present in all membranes, nerve tissues, bone marrow and the vital organs, and we cannot lose this fat without compromising physiological function and health. Storage fat (located mostly in white adipose tissue), on the other hand, is our main form of energy reserve; in most people, the fat energy reserves are at least 30 times the amount that is stored

Table 8.1 Body-fat percentages for men and women aged 18–40 and their classification and the typical values for elite footballers

Men	Women	Classification
3–5%	10–13%	Essential body fat
5–10%	8–15%	Athletic
7–15%	13–20%	Footballers
11–14%	16–23%	Good
15–20%	24–30%	Acceptable
21–24%	31–36%	Overweight
Over 24%	Over 36%	Obese

Note that these are rough estimates. The 'athletic' values are those found in elite sportspersons such as distance runners, cyclists and tennis players for whom low body fat is an advantage.

as carbohydrate (mostly in the form of glycogen in the liver and muscles). Fat is stored in the body mainly as triglyceride inside cells called adipocytes, which make up white adipose tissue. Body fat stores accumulate when more dietary energy than we need is consumed, and decrease when more energy is expended than consumed. Essential body fat is approximately 3–5% of body mass for men and 10–13% of body mass for women. It is thought that the reason why women have more essential body fat than men is because of childbearing and hormonal functions. Women store more fat under the skin and on their hips, buttocks and thighs than men who tend to deposit excess fat in the torso and particularly in the belly region.

IS THERE AN IDEAL BODY COMPOSITION FOR A FOOTBALL PLAYER?

The optimum physique, in terms of lean muscle mass and fat mass levels, varies according to an individual player's physiology, their overall build, their playing position and their style of play. Therefore, there is no single ideal value for body weight, muscle mass or percentage body fat against which targets or judgements can, or should, be made. Mean percentage body-fat levels in elite male players measured by DEXA, typically range from 7–15%, although lower and higher values have also been recorded. Goalkeepers are typically taller and heavier with body fat a few percentage points higher than outfield players. Elite senior male players have, on average, higher muscle mass than players in Under-21 and Under-18 teams, although differences in body-fat percentage are usually small. Over the course of a season, on average, body fat levels tend to fall, and lean muscle mass increases slightly.

CHANGING A PLAYER'S BODY COMPOSITION

Nutrition can have a profound impact on a player's body composition, which in turn, may impact their performance. There are different time points throughout the season where players may need to manipulate their dietary intake to maintain or modify their current body fat and lean muscle mass. This may be needed during pre-season or rehabilitation from injury where nutrient intake may need to be modified to match the altered energy expenditure and training or recovery goals. This relationship is very important to the player's health and performance, as it is often not reflected in body mass measurements alone.

The sports nutritionist and other members of the performance support team need to work closely together to plan out how the interaction between diet and training will change body composition. For some players, an increase in muscle mass may be desired in order to improve strength and power. This may be instigated by the manager if he thinks the player gets knocked off the ball too easily, is weak in the tackle, could jump higher or is just not quick enough. During long injury lay-offs, especially when the player may be immobilised to allow healing of a bone fracture, knee ligament injury, ankle sprain or muscle tear, the preservation of lean muscle mass is crucial. For other players, the aim may be to lose some excess weight, as having too much body fat will negatively affect a player's power-to-weight ratio, acceleration capacity and endurance. Again, this may be because of the manager's own perception of the player as being too fat, overweight, slow, lazy or just can't last a full 90 minutes. However, players may also choose to manipulate their body composition to achieve a desired physique – usually a leaner and/or more muscular appearance – but this could potentially conflict with the player's performance goals. Therefore, each individual player's body composition goals should be agreed between the player and the performance team.

Another potential risk in a sport with a big emphasis (or perceived emphasis for the players) on body image is the development of eating disorders (e.g. anorexia nervosa and bulimia nervosa) that manifest due to a compulsive desire to lose weight and look thin. This may be achieved by just eating less (not easy when players are under constant scrutiny) but, more frequently, involves purging by vomiting in secret or using laxatives so that less of the food (and the calories it contains) is absorbed. This can lead to the condition known as relative energy deficiency in sport (RED-S). This is generally far more common in female players in an attempt to conform to various self-imposed expectations or demands from others, and was previously known as the 'female athlete triad' and later introduced as RED-S to make it applicable for both male and female athletes with or without disordered eating or eating disorders. Although football is not considered one of the high-risk sports for RED-S, suspicions should be raised for female players who have menstrual dysfunction and a tendency for stress fractures. Among male players, RED-S can manifest as a loss of aggression and libido (extremely unusual in my experience) as a result of low levels of testosterone, which can also increase the risk of bone injuries.

How a player goes about losing some excess weight (with appropriate advice, supervision and monitoring) can also have an impact on their health. For the general public, losing weight means having to change your diet, eating fewer calories and also trying to fit more exercise into your daily routine. Footballers are very active individuals much of the time so increasing training volume is not usually an option (except in pre-season) due to the risk of burnout, and so any weight-loss goals must usually be achieved by decreasing daily food intake. Although weight loss may be desirable for performance and/or health reasons, if it is done incorrectly (e.g. eating insufficient protein or cutting out major macronutrients or food groups from the diet), it can often be accompanied by a reduction in muscle mass, and it may reduce liver and muscle glycogen stores (the body's main carbohydrate fuel reserves) as well, which will make doing any moderate- to high-intensity exercise feel harder and result in an earlier onset of fatigue. Furthermore, trying to lose too much weight too quickly can also result in chronic fatigue, irritability, depressed mood and an increased risk of injuries and illness. Too much emphasis on losing weight can also lead to the development of micronutrient deficiencies and, as previously mentioned, the development of eating disorders, which are harmful to health as well as performance. So great care should be taken in managing the player at any level – from senior pro to academy junior – who is seeking to lose some excess weight.

ACHIEVING WEIGHT LOSS IN PLAYERS WITHOUT NEGATIVELY IMPACTING THEIR PERFORMANCE

Weight loss requires a negative energy balance, which means that an individual's daily dietary energy intake must be lower than their daily energy expenditure. The size of the average daily energy deficit over a period of time (i.e. days, weeks or months) will be the major determinant of how much weight is lost. A commonly quoted estimate is that 1 lb (0.46 kg) of fat should be expected to be lost for a 3,500-kcal energy deficit. This is an average value, and it will not be the same for everyone as it depends on genetics, the magnitude of any adaptive reduction in metabolic rate, the amount of weight loss, the duration of dieting and the individual's initial body fat mass. Larger than average cumulative energy deficits are required per pound of weight loss for people with greater amounts of initial body fat, according to weight-loss studies in lean, moderately overweight and obese subjects. In other words, weight loss by dieting is harder the fatter you are at the start. Professional footballers are very unlikely to be more than a few kilograms overweight and this amount of excess weight can easily be lost within a few weeks without having to resort to drastic dieting. Daily energy expenditure on training days has been estimated, on average, to be about 3,000 kcal for professional male players. To be in energy balance, players would have to consume 3,000 kcal per day in food and beverages. Therefore, a footballer could achieve a daily 1,000 kcal energy deficit by reducing their energy intake to 2,000 kcal and that should result in a loss of 2 lb (0.9 kg) of body fat per week.

Readers will no doubt be aware that there are many diets out there. It makes no sense for footballers who want to lose weight to go on diets with extreme macronutrient composition (e.g. very low-carbohydrate diets, known as keto diets or virtually fat-free diets). All successful weight-loss diets have one thing in common: they aim to reduce daily calorie intake because, despite what you may have heard from other sources, that is the only way that diets can produce effective, sustained weight loss. But many diets are criticised by experts for being too restrictive, not providing enough of some essential nutrients, not being easy to adhere to and being unhealthy. Among the diets that are not the best choice for your health, I would include many of the 'fad' diets and other diets that require complete elimination of specific food groups or macronutrients. Although these types of diet can be effective for weight loss if you stick with them for 6 weeks or more, they are not best ones for your overall health. If safe, healthy and effective weight loss is of interest to you then try reading my book *The Pick 'n Mix Weight Loss Diet* (published by Meyer & Meyer Sport, 2020).

As discussed in previous chapters, carbohydrate is an important fuel for both training and match play, so it would be silly for a footballer to go on a very low-carbohydrate diet. Some diets encourage the elimination of all fat-containing foods because fat is the macronutrient with the highest energy content per gram (9 kcal/g compared with only 4 kcal/g for protein and carbohydrate). While reducing the fat content of your diet can be an effective means of achieving weight loss, cutting fat out altogether will likely lead to becoming deficient in the essential fatty acids linoleic and alpha-linolenic acid, which are needed for the formation of healthy cell membranes, proper development and functioning of the brain and nervous system, hormone production, regulation of blood pressure, liver function, the immune response, inflammation and blood clotting. They also support healthy skin and hair. The fat-soluble vitamins A, D, E and K will also be in very short supply on a virtually fat-free diet and that produces other health concerns. For these reasons, the fat content of the diet should not be reduced below 20 g/day or 10% of daily energy intake.

Players wanting to lose weight should not reduce their normal protein intake (i.e. about 1.6 g/kg BM/day) as protein is needed to maintain lean body mass and for muscle adaptation and repair. Protein is also more satiating than carbohydrate and fat, so hunger pangs are less on a high-protein diet. Furthermore, excess protein intake does not get converted to body fat as readily as excesses of dietary carbohydrate or fat.

As a normal daily energy intake to maintain energy balance for a footballer is about 3,000 kcal (see chapter 5 for further details), a diet containing 30% fat has 900 kcal in the form of fat; reducing this to just 20% fat (600 kcal) results in a saving of 300 kcal. More extreme reductions in dietary fat are not recommended for the reasons previously explained. A moderate reduction in dietary fat is best achieved by eliminating foods with high-fat content from the diet. That means cutting out fatty meats, sauces, cheese, creams, pizza, cakes and cookies and substituting some foods or beverages with lower fat alternatives (e.g. skimmed milk, low-fat yoghurt and reduced fat coleslaw). To achieve a 1,000 kcal energy deficit per day, another 700 kcal has to be removed from the daily energy intake and this can be achieved by reducing the carbohydrate intake from about 375 g (that's 5g/kg BM for a 75 kg player) to around 200 g per day. This moderate reduction in daily carbohydrate intake can be achieved by swapping the consumption of some starchy foods, such as potato, pasta, rice and bread, for non-tropical fruits and

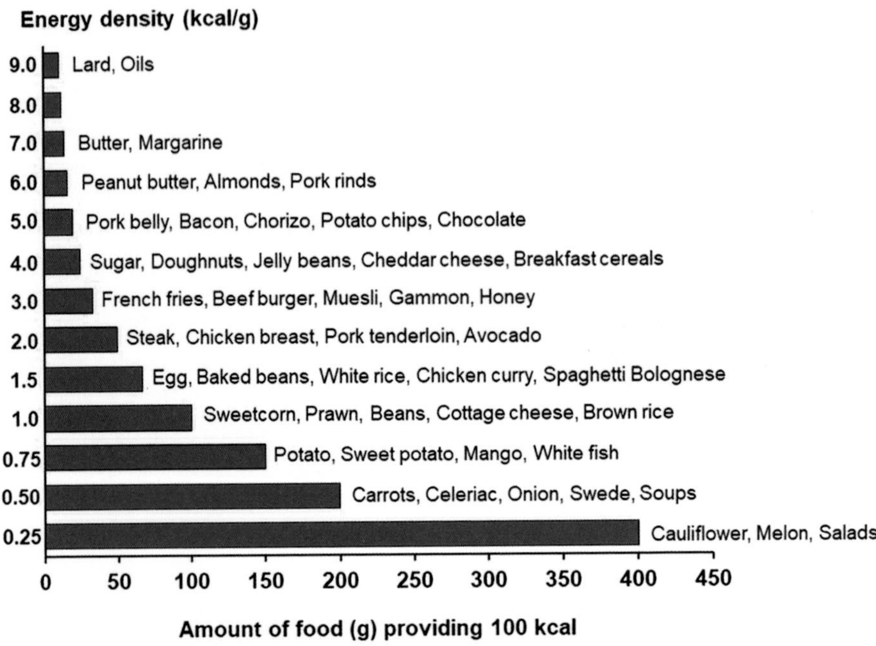

Figure 8.1 Energy density (kcal/g) of some common foods and the amount of food (in grams) that provides 100 kcal.

non-starchy vegetables, such as asparagus, broccoli, cauliflower, green beans, spinach, or salad leaves with tomatoes, onion, celery etc. Gourds (a fleshy, typically large fruit with a hard skin) including aubergine (eggplant), squash, marrow, melon, and courgette (zucchini) are a particularly good choice as all have a low energy density (less than 0.5 kcal/g). The energy density of some common foods is illustrated in figure 8.1. Using the principles of energy density, it is possible to achieve a lower calorie intake, which will help towards weight loss, whilst allowing generous, voluminous portions of food that provide an overall balanced healthy diet that is high in protein, fibre, micronutrients and phytonutrients with minimal impact on appetite.

BUILDING MUSCLE MASS IN PLAYERS THROUGH CHANGES TO DIET AND TRAINING

Many footballers may decide that they want to increase their muscle strength and power at some point in their careers, and this can only be achieved by increasing the muscle mass of the limbs involved in the activity. For outfield players, this would mean targeting the thighs and calves; for the goalkeeper or a long throw-in specialist, it might mean the

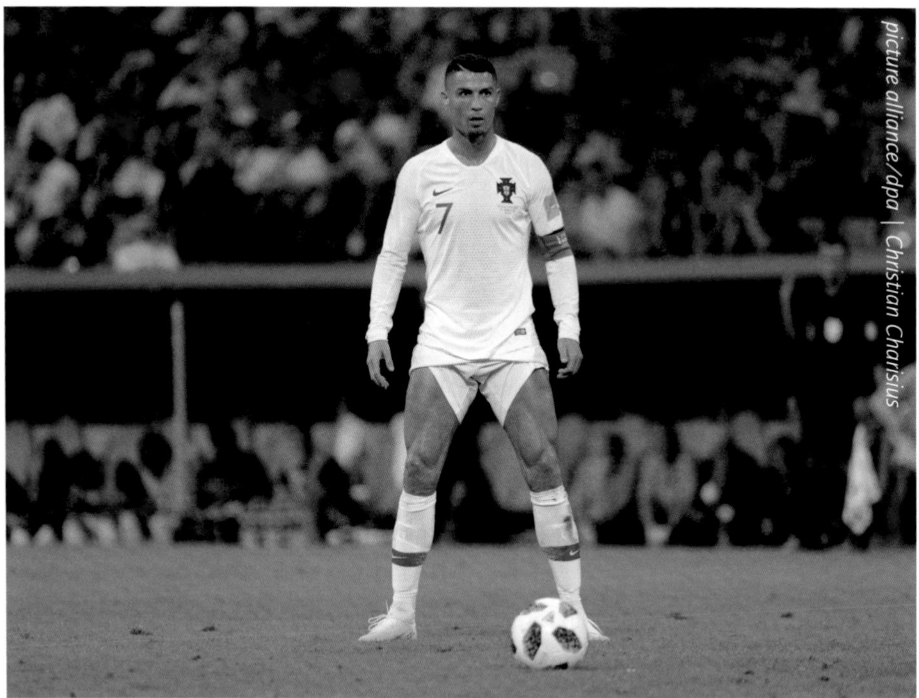

Photo 8.3 Cristiano Ronaldo, one of the best players in the world for the past decade, always seems to like showing off his lean, muscular legs and torso.

upper arm or forearm muscles to improve ball throwing. Often, it will be the manager or coach who perceives that a player may benefit from having some more muscle so young players, and those with a naturally slimmer build, are often the targets; especially those players who are perceived to get 'knocked off the ball too easily' or are 'weak in the tackle'. Body core strength and stability are also important for resisting physical challenges on the pitch, so improving abdominal strength (e.g. by doing repeated sit-ups) may also be targeted. I have yet to meet a player who does not like to show off their 'abs' if they have developed a nice 'six-pack'!

The first point to remember, if the aim is to build up your muscles in particular body areas, is that peripheral adaptations to resistance training are site-specific so the muscles that you want to get bigger and stronger are the ones that need to be trained. To achieve significant increases in muscle mass, the individual needs to engage in regular training bouts of high-load resistance training. Generally, lifting heavier loads over longer durations stimulates greater improvements in muscular hypertrophy and the greatest effects are seen when sets are done to the point of contraction failure or fatigue. However, it is important to incorporate a variety of training intensities into the muscle-building programme. The one-repetition maximum (1RM) is the maximum weight that can be lifted (or the maximum amount of force that can be generated) in one maximal contraction. If the aim is to do five repetitions of a weight before contraction failure (which is called a 'set') it is likely that the weight being lifted will be about 85% of 1RM and this is the best for pure strength gains; about 3 minutes rest should be allowed between successive sets. For 10RM, it will be 70–80% of 1RM, which is best for hypertrophy (with 1–2 minutes rest between sets). For an effective resistance training session for footballers, it is recommended to use 12–20 repetitions per set at 40–60% of 1RM with a 1-minute rest between sets. About five or six sets may be completed in a single training session lasting about 15 minutes, with just a few additional heavy load training sets at 1–5RM under careful supervision to limit the risk of injury. This is the sort of training that Cristiano Ronaldo has done to achieve his impressively fit-looking physique. Even so, it is important to realise that building muscle is a relatively slow process. With appropriate lower-limb resistance training and good nutrition, a realistic goal is to expect muscle mass gains of 0.5–1.0 kg per month. As with other forms of exercise, it is recommended that a low- to moderate-intensity exercise warm-up of the muscles is performed before the resistance bout. If it is planned to perform any high-intensity endurance training sessions on the same day, it is best that these take place in the morning, and at least a few hours of recovery is allowed before a resistance-training session in order to limit interferences and excessive muscle fatigue. The latter always increases the risk of injury.

Muscle hypertrophy is mostly achieved through the generation of more myofibrils (the contractile elements in the muscle fibres), which are composed of protein. Positive muscle protein balance (i.e. net tissue protein gain) is only achieved when the rate of new muscle protein synthesis exceeds the rate of existing muscle protein breakdown. Therefore, muscle mass increases can only be achieved through doing appropriate resistance training and also having an adequate protein intake. Research in sport nutrition conducted in the past two decades has shown that the timing, amount and composition of protein ingested can be manipulated to optimise resistance training adaptation. These factors and some of the other factors that may influence the muscle anabolic response to resistance training are illustrated in figure 8.2. For timing and amount, it appears optimal to ingest protein in the immediate post-workout period in amounts of about 0.4 g/kg BM (typically 25–30 g). This is a sufficient dose to promote a marked rise in muscle protein synthesis, but bigger doses of protein will not produce much bigger increases than this. The protein of choice is one that is readily digestible and with a high leucine content because this essential amino acid is a direct stimulator of protein synthesis. Whey protein is considered ideal, but skimmed milk and eggs (particularly the white part) are suitable substitutes. For vegetarian or vegan players, soy protein isolate is the best option.

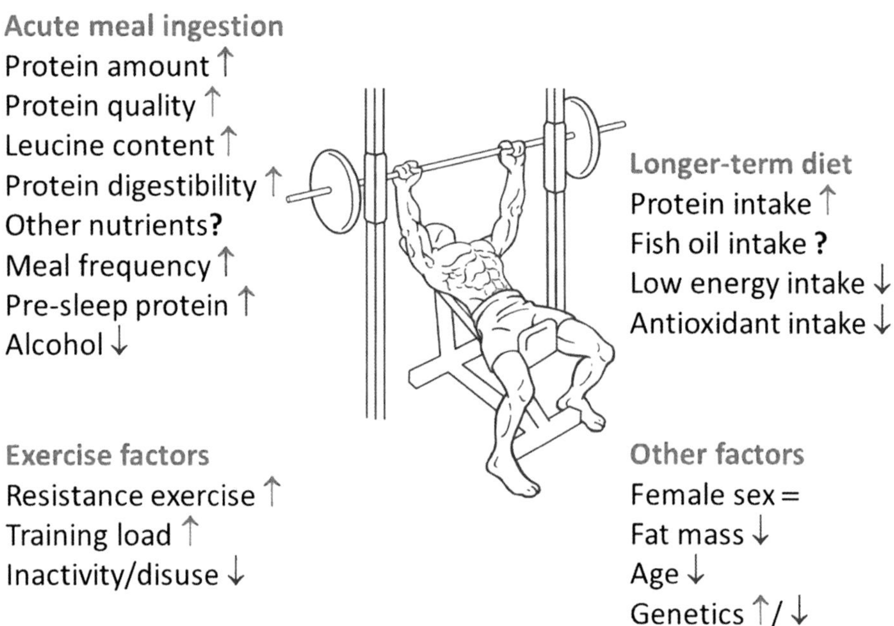

Figure 8.2 Factors that can influence the muscle protein synthesis and net tissue protein gain response to resistance training.

If undertaking the resistance exercise session in the morning, the player should eat up to three other meals distributed throughout the day (each containing protein at a dose of 0.4 g/kg BM) with the aim of achieving a total dietary protein intake of about 1.6–2.0 g/kg BM/day. Tables 5.4 and 5.5 in chapter 5 list some suitable food choices that can be combined to achieve the desired amounts of protein and leucine. Eating fewer meals with more protein is not as good as eating this optimal dose. Eating much more than 1.6–2.0 g/kg BM/day is unnecessary as it will not produce greater daily gains in muscle mass. If undertaking a resistance exercise session in the late afternoon or evening, it is advisable to ingest some protein immediately before bedtime to maximise the anabolic response during overnight sleep. Ingesting a 0.4–0.5 g/kg BM dose of protein before bedtime appears to amplify both acute overnight muscle protein synthesis and training adaptations. Adequate energy is also needed to support these processes so players should aim to maintain daily energy balance. Other protein consumed during the day should be mostly lean high-quality protein containing all the essential amino acids in approximately equal proportions. This will predominantly be protein from animal sources including beef, ham, lamb, poultry and fish, but can be supplemented with soy, beans, cheese, nuts and bread. If high leucine sources of protein are unavailable, then adding a 3 g leucine supplement to the post-exercise meal can be considered. The addition of any other individual amino acid is ineffective in promoting the resistance exercise-induced anabolic response. Creatine supplements (3–5 g/day) can also be considered as there is evidence that creatine can also augment muscle hypertrophy with appropriate resistance training and dietary protein intake.

Alcohol should be avoided as it has been shown to impair muscle protein synthesis. Finally, it is known that lack of sleep can contribute to a negative protein balance by reducing mechanisms that promote muscle protein synthesis and stimulating those causing muscle protein breakdown. Therefore, it is important to ensure that the player gets adequate sleep (a minimum of 7 hours) at nighttime.

BODY COMPOSITION NUTRITION

Body fat

- There is no single body mass or % body fat value that fits all players
- Minimum healthy essential body fat values are 3-5% in men & 10-12% in women
- Typical body fat in professional players is 7-15% in men & 13-20% in women
- For weight loss purposes players should maintain their protein intake at ~1.6 g/kg BM/day & reduce both their carbohydrate & fat intakes by ~30-40%

Measurements

- Dual X-ray absorptiometry (DXA) provides the most accurate measure of body composition for football players
- Anthropometry (e.g. skinfold thicknesses) provides a reliable, practical & accessible alternative when conducted by someone with appropriate training in the technique
- Body mass & bioelectrical impedance measurements are useful for weekly monitoring of players

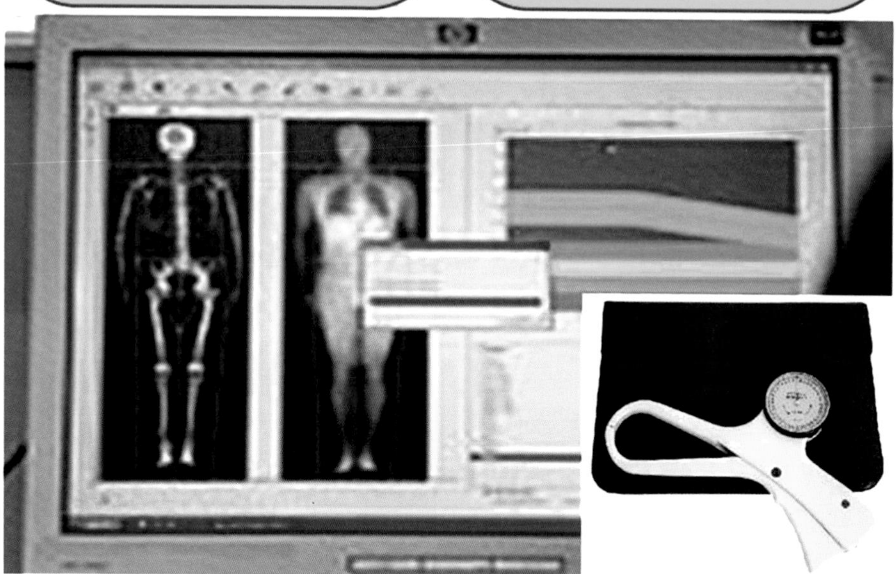

Infographic 8 Body composition and nutrition in football.

CHAPTER 9

Injury and Rehabilitation Nutrition

- Injury Rates in Professional Football
- Can Nutrition Help to Speed Up Healing From Injuries?
- Nutritional Strategies to Reduce Muscle Loss and Assist Rehabilitation From Injury

Injuries are an unavoidable aspect of regular participation in football where frequent physical contact, tackles, jumps, falls, high-speed running, twisting, turning and collisions (both accidental and deliberate fouls) are a frequent occurrence in both training and/or competitive matches. Injury risk is increased as players become fatigued and training or competition load are increased and the time for recovery between matches is reduced. When a player becomes injured, it can require several weeks or months to heal, recover and return to match fitness. Nutrition can play a crucial role in speeding up the process of rehabilitation and this is the main focus of this chapter.

INJURY RATES IN PROFESSIONAL FOOTBALL

The total number of injuries that resulted in players being unavailable for selection for matches was 764 during the 2018–19 English Premier League season (an average of 38 injuries per club) which resulted in total costs of over £220 million and well over 1,000 player-days lost for the majority of clubs. The clubs most affected by injuries throughout the season were West Ham (2,003 days out), Arsenal (1,771 days out) and Tottenham (1,652 days out); these three clubs also topped the list for average unavailability of players each match day. In 2018–19, knee injuries were the most common cause of lay-offs (114), they caused the longest absences (58 days per injury), and were the costliest in terms of wages paid to players who could not play. That followed two seasons in which hamstring injuries had been the most common. Other common injuries affected the ankles, groin, hip/thigh, foot, shin/calf and back. On average, over the course of a season, players lose 8 days per injury. The annually recorded data show that footballers are nearly seven times more likely to be injured during a competitive game than in training or match practice.

Many injuries result in prolonged periods of limb immobilisation to reduce further potential damage and allow repair of bone, skeletal muscle and connective tissue. Immobilisation results in muscle disuse and loss of muscle mass due to increased periods of negative muscle protein balance resulting from decreased basal muscle protein synthesis (which is usually stimulated by exercise) and the development of anabolic resistance to dietary protein ingestion (i.e. it becomes harder to get the desired amount of muscle hypertrophy with the usual dietary protein intake). Muscle loss is most profound in the first few weeks of limb immobilisation. The extent of muscle loss during injury strongly influences the level and duration of rehabilitation required to get back to match-ready fitness.

CAN NUTRITION HELP TO SPEED UP HEALING FROM INJURIES?

When an injury occurs, support teams are faced with the challenge of bringing a player back as quickly and safely as possible. Nutrition may aid in optimising the healing and rehabilitation process, and facilitating the desired rapid return to availability for team selection.

Most injuries rapidly trigger inflammatory processes that initiate wound healing and tissue repair. Care should be taken to ensure sufficient energy and protein intake and avoid deficiencies in calcium, vitamins C and D, copper, manganese and zinc, all of which may impair the initial healing process. Alcohol intake should be avoided for the same reason.

Inflammation initially promotes blood flow to the injured area and an influx of white blood cells into the tissue to remove damaged tissue, fight potential infection and initiate the healing process. However, excessive or prolonged local tissue inflammation in response to an injury can contribute to the subsequent deconditioning of the muscle and/or tendon. Several 'nutraceuticals' including some phenolic compounds, curcuminoids and omega-3 fatty acids have been proposed as potential strategies to limit the acute inflammatory process, but direct evidence of their anti-inflammatory effects in humans is lacking. Furthermore, reducing post-injury inflammation has not been shown to influence tissue deconditioning, and could actually be counterproductive to the healing process. Therefore, current evidence does not support the use of any nutritional strategies that might limit acute (i.e. short term) injury-induced inflammation.

NUTRITIONAL STRATEGIES TO REDUCE MUSCLE LOSS AND ASSIST REHABILITATION FROM INJURY

After the initial wound healing response comes rehabilitation, which requires a period (anywhere from days to months) of whole body bed-rest (some of which may be spent in hospital) and/or local limb disuse (sometimes involving immobilisation, especially for bone fractures and knee ligament injuries) and/or reduced activity (i.e. a reduction in the training load or complete absence from training). During this time, rapid muscle, tendon and bone deconditioning can be expected due to the absence of the usual mechanical stimulus that maintains these structures. Quite literally, a player has to 'use it or lose it'. The muscles are the most susceptible to disuse, with atrophy and deconditioning (e.g. reduced force-generating and oxidative capacities) evident after only a few days. Tendon metabolic and functional properties begin to decline after about two weeks, and progressive bone demineralisation and weakening begins in the first few weeks of unloading and reduced physical activity.

Nutritional strategies can, to some degree, limit the muscle loss and decline in functional capacity that occurs in the injured player. During rehabilitation and recovery, nutritional needs are very much like those for any healthy athlete desiring muscle hypertrophy to increase strength and power. Daily protein intakes of 1.6–2.5 g/kg BM are recommended to support maintenance of muscle mass during disuse. This should be achieved by the regular (4–6 times per day) consumption of meals containing 25–30 g of rapidly digested protein with high leucine content (2–3 g) and spread evenly across the day (every 3–4 hours). Given that the injured player has greatly reduced physical activity levels, maintaining muscle mass whilst simultaneously avoiding gains in fat mass can become challenging, so selecting protein sources with relatively low-fat content (e.g. grilled lean beef steak, oven-baked fish, seafood, beans) and avoiding other fatty foods as well as reducing carbohydrate intake to just meet resting needs is important.

Although the energy requirements of the injured player will be less than those who are healthy and in full training, they are not quite as low as in a healthy but sedentary person. You may recall from chapter 3 that the daily resting energy expenditure of a person can be estimated based on their sex, age, body weight and height, and is approximately 2,000 kcal/day for men and 1,900 kcal/day for women. You might think that this is what the injured and effectively immobilised player needs to maintain energy balance, but the tissue/wound recovery processes have additional energy costs and it is important that this is taken into account to ensure that the player stays as close to energy balance as possible, because this, as well as high-protein and adequate micronutrient intake, is crucial for rapid and effective healing and recovery from injury. Avoiding drastic reductions in energy intake is supported by a recent case study, which reported an average daily energy expenditure of 3,100 kcal – which is only about 10–15% less than the energy expenditure of outfield players in full intensive training – during the first 6 weeks of rehabilitation from an anterior cruciate ligament injury in an elite English Premier League player. Bearing in mind that the majority of absences from training or competition due to injuries will be less than one month, it is prudent to follow the aforementioned guidelines while the player is away from normal training, and move back towards nutritional recommendations to support optimal training performance (as described in chapter 5) as the player approaches the increased likelihood of return to play.

INJURY & REHAB NUTRITION

Short-term

- During the acute post-injury phase care should be taken to maintain energy balance, protein intake and avoid micronutrient deficiencies to facilitate wound healing & repair
- Although immobilisation or bed-rest will mean absence from training, energy requirements are higher than for a healthy sedentary individual due to the needs of activated immune cells & tissue repair

Longer-term

- Maintaining energy balance & protein intake (1.6-2.2 g/kg BM/day) are the nutritional priorities to limit tissue deconditioning associated with reduced physical activity during recovery from injury
- Distributing 20-30 g of leucine-rich (2-3 g) protein-containing meals throughout the day may further minimise loss of muscle mass & tissue deconditioning

I'll eat anything you want me to if it will get me back playing again tomorrow

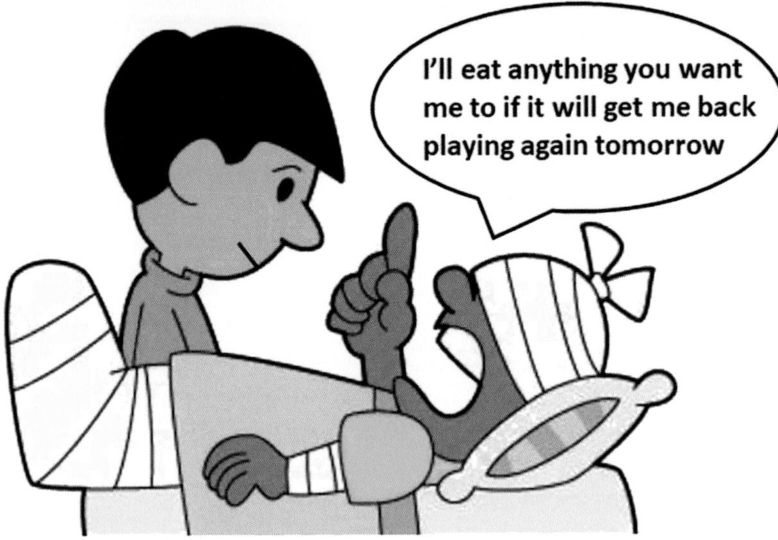

Infographic 9 Injury and rehabilitation nutrition.

CHAPTER 10

Special Considerations

- Nutrition for Elite Female Players
- Nutrition for Youth Players
- Nutrition for Match Officials
- Diabetic Footballers
- Nutrition During the Off-Season
- Nutrition During the Pre-Season
- Nutrition for the Retired Player
- Nutrition for Managers, Coaches and Support Staff

The main focus of the book, so far, has been on the elite male player during the competitive season for whom the nutritional recommendations are fairly well established. But there is also a need to consider the different nutritional needs during the off-season and pre-season training, and of others participating in the beautiful game including the elite female footballer, the academy youth player and the on-pitch match officials. A few elite players may be Type 1 diabetics, which has an influence on their nutritional needs, particularly in relation to the amount and timing of their carbohydrate intake. Most players retire from the professional game (barring career-ending injuries) in their 30s and will need to adjust their nutrition accordingly to a less-active lifestyle to avoid becoming overweight, which is a major risk factor for metabolic and cardiovascular diseases. These other populations and scenarios are discussed in this chapter. As we always should, let's put the ladies first.

NUTRITION FOR ELITE FEMALE PLAYERS

Now first of all, I must say that when I was a young lad, the girls did not play football. They played lots of other sports such as athletics, gymnastics, netball, tennis and hockey. Come to think of it, in my youth, not many boys played hockey and no men that I know of ever play netball. I have heard some people say that the reason women don't play football is that 11 of them would never wear the same outfit in public at the same time (strictly that should be 10 because the goalkeeper wears a different kit to the outfield players). Joking apart, female professional football is here to stay, and the standards of both skill and fitness have progressively improved over the years. How long, I wonder, before we could see an elite female player become part of a team in professional (currently exclusive) male football? The rules may change in the future to allow the best players – no matter if they are male or female – to participate in mixed-sex competitive matches. After all, some sports (e.g. tennis, badminton) have mixed-sex (i.e. doubles) matches at the elite level, so why not football? Certainly, at junior level there are many female players who are better technically and physically than the boys. Just a thought, but maybe one day we will be cheering a Christine Ronaldo from the stands of a Premier League stadium, as much as the Manchester United fans cheered her male name-sake, Cristiano! Enough speculation for now; let's get back to the science...

Elite female players are generally smaller and lighter than their male counterparts. The physical characteristics of female players competing in the national team or highest national league have been reported to range between 19 and 26 years of age, 1.61–1.70 m in stature, with a body mass of 56.6–65.1 kg and a body fat percentage of 14.5–22.0%.The range of values for age, stature and body mass among 552 players from 24 countries participating in the 2019 FIFA World Cup is a little wider than this: for age the range was 16–41 years, for stature 1.48–1.87 m, and for body mass 46–88 kg indicating a wide range of body shapes and sizes among top-level female football players, just as there is for males. Therefore, attempting to set specific anthropometric and body composition targets for female players is currently unjustified.

Observations of match play for outfield international-level female players indicate that they generally cover approximately the same average total distance as their elite male counterparts, but they cover less distance running at high speeds. The average female player also has a lower body mass than the male player so their overall energy and carbohydrate requirements are proportionally less, although not very different when comparisons are made on the basis of per kilogram body mass.

Estimations of daily exercise energy expenditure (i.e. the total amount of energy expended during a day when physically active rather than resting) have been reported for female players and indicate that on rest days it amounts to less than 50 kcal, whereas on intensive training days it amounts to about 800 kcal and up to 900 kcal on match days. Since the average daily resting expenditure of the average player weighing 60 kg is about 1500 kcal, this suggests that daily energy requirements on intensive training and match days are about 2,300–2,400 kcal. Several surveys of what elite female players are actually eating reveal that undereating (and therefore underfuelling) is considerably more prevalent than in their male counterparts. In 2021, Jordan Nobbs, the Arsenal and England women's striker said, 'One of the most important things I have learnt is to eat more. And I think now 70% of my focus is more towards nutrition than actually the way I train.'

Recommendations for daily protein intake are the same as they are for males (i.e. around 1.6 g/kg BM) and fat should provide 20–35% of total dietary energy intake. Recommendations for match-day food intake before and after matches, and for ergogenic supplements (if desired), can also be considered to be virtually identical to those for males on a per kilogram body mass basis. During training and matches, sweat rates in male players have been reported to range from 0.5 to 2.5 L/hour, depending on individual differences and environment conditions or clothing worn. Lower sweat rates are generally reported in female players because of lower body mass, fewer and smaller sweat glands in the skin and lower absolute work rates. Just as for the male players, fluid intake should still be individually prescribed to limit losses to no more than 2% of body mass.

DIFFERENCES IN MICRONUTRIENT NEEDS

Because of blood loss during menstrual bleeding, women require about twice as much iron as men (table 10.1). The recommended daily intake for iron in the UK is 14.8 mg/day for females and 8.7 mg/day for males. Due to regular monthly blood loss (and possibly due to a lower consumption of meat), post-pubertal female footballers are at a higher risk of iron deficiency than their male counterparts. Iron is an essential component of haemoglobin and myoglobin, which are involved in oxygen transport, and iron is also an essential constituent of several enzymes and cytochromes involved in aerobic metabolism. Therefore, iron deficiency, even in the absence of anaemia (i.e. below normal blood haemoglobin concentration), can result in lethargy and reduced performance. Iron deficiency can be identified through blood screening, and iron status should be monitored at least twice per year in female players (and probably more frequently when

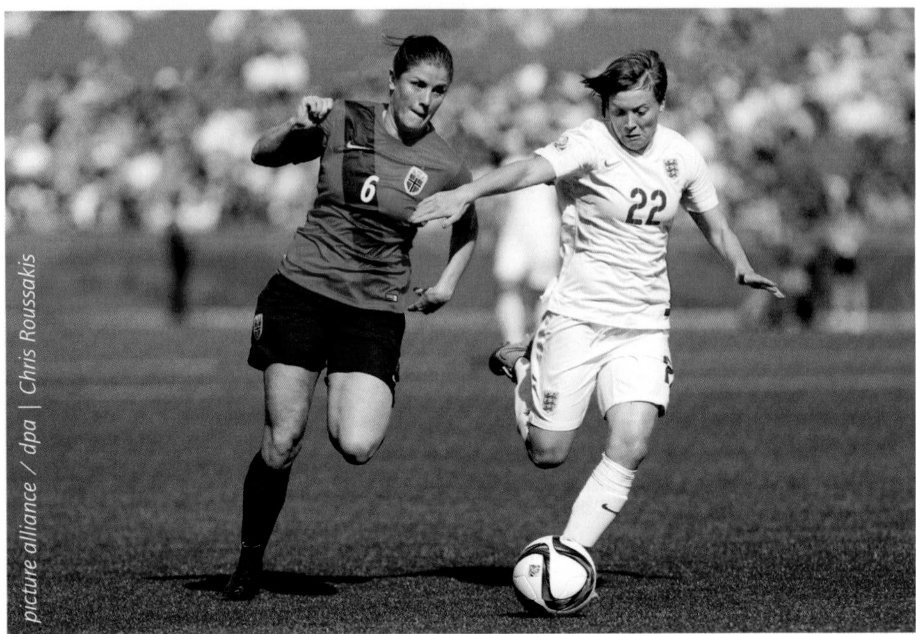

Photo 10.1 In match play, elite female players generally cover approximately the same average total distance as their male counterparts, but they cover less distance running at high speeds. Female players have lower overall energy and carbohydrate requirements than men, although differences are fairly small when expressed per kilogram body mass.

Table 10.1 Recommended daily intakes for iron and calcium in males and females in the UK

	Age (years)	RDA for Iron (mg)	RDA for Calcium (mg)
Males	19–50	8.7	700
	15–18	11.3	1,000
	11–14	11.3	1,000
Females	19–50	14.8	700
	15–18	14.8	800
	11–14	14.8	800

From Dietary Reference Values for Food Energy and Nutrients in the United Kingdom: Report of the Panel on Dietary Reference Values of the Committee on Medical Aspects of Food Policy. *London: Her Majesty's Stationery Office, 1991.*

iron deficiency has been detected in recent monitoring). The cut-off values for establishing anaemia are blood haemoglobin levels below 115 g/L for females or less than 125 g/L for males, whereas iron deficiency for both sexes is defined as serum ferritin below 35 μg/L and normal (i.e. not yet affected) blood haemoglobin concentrations.

Other micronutrients of particular concern for female players are calcium and vitamin D. Deficiencies of these two essential micronutrients can be harmful to both the health and performance of the player. and lack of sufficient vitamin D and/or calcium can make bone fractures more likely. This is particularly important for females who are in negative energy balance because in this situation, menstrual cycles can be less frequent or absent altogether – a condition called amenorrhoea. This results in reduced levels of the female sex steroid hormone oestrogen, which is important for bone development and growth. Female players with a relative dietary energy deficiency have higher incidence of stress fractures, and it is important that players get adequate amounts of calcium (table 10.1) and vitamin D. The RDA for vitamin D in the UK is 10 μg or 400 IU per day for both males and females of all ages. As for the male players, if a deficiency is observed (it can be detected using a blood test) or anticipated (e.g. in the winter months) then a supplement of 2,000 IU/day of vitamin D3 is recommended.

POTENTIAL CONCERNS ABOUT INADEQUATE ENERGY INTAKE IN FEMALE FOOTBALLERS

In many sports, including football, both male and female athletes may try to lower their body-fat content in an attempt to improve power-to-weight ratios. For female athletes, this often means they are challenging the boundaries of their biological predisposition and when a substantial negative energy balance is sustained for more than a few months, or body fat is reduced to levels below 10–12%, various body functions may be impaired, and menstruation may disappear, as discussed. If this situation is kept up for a long time, it will result in a number of other health complications and the clinical syndrome known as the female athlete triad since renamed as relative energy deficiency in sport (RED-S) because the condition can be applicable in both male and female athletes, and games players with or without disordered eating or eating disorders. In females, the classic characteristics of the syndrome are low energy availability with or without disordered eating, the absence of menstruation (and hence temporary infertility) and low bone density. The broader syndrome of RED-S refers to impaired physiological functioning caused by relative energy deficiency (i.e. regularly consuming considerably fewer calories than the daily energy requirement) and includes, but is not limited to, impairments of metabolic rate, menstrual function, bone health, immunity, protein synthesis and cardiovascular health.

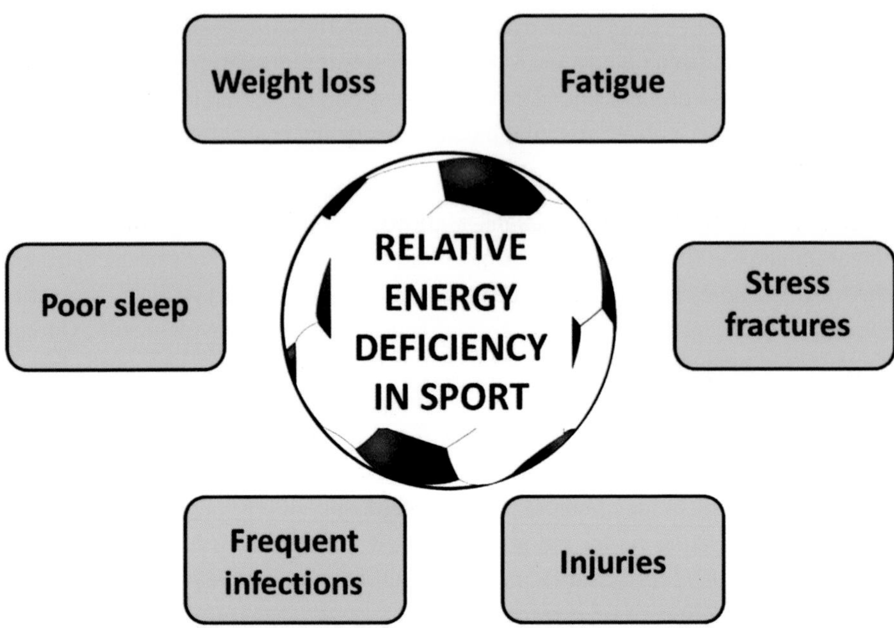

Figure 10.1 Common signs of Relative Energy Deficiency in Sports (RED-S) include weight loss, fatigue, stress fractures, injuries, increased infections and reduced sleep quality.

In common with the female athlete triad, the underlying cause of the symptoms of RED-S remains low energy availability. However, whilst the triad exclusively describes the impact of low energy availability on menstrual dysfunction and bone pathology, RED-S identifies a number of other body systems that are negatively impacted. For this reason, RED-S is considered to be a more appropriate term that describes the potential health and performance consequences affecting both female and male athletes. Other common signs of RED-S (figure 10.1) include weight loss, fatigue, stress fractures, injuries, increased infections and reduced sleep quality. The eating habits of an individual suffering from RED-S can appear to be normal when in the public gaze but may be followed by self-induced vomiting and/or use of laxatives in secret.

Eating a diet lacking in total calories and/or specific micronutrients is more prevalent in female athletes and games players than their male counterparts. Ultimately, this will result in compromised recovery, adaptation and diminished sporting performance. A player's dietary strategy should aim to match nutrient intake to the energy demands of daily living, training and competition, with consideration for their body composition goals. An excessive energy deficit can result in many health-related issues, with menstrual dysfunction and poor bone health a major concern to female players that can have not only implications for their sporting career but also later in life when reduced bone density accelerates following the menopause and further increases the risk of fractures. Whilst disordered eating, low bone-mineral density, menstrual dysfunction and body image issues are known to be more prevalent among female players, adequate knowledge of these factors among coaches and players is generally lacking.

The contribution of low energy availability to bone health and injury rates is one of the key reasons for concern when ensuring that players avoid sustained energy intake/expenditure mismatches, and it has been identified as a problem in males as well as females. For example, one recent study of male and female endurance runners found a five-fold increase in bone injury rates with RED-S in 37% of females (with amenorrhoea) and 40% of males (with low serum testosterone). Factors that may contribute to low the development of RED-S include not only changes in body mass and composition resulting from disordered eating but also increases in training volume/intensity without associated changes to fuelling (i.e. energy and carbohydrate intake).

The management of body composition in football requires knowledge and skills in how to approach a player with unrealistic aims, expectations or methods regarding lower body-fat content, how to present and discuss the results of body composition assessments, and when to raise the alarm and engage other support staff to prevent RED-S or eating disorders developing. It is also recommended that team protocols are standardised to ensure that body weight and composition monitoring of all players is undertaken regularly; that body composition data are integrated with other test parameters (e.g. fitness, strength, sprint speed etc.); and that team support staff are aware of the health risks associated with RED-S and disordered eating.

Female players consuming a very low energy diet will be eating insufficient amounts of some, or all, of the macronutrients (i.e. carbohydrate, fat and protein) and are also at risk of developing essential micronutrient deficiencies. Female players attempting to lower body weight through a reduced dietary energy intake need to maintain their habitual protein intake, otherwise they are likely to lose some lean muscle mass as well as fat mass. Where a player is identified as having an eating disorder, treatment will likely require the intervention of a psychologist and other sports medicine professionals trained in the treatment of the condition. As with most nutrition-related conditions that are potentially harmful to health, prevention (through sound education in the principles of healthy eating) is preferable to finding a cure. The team support staff including coaches, nutritionist, psychologist etc., can play a key role in supporting, educating and referring players to appropriate resources to help them achieve their performance, body composition and nutrition goals. Education received from a trusted source can ensure the player doesn't go searching the internet for themselves and perhaps stumbles upon unreliable, inaccurate and potentially harmful information.

Athletes from many sports – and football is no exception – may feel they are under pressure to maintain or improve their body shape, composition or weight and, therefore, how that information about nutrition, and its impact on body composition and performance, is conveyed is critical. Individuals can often be very sensitive about such topics and so they must be discussed in an appropriate manner with support, education and compassion. The members of the support team need to be consistent in the messages they provide to the players on these topics – and this applies to both female and male players – to ensure the engagement and trust of the players.

NUTRITION FOR YOUTH PLAYERS

Nutritional support, as with adult footballers, is key to ensuring that elite junior players (i.e. professional, under-18 years of age) can cope with training and match-play demands. An additional goal is to educate young players about the importance of good nutrition, not only for football performance but also for growth, health, recovery, training adaptations and body composition in the expectation that they will commit to a lifelong buy-in to good nutritional choices. Young players' bodies are growing and maturing, which has an important impact on their nutritional requirements. Body metabolism is also a little different in young players compared with adults, as the youngsters tend to be more reliant on fat oxidation as a source of energy for exercise. The RDAs of some essential micronutrients (e.g. calcium and phosphorus for both males and females, and iron for males) are higher for junior players than adults (see table 2.6) because of the extra needs for growth, although it should be recognised that some 15–18-year-old players can be physically, if not always emotionally, mature. As with adult players, emphasising a 'food first' philosophy and healthy food choices are essential when educating junior players. Some may be living away from their parents for the first time in their life, many may be incapable of cooking for themselves and might not have a good understanding of the importance of good nutrition for performance and health. The academy sport nutritionist has an important role to play in their education and to provide solutions to these issues.

In an academy at a professional football club, a typical week for players from the age of 12 upwards is likely to include four training days, one match day and two rest days. On a typical training day, players will take part in on-pitch sessions, video analysis sessions, tactical talks and various sport science activities such as gym work, yoga and occasional strength and fitness testing. In a typical week, the total weekly training and match volume (i.e. duration and total distance covered) is about 330 minutes and 20 km for players under the age of 14, rising to 410 minutes and 26 km in the 15–18 age group. Weekly high-speed running distance also increases progressively from 220 metres in the

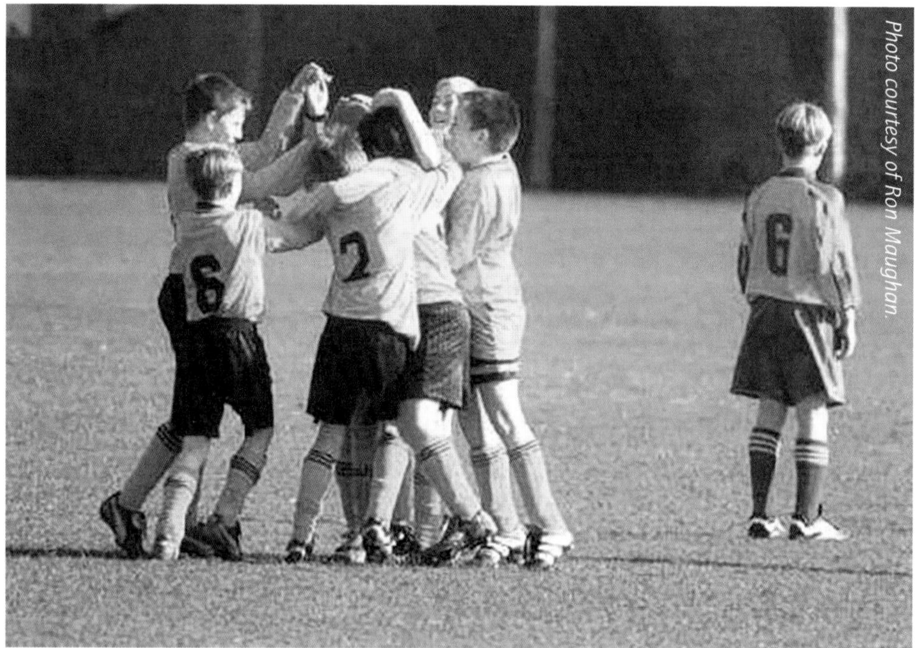

Photo 10.2 Junior players have different nutritional requirements to adult players as they are in a phase of rapid growth and development. Meeting energy requirements on training days can be a challenge for junior players as academy training sessions usually take place in the evening after a full day at school.

under-12s to 1,000 metres in the under-18s. These data are from an English Premier League club academy. It is important to realise that these activities come on top of (and usually following) a full day of school education, which may include some physical education (PE) and recreational sport activities. For junior players, this can commonly amount to a 12-hour working day. These demanding schedules are clearly a challenge for both the academies and their players – particularly when it comes to feeding them.

Given that a key role of sports science staff within an academy is to promote the health, growth, maturation and physical development of the players, as well as their on-pitch performance, it is vital to understand the energy requirements of these players. If a young player fails to meet their energy requirements with an appropriate energy intake on a regular basis, it can have a catastrophic effect on both their health and performance. While the sport of football is not one of the sports that overemphasises leanness, some studies that have monitored self-reporting of food intakes in young players have indicated that boys and girls may frequently not meet their extra dietary energy needs, which could have a negative impact on their growth, bone development and general health, as well as being detrimental to participation in football training and match play. Some professional clubs have observed higher than expected rates of bone fractures in junior players, which could be associated with inadequate intakes of energy and/or protein, calcium and vitamin D. Energy deficits are generally greater on match days and heavy training days, which may affect both their performance and recovery. Individuals up to the age of 18 are likely to be in full-time education (e.g. school or college), which means that football training with a club takes place in the evenings on weekdays. Some young players may have to travel to the club academy training ground straight after school, meaning that they have had limited time to eat and drink before training begins. Some professional clubs have addressed these issues by providing convenient sports foods such as a high-energy milk shake (providing up to 1,000 kcal) with added carbohydrate and whey protein for consumption on arrival at the training ground.

Some recent studies have measured changes in body composition and resting metabolic rate (RMR) in a cohort of male English Premier League academy soccer players from age groups ranging from the under-13s to the under-23s. Increases in body size, body mass, lean (fat free) body mass and RMR were recorded between ages 12–16, highlighting the need to increase daily energy intake to support healthy growth and maturation. Fat mass appears to change very little from the under-13s to the under-23s, with increases in body mass driven mostly by increases in lean mass (i.e. muscles, bones and organs), which approximately doubles from about 30 kg to over 60 kg during these years of growth and maturation. The RMR increased from 1,655 kcal/day in the under-13s to 2,042 kcal/day in the under-16s and 1,941 kcal/day in the under-23s (figure 10.2). Clearly, the largest differences in lean body mass and RMR typically occur between the under-13s to the under-16s, suggesting this is a key period for growth, maturation and physical development during which energy requirements are progressively increasing. These are average values and, in this study, there were large inter-individual differences between players within each age group, highlighting the need for an individualised approach to the nutritional management of junior players.

The total daily energy expenditure of players has also been observed to increase progressively as they progress through the academy pathway (figure 10.2), likely a result of players growing, increasing their muscle mass and engaging in increased physical loading. For example, average daily energy intakes of under-13, -15 and -18 male players (measured using the gold standard doubly labelled water method) were found to be 2,859, 3,029 and 3,586 kcal/day. For some players (evident in all age groups), total energy expenditure was actually greater than that previously observed in adult Premier League players (approximately 3,600 kcal/day).

As already mentioned for female players, RED-S may affect some players and this can also be an issue for both junior female and male players, with deleterious effects on hormonal and immunological functions, as well as on bone development and the risk

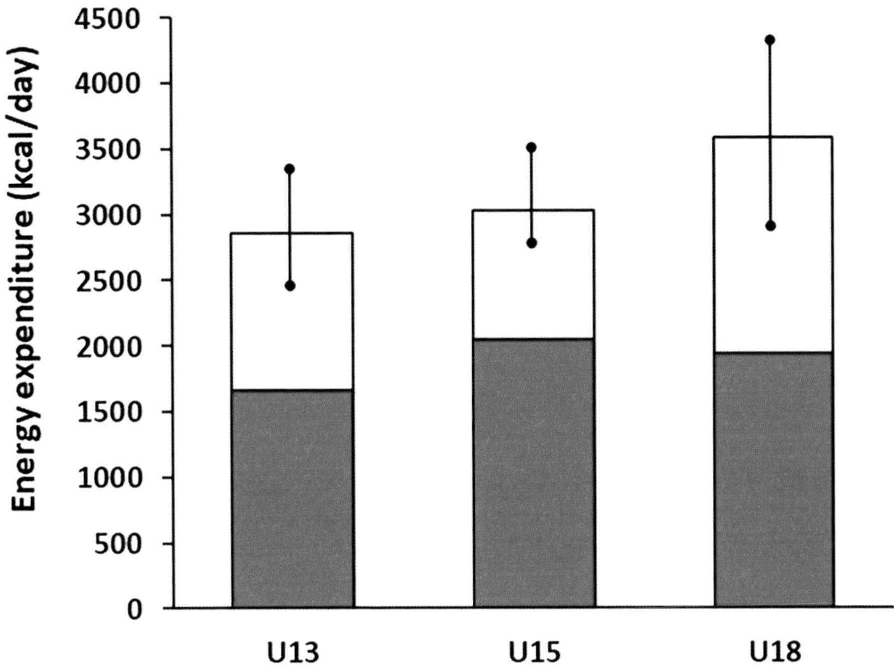

Figure 10.2 Average total daily energy expenditure and RMR (red columns) in academy players according to age group. The bars indicate the upper and lower values for total daily energy expenditure among the eight players that were measured in each age group highlighting the wide range among individual players. Data from Hannon et al. (2021).

of developing eating disorders. Therefore, it is important that young players should be evaluated when joining a football academy and monitored periodically thereafter using appropriate charts to examine changes in height-for-weight, weight-for-age, BMI-for-age and body composition. The academy nutritionist has an important role to play in both the monitoring and nutrition support, and education of young players whose bodies are constantly changing. Recent important research on the physical loads and nutritional needs of academy players has highlighted the need for appropriate nutrition support at all stages of the academy pathway, and not just towards the professional development phase.

MACRONUTRIENT REQUIREMENTS FOR JUNIOR PLAYERS

Daily carbohydrate recommendations for junior footballers are similar to those of senior players when expressed as g/kg BM, and the amounts will depend on the daily training load, with carbohydrate ingestion spread strategically over the day to enable good training performance and adequate recovery afterwards. For very low-to-moderate daily training, about 3–6 g/kg BM/day will be appropriate, and for high training loads, 6–8 g/kg BM/day is recommended.

Just as for the senior players, the aim is to provide sufficient carbohydrate to optimise glycogen stores and deliver glucose as energy for repeated high-intensity sprints and performance. During prolonged training sessions and 90-minute matches, some carbohydrate intake during rest intervals (for training) or half-time (for matches) may be favourable, as feeding carbohydrate (30–60 g/hour) during intensive physical activity can spare the body's own carbohydrate reserves (i.e. liver and muscle glycogen) and could help delay fatigue and improve performance.

Protein needs increase during adolescence due to the extra protein needed for growth and, in particular, for increases in lean body (muscle) mass. Intensive football training also increases the protein requirements to allow muscle repair and adaptation to the training stimulus, so a daily intake of up to 1.6 g/kg BM for junior players – essentially the same weight-specific amount as for senior players – is appropriate. This level of protein intake can be easily achieved by consuming appropriate amounts of high-protein foods (e.g. meat, poultry, fish, dairy produce, beans and pulses) without the need for supplements. The best strategy for optimising the distribution of protein intake over the day is to aim for 0.3–0.4 g/kg BM with each meal, although most reports of actual protein intake in junior players indicate that the highest amount of protein intake is usually in the evening dinner, with a moderate intake for lunch and a relatively low intake for breakfast. Recommendations to junior players should emphasise a balanced distribution of protein in meals over the course of the day to optimise muscle, tendon and bone development. Any junior players who are temporarily on reduced calorie diets to lose weight, or players who are choosing to consume vegetarian or vegan diets, should be regularly evaluated using 7-day weighed food intakes or food frequency questionnaires to determine if they are achieving a sufficient protein intake.

As for senior players, the daily energy intake from fat should be 20–35% of total energy intake, and daily cholesterol intake should not exceed 300 mg. These recommendations are essentially the same as for non-athletic adolescents and adults.

MICRONUTRIENT REQUIREMENTS AND SUPPLEMENTS FOR JUNIOR PLAYERS

Due to concerns about becoming overweight, some junior players may intentionally limit their intake of dietary fats to only 10–20% of total energy intake, but this should be discouraged as it could result in the development of micronutrient deficiencies including iron, calcium and vitamins A, D, E and K.

An adequate intake of calcium is critical for bone mineral growth and health, and it is important to understand that an adolescent player's daily calcium intake should be 500–800 mg higher than the 700 mg RDA for adults. Cow's milk (no matter if it is whole, semi-skimmed or skimmed) is an excellent source of calcium as it contains about 300 mg per 250 mL serving. An inadequate vitamin D intake is known to increase the risk of stress fractures among adolescents, especially those involved in daily high-impact activities. The RDA for vitamin D for adolescents is the same as for adults, at 400 IU (or 10 μg) per day in the UK and 600 IU (or 15 μg) per day in the US, but this may be difficult for young players to achieve through dietary sources alone, meaning that an inadequate vitamin D status may develop, particularly during the winter months when the sunlight strength becomes insufficient to allow the production of vitamin D in the skin. For these reasons, the assessment of bone health (by densitometry) and vitamin D status (by blood sample analysis) may be useful, particularly for individuals who have had previous bone injuries or are of a relatively slight build, since collisions and intense efforts are frequent in football. A daily vitamin D3 supplement of 1,000 IU (25 μg) in the winter months is considered appropriate to maintain vitamin D status at peak end-of-summer levels for junior players.

Iron requirements are higher during adolescence in boys (11.3 mg/day) compared with younger boys and senior male players (8.7 mg/day). In girls, after the start of menstruation, the requirements are even higher to replace monthly blood loss: from the age of 11 the iron requirement for females is 14.8 mg/day (in the US it increases further to 18 mg/day after the age of 18) until the menopause. A deficiency of iron in the body may impair high-intensity and endurance performance due to the important role of iron in oxygen transport and aerobic metabolism. Iron is also important for a robust immune function. To achieve adequate daily intakes according to age and sex, junior players should be encouraged to ingest non-haem iron-containing foods with vitamin C and avoid drinking tea and coffee at meal times, as these beverages contain compounds that can inhibit iron absorption. The iron status of junior football players should be measured several times during the season by the medical/science support team (or by paying for hospital laboratory testing). Measurement of the players' serum ferritin and blood haemoglobin concentrations can give a reliable indication of iron status and establish the presence of iron deficiency, anaemia or both. Iron supplementation should only be given if a deficiency is confirmed.

Other supplements for junior players are generally discouraged. Although the youngsters may want to copy what the senior pros are taking (e.g. creatine, caffeine, β-alanine, nitrate, probiotics, etc.), it is more important, at this early stage in their potential football careers, that they focus on eating a healthy, well-balanced and diverse diet. Sports drinks, carbohydrate gels and possibly beetroot juice (a good natural source of dietary nitrate) can be considered as possible exceptions to this general rule. This should be a decision for the club academy nutritionist and medical staff, based on an evaluation of the specific needs of individual players, the team and local policies. It is an ongoing concern that many adolescents consume supplements, often because they are simply following mass media trends (e.g. for high-energy caffeinated drinks) and misinformation provided by manufacturers or suppliers, often from internet sources. Sometimes, it can be the parents or coaches who may have erroneous beliefs and wrongly supply their offspring or charges with unnecessary supplements, which in many cases may do more harm than good.

Just as for adult athletes, mild dehydration (i.e. more than 2% body mass loss) is known to impair high-intensity exercise performance in trained athletic boys. Although sweat rates when exercising in the heat are generally lower in young athletes compared with seniors, there is still a significant risk of dehydration, which impairs the ability to limit rises in body temperature and increases the risk of exertional heat illness. This can be a challenge in junior football tournaments where successive games may be played with limited time for recovery. The monitoring of body mass and urine osmolality can help to estimate hydration status and it is important to ensure that junior players are well hydrated before beginning training sessions and competitive matches, especially in warm weather.

NUTRITION FOR MATCH OFFICIALS

The on-pitch match officials are, of course, the referee and the two individuals who run the sidelines. The physiological and energy demands of football refereeing have some similarities to playing the game, in that the physical activity is intermittent and relatively high intensity. At the highest levels of the game, football referees maintain about 80–90% of their maximum heart rate and 70–80% of their aerobic capacity (maximal oxygen uptake) during competitive matches, while expending up to 1,200 kcal. These values are fairly similar to those of the players (see chapter 4 for details) although, on average, players expend about 400 kcal more during a 90-minute match. Referees are generally older and have higher percentage body fat than players, and unlike the players, referees are not involved in body contact (unless by accident), but they must keep up with the game whatever the imposed tempo, which limits their chance to recover after demanding phases of the match. The amount of high-intensity activity that referees perform is similar to that reported in midfielder players, but referees cover a shorter total sprint distance, with generally fewer, but longer, individual sprints during a match. Referees are often criticised by managers (usually the losing ones) after a game for what they perceive as mistakes in crucial decisions; referees also have to maintain full concentration throughout the 90 minutes. One major concern is that the physical and physiological demands can impact cognitive performance in decision making. Good nutrition choices before the match and during the half-time interval can help them cope with these demands.

Guidelines for nutrition for on-pitch match officials, on match days, before kick-off and during the half-time interval, should essentially be the same as those for players, with an emphasis on consuming appropriate amounts of carbohydrate and fluids. In general, match officials do not need dietary ergogenic aids, although caffeine in doses up to 3 mg/kg BM could be considered to facilitate maintenance of cognitive function in the later stages of the game. This could be in the form of a strong cup of coffee ingested one hour before kick-off and/or another coffee or caffeinated chewing gum during the half-time interval. As already mentioned, elite football referees have lower energy needs compared with outfield players on match day and so will require fewer calories in their post-match meal. Fluid replacement should be based on sweat losses, as it is for players. During training, total energy and carbohydrate intakes for referees who are not full-time professionals, should be appropriate to the individual training load and increased only around match days, during periods of intense training, or when engaged in other occupations with a high-energy demand. Specific nutrient recommendations are generally similar to those for players: protein intake should be 1.2–1.6 g/kg BM; fat should be 20–35% of total dietary energy intake; and a healthy, well-balanced diverse diet should be consumed to ensure adequate intake of essential micronutrients, fibre and phytonutrients.

DIABETIC FOOTBALLERS

Diabetes mellitus is a metabolic syndrome consisting of two main groups, Type 1 and 2, which are characterised by a complete lack of insulin production (Type 1) or a combination of relative insulin deficiency and insulin resistance (Type 2). About 90% of people with diabetes have Type 2 diabetes. It can develop slowly, usually over the age of 40 and usually in people who are overweight and sedentary, so it can become a health issue for some retired players and current managers as well as older amateur players and football fans. Individuals with diabetes mellitus may take part in football for health promotion, disease management or simply for their enjoyment of recreational or competitive sport. Type 2 diabetes is not a concern for players in the professional game, as most are under 40 years of age, not overweight and have a lower-than-average percentage body fat. Having said that, Type 2 diabetes can develop in some players after retirement and could also affect some older managers and coaches during their careers, particularly those who are over 50 years of age and somewhat overweight. In contrast, Type 1 diabetes mellitus results from a highly specific immune-mediated destruction of the insulin-producing β cells in the pancreas, resulting in chronic elevated blood-glucose concentration (known as hyperglycaemia) due to the absence of insulin production. The condition usually occurs in early childhood and it is a chronic disease that can lead to many serious complications if not properly managed. The diabetic person and physician must work together to optimise glucose control involving both insulin administration and modifications to the diet: primarily reducing total calorie and high-GI food intake.

Exercise has numerous health benefits (further details about this can be found in the next chapter) and both Type 1 and Type 2 diabetics should take advantage of these benefits. Individuals with Type 1 diabetes are capable of undertaking a wide array of exercise activities and there are no contraindications to most sports for diabetic people. Indeed, competition at the highest level is possible. Examples of outstanding sportsmen with Type 1 diabetes include Gary Hall Jr and Sir Steven Redgrave. Hall is an American former competition swimmer who represented the US at the 1996, 2000 and 2004 Olympics and won ten Olympic medals. He is a former world record-holder in two relay events. Redgrave is a retired British rower who won gold medals at five consecutive Olympic Games from 1984 to 2000. He also won three gold medals at the Commonwealth Games and nine World Rowing Championship gold medals. Redgrave is the most successful male rower in Olympic history and the only man to have won gold medals at five Olympic Games in an endurance sport. In professional football, some diabetic players who have had full and successful careers include Gary Mabbut (Tottenham Hotspur 1982-1998), José Ignacio (Nancho) Fernández who won La Liga with Real Madrid and the World Cup with Spain, Borja Mayoral who also played for Real Madrid, and former Glasgow Celtic players Danny McGrain and Scott Allan (currently playing for Hibernian).

For individuals with Type 1 diabetes, injecting too much insulin, skipping meals, eating less than normal or exercising more than usual can lead to low blood glucose (hypoglycaemia). Exercise uses up energy and there is a rapid and large increase in the uptake of glucose by the working muscle that is independent of insulin action. Therefore, exercise can quickly cause the blood-glucose concentration to drop if the diabetic has not eaten correctly beforehand. For these individuals, the main risk with prolonged exercise is that it may cause a fall in the blood-glucose concentration below the normal range. If the fall is too drastic and sustained, it can lead to feeling fatigued, pale skin, and an inability to concentrate or think clearly, followed by fainting, loss of consciousness, seizure and coma; if not corrected it can be fatal. The early symptoms of hypoglycaemia are shakiness, dizziness, sweating, hunger, irritability or moodiness, anxiety or nervousness and headache.

When engaging in high-intensity intermittent exercise such as football match play and training, individuals with Type 1 diabetes may develop hyperglycaemia – a sustained elevation of the blood-glucose concentration above normal. The hormonal response to high-intensity exercise is pretty much the same as in healthy people, as elevated adrenaline promotes glucose release from the liver, which in the presence of low insulin levels, results in mild hyperglycaemia during exercise. However, insulin levels do not rise in diabetics as they would after exercise in healthy individuals, meaning that there is then the potential problem of sustained post-exercise hyperglycaemia.

A problem that is common to both short-term intense exercise and more prolonged endurance exercise, is the development of late-onset post-exercise hypoglycaemia, which can occur 6–15 hours post-exercise. This may be due to the exercise-induced recruitment of GLUT-4 glucose transporters to the cell surface, which facilitate glucose uptake into the muscles for glycogen resynthesis. Although this is an important process for the replenishment of depleted muscle glycogen reserves and the performance of subsequent exercise, in diabetic individuals it causes hypoglycaemia, and can often occur during sleep (particularly if the exercise was performed in the afternoon) when it is much less likely to be recognised or acted upon.

To minimise the risk of hypoglycaemia during prolonged exercise, the usual recommendation is to consume a low-fat, high-carbohydrate (at least 1 g/kg BM and low-GI) meal 1–3 hours before exercise, and to reduce the usual post-meal insulin dose by 30–50%. The individual should check their blood-glucose level about an hour before exercise to make sure it is within the usual target range before participating in prolonged physical activities. If the blood-glucose concentration is too low, a small meal or snack containing 15–20 g carbohydrate should be consumed before starting exercise. Suitable snacks include cereal bars, fresh or dried fruit, fruit juice, pretzels and biscuits; alternatively, 15–20 g of glucose tablets or 250–350 mL of a typical sports drink (containing 6 g CHO/100 mL) can be ingested. If the exercise is going to last for an hour or more, additional carbohydrates should be ingested during the workout. During such exercise, 30–60 g CHO/hour should be ingested; or more than this if the insulin dose was not reduced after the last meal before exercise. Exercise gels, sports drinks, cereal bars and candy bars can provide the body with a rapidly available source of glucose during exercise.

After prolonged exercise, it is important to restore the liver and muscle glycogen stores to reduce the risk of subsequent hypoglycaemia. Carbohydrates should always be available during training sessions and in the recovery period afterwards. The usual nutrition guidelines for post-exercise recovery used by non-diabetic players can be followed, which means, for example following a 1- to 2-hour training session or a 90-minute match, having a low-fat, high-carbohydrate (1–2 g/kg BM and high-GI) meal containing 0.4 g/kg BM protein within the first hour or two after finishing exercise. This can then be followed by appropriate insulin administration for blood-glucose management. The usual bolus insulin dose at this time could be halved to reduce the risk of delayed nighttime hypoglycaemia. Moderate- or high-intensity exercise in individuals with Type 1 diabetes can cause blood glucose to drop for up to 24 hours after exercise. Therefore, the blood-glucose concentration should be checked immediately after exercise and every 2–3 hours afterwards until it is time for bed. If blood glucose is low, then a carbohydrate snack should be ingested. Reducing the evening insulin dose by ~20%, or consuming a bedtime snack without insulin, may also help prevent nocturnal hypoglycaemia after exercise.

Footballers with diabetes need to be advised of their most appropriate diet to maximise performance and reduce fatigue. Energy and macronutrient needs, especially carbohydrate and protein, must be met – just as they are for non-diabetic players – to allow hard training, promote adaptation and maintain health. With proper modifications of insulin dose and diet, plus careful blood-glucose monitoring, players with Type 1 diabetes can train and play competitively safely and regularly. At the elite level, individualised management strategies should be created with close cooperation between the Type 1 diabetic player and their healthcare team (including a physician and dietitian).

NUTRITION DURING THE OFF-SEASON

When the competitive football season ends, players will have usually free time to relax, spend time with their families and go on holiday. However, before they leave their club, most will be given a prescribed programme of physical activity in order to maintain a base level of aerobic fitness and reduce the risk of weight gain. The off-season is also a time when a player can work individually, or with a personal trainer and/or nutritionist, to modify their body composition. For example, they may do more resistance training to increase muscle strength and core stability. Their nutrition in the off-season should be modified accordingly. It is likely that their weekly training load will be somewhat lower than during the competitive season and pre-season, so consequently, they will need to lower their energy and carbohydrate intake but generally maintain a daily protein intake of at least 1.2 g/kg BM and continue to get around 20–35% of their dietary energy from fat, mostly in the form of PUFAs. A healthy, well-balanced and diverse diet should be encouraged, and bad habits such as dining in fast-food restaurants, eating takeaways and drinking alcohol should be positively discouraged. The main, and rather obvious aim, other than to work on their perceived weaknesses, is to be able to return for pre-season training in a fit and healthy condition and not to become overweight by more than a few kilograms.

NUTRITION DURING PRE-SEASON

Traditionally, when players return for pre-season, they will undergo a battery of fitness tests, body weight and composition assessments, and health checks (including blood tests) followed by a programme of 4–5 weeks of intensive training with weekly training loads around 20–30% higher than in the competitive season. Obviously, this increases daily energy and carbohydrate needs, and also offers an opportunity for players to lose any excess weight gained during the off-season. Daily carbohydrate intake typically will be 5–8 g/kg BM and be adjusted to the daily training load, or it may be lower than this for some players who need to lose some weight or lower body-fat content. Protein intake may be increased to 1.6–2.2 g/kg BM/day to optimise training adaptations. Pre-season training is designed to induce physiological adaptations, mainly related to recovering aerobic fitness and endurance back to levels at the end of the previous season. Improvements in muscle strength, sprinting speed, jump height and flexibility may also be sought according to individual needs or the coach/manager's perception of such needs.

Some clubs take their first team squad to a training venue located at altitude (typically 2,000–3,000 m above sea-level) as this induces adaptive increases in blood haemoglobin content and the number of red blood cells in the circulation, which can give a further boost to aerobic capacity. The consumption of iron-rich food sources (e.g. red meats, liver, poultry, seafood, eggs, legumes, broccoli and leafy green vegetables) can be encouraged to help achieve this. It also allows a period of time during which the coaches, players and support staff are working, living, eating and socialising together, away from family, commercial and media distractions. This allows the integration and bonding of both existing squad players and new signings.

After this intensive period of pre-season training, clubs usually arrange a series of friendly matches for players to develop what the managers refer to as 'match fitness'. There seems to be a general consensus among the football community that off-pitch training alone does not sufficiently prepare a player for optimal performance in a match, and that actual match-play time is needed for this. This is true in many sports involving skill, coordination and decision making as these, what could be called 'sport-specific attributes', can only really be attained and practiced by participation in the actual sport, ideally in a competitive (match play in the case of football) situation. Some of the top clubs may participate in international tournaments during pre-season and this may bring other complications such as long-haul travel, jet lag and environmental (e.g. heat) acclimatisation issues, which may interfere with some of the training goals. Sometimes in top-level professional football, the desires of the money men (i.e. owners, financial directors and commercial staff) appear to outrank the desires of the coaching staff and the players themselves.

NUTRITION FOR THE RETIRED PLAYER

With a few exceptions, most players retire in their mid-30s. For some, it can be at an earlier age if they suffer a debilitating injury or an illness such as cancer. The change in lifestyle from being an active footballer to being retired and suddenly having a lot of free time can be profound. Obviously, one of the biggest changes is likely to be the reduction in average weekly energy expenditure in the absence of regular training and match play. If food energy intake is not adjusted accordingly downwards, the retired player can soon become overweight, which increases the risk of developing chronic diseases such as Type 2 diabetes and coronary heart disease in their later years. Retired professional players should be encouraged to keep doing forms of exercise that they enjoy (e.g. amateur football, golf, tennis, swimming, gym work and playing with their children) and to appreciate – and adhere to – the main principles of healthy eating. Failure in this (sometimes accompanied by addiction to alcohol, which is another major contributor to weight gain and ill health) can lead to premature death, as exemplified by the passing of two of the geniuses of the game, namely George Best and Diego Maradona who died at the ages of 59 and 60, respectively. I recall one BBC television interview with George, which was recorded only a few months before he died. When asked how he had managed to fall on hard times after being a star player, he said: 'I spent a lot of money on booze, birds and fast cars. The rest I just squandered.' Previously, he had also been heard to quip: 'I've stopped drinking, but only while I'm asleep' and 'In 1969 I gave up women and alcohol – it was the worst 20 minutes of my life.' If retired players want to live a long and healthy (and nowadays an even more wealthy) life, they need to avoid that kind of mindset!

Here, I provide an extensive list of evidence-based recommendations on how a retired player, or anyone for that matter who is not highly physically active, can eat a healthier diet. I have put this list of recommendations together from information provided by the *Dietary Guidelines for Americans 2015–2020*, the 2016 *Eatwell Guide* from the UK and guidelines published by organisations and institutions in various other countries. In this bulleted list, the recommendation is first stated, and then the reason(s) why this recommendation is given is briefly summarised.

- *Recommendation:* Follow a healthy-eating pattern across the lifespan. *Why?* Healthy-eating patterns (i.e. the combination of foods and drinks that a person eats over time) ensure a diet that is balanced, nutritious and unlikely to be fattening. Such diets are an important contributor to health. Healthy-eating patterns include a variety of nutritious foods such as vegetables, fruits, grains, low-fat, and fat-free dairy, lean meats and other foods high in protein and plant-based oils (e.g. rapeseed oil for frying, extra virgin olive oil for salad dressings), while limiting saturated fats, *trans* fats, added sugars and salt. A healthy-eating pattern can be tailored to meet a person's taste preferences, traditions, culture and budget.

- *Recommendation:* Eat a wide variety of nutrient-rich or nutrient-dense foods. *Why?* By eating a variety of foods from within and between each food group, people will likely ingest adequate amounts of all essential nutrients. The term 'nutrient-dense' indicates the essential nutrients and other beneficial substances in a food have not been 'diluted' by the addition of calories from added solid fats, sugars or refined starches, or by the solid fats that are naturally present in the food. Thus, nutrient-dense foods are those that provide vitamins, minerals and other substances that contribute to adequate nutrient intakes or may have positive health effects, but contain little or no solid fats, added sugars, refined starches and salt. Ideally, these foods should be in forms that retain naturally occurring healthy components, such as vitamins and dietary fibre. All vegetables, fruits, whole-grain products (bread and cereals), fish, seafood, eggs, legumes (beans and peas), unsalted nuts and seeds, fat-free and low-fat dairy products, and lean meats and poultry can be considered to be nutrient-dense foods. These foods contribute to meeting food group recommendations within the desirable calorie and sodium limits. In contrast, many processed foods, sauces, pastries and ready meals are not nutrient-dense because they contain substantial amounts of undesirable high calorie items and often include added sugars and salt.
- *Recommendation:* Eat a diet rich in vegetables, fruits, and whole-grain and high-fibre foods. People should eat at least five portions of fruit and vegetables daily. *Why?* Consuming vegetables, fruits, and whole-grain and high-fibre foods will help to achieve the recommended carbohydrate intake and increase fibre intake, which is good for digestive and cardiovascular health. In addition, these foods contain relatively large amounts of phytonutrients, which have some beneficial health effects. Epidemiological studies have generally shown that diets high in whole-grain products, fruits, legumes and other vegetables, have significant health benefits.
- *Recommendation:* Eat a variety of healthy protein foods. *Why?* Consuming a variety of high-protein food sources including fish, seafood, lean meats and poultry, eggs, legumes, soy products, and nuts and seeds that provide 10–15% of daily calories should ensure that daily protein requirements are met while avoiding excessive fat intake. Eating a diverse range of high-protein foods gives your body other important nutrients, including iron, zinc and other important minerals and vitamins (particularly B-group vitamins). Furthermore, research has shown that consuming about 25 g of protein in each of your three or four main meals per day helps build muscle with resistance training and maintains muscle mass (i.e. delays sarcopenia) in people aged over 50.

- *Recommendation:* Choose a diet moderate in total fat but low in saturated fat, trans fats and cholesterol. *Why?* Apart from the essential fatty acids linoleic and alpha-linolenic acid, there is no specific requirement for fats. Too much saturated and trans-fat intake is linked to cardiovascular disease. But some fat is needed to help with the intake of the fat-soluble vitamins A, D, E and K. Because most foods contain some fats, the intake of these vitamins is usually not a problem. To lower total fat intake, dairy products that are fat free or low in fat (e.g. semi-skimmed milk; low-fat yoghurt) are recommended. The standard recommendation (over the course of one week) is to have an intake of saturated fat below 10% of total energy intake, limit cholesterol intake to 0.3 g or less per day, and keep *trans*-fat intake to a minimum.
- *Recommendation:* Eat fewer commercially prepared processed foods, baked goods and avoid fast foods. *Why?* These foods are generally high in energy and fat and may contain a significant amount of *trans*-fatty acids, which are harmful to cardiovascular health. Consumption of small amounts of oils is encouraged, including those from plants: canola, corn, olive, peanut, rapeseed, safflower, soybean and sunflower. Oils also are naturally present in nuts, seeds, seafood, olives and avocados.
- *Recommendation:* Cut back on beverages and foods high in calories and low in essential nutrients. *Why?* Beverages such as soft drinks, and foods with added sugar, contribute significantly to energy intake but don't add useful nutrients. High levels of added sugar intake are associated with high blood triglyceride concentrations, obesity, insulin resistance and increased incidence of dental cavities. The US National Academy of Sciences has advised that added sugars should make up no more than 25% of the total daily energy intake but that reducing this to 10% may be a healthier alternative. Indeed, the *Dietary Guidelines for Americans 2015–2020* recommends that less than 10% of daily calorie intake should come from added sugars, and in the UK, this has been reduced to no more than 5%.
- *Recommendation:* Use less sodium and salt. *Why?* Salt is simply sodium chloride (NaCl), and consuming too much sodium increases water retention, blood volume and consequently raises blood pressure, which itself is a risk factor for cardiovascular disease including atherosclerosis, coronary heart disease and stroke. However, salt should not be absent from the diet altogether because its constituents – sodium and chloride – are both essential nutrients and their recommended daily intakes are 1.5 g of sodium and 2.3 g of chloride, which equates to 3.8 g of salt per day. Salt is present as an additive in many processed foods including bread, cheese, pizza, soups, sauces, canned vegetables, smoked and cured meats, as well as in salted nuts, potato chips and pretzels. Salt is also found in natural products including meat, poultry, fish and seafood. As an upper limit, healthy adults are generally

advised to ingest no more than 6.0 g of salt (2.3 g sodium) per day, but most people currently consume, on average, about 8.5 g salt per day (3.4 g of sodium), which is equivalent to about one and a half teaspoons of salt. People should choose foods with little salt, prepare food with minimal amounts of salt, and add no more than a pinch of table salt to their food on the plate as a condiment, particularly if most of the food is plant-based as it has lower sodium content than animal produce. Although this can be cut out altogether, you'll find that if you stop adding salt to your food, your taste buds will adapt to it, and soon you won't miss it.

- *Recommendation:* Do not consume more than 500 g of red meat per week. It is also recommended to limit intake of processed meat. *Why?* Evidence derived from numerous large-scale prospective epidemiological studies and their meta-analyses shows that regularly consuming red meat (beef, lamb and pork) and processed meat (including bacon, ham and salami) increases colorectal cancer risk by 20–30%.
- *Recommendation:* Drink alcohol in moderation. *Why?* Alcohol is a nonessential nutrient but contains 7 kcal/g. It can add significant energy to total daily intake without adding nutrients. One 750 mL bottle of red wine, for example, contains 600 kcal. Current evidence suggests that light-to-moderate alcohol intake (one standard drink per day) will cause no real risk for healthy adults and may be of benefit by reducing the risk of cardiovascular disease. For females, alcohol should be avoided during pregnancy. Current guidelines recommend drinking up to one drink per day for women and up to two drinks per day for men. A standard drink is defined as 360 mL (12 fl oz) of regular strength beer (5% alcohol), 150 mL (5 fl oz) of wine (12% alcohol) or 45 mL (1.5 fl oz) of spirits (40% alcohol).
- *Recommendation:* Avoid excessive intake of questionable food additives and nutrition supplements. *Why?* Although most food additives used in processed foods are safe, it is often recommended to avoid these additives. In addition, although nutritional supplements are often claimed to have various positive health effects or performance benefits, some negative effects may occur. Nutrition supplements are not under strict regulation and may contain substances that are not listed on the label, and therefore pose a greater risk to health.
- *Recommendation:* Practice food hygiene and safety. *Why?* Food should be stored appropriately to avoid accumulation of bacteria. This practice often means refrigerating perishable foods and not storing foods for too long. Food should be cooked to a safe temperature to kill microorganisms, but people should be aware that excess grilling of meat can produce carcinogenic substances called heterocyclic amines. To avoid microbial foodborne illness, when preparing food, it is important to have clean hands, cutlery and work surfaces. Fruits and vegetables should be washed in cold running tap water, but meat and poultry should not be washed or

rinsed. People should avoid raw or partially cooked eggs or foods containing raw eggs, raw or undercooked meat and poultry, unpasteurised juices and milk, or any products made from unpasteurised milk.

- *Recommendation:* Cook food in ways that preserve the integrity of nutrients and remove some of the fat. *Why?* The way that we cook food influences its nutrient and energy content. Grilling or roasting meat, poultry and fish, and discarding the fat, is better than pan-frying or deep-fat frying. For example, a whole chicken weighing 2 kg (4.4 lbs) contains about 400 g of fat and most of this will be lost if you cook the bird in a roasting bag in a hot oven for two hours. Losing the fat by this method of cooking makes the meat much healthier to eat as it is now low in fat but still high in protein. Steaming rather than boiling vegetables will retain more of the vitamins and phytonutrients. Remember that some vegetables are good to eat raw such as grated carrot, diced onion, celery, cucumber, tomato and salad leaves.

For a much more detailed explanation of healthy eating and which foods to avoid, see my evidence-based healthy lifestyle guidebook *Eat, Move, Sleep, Repeat* published by Meyer & Meyer Sport in 2020. The most important things to remember are to have a varied, well-balanced and diverse diet that includes all the major food groups, has no extremes of macronutrient composition and above all, practice moderation in everything you eat and drink (including not exceeding 14 units of alcohol per week). Figure 10.3 shows a food pyramid that illustrates some of the more important principles of healthy eating.

Healthy eating does not have to be complicated. Here is a list of 10 top tips to follow to ensure that your diet will be a pretty healthy one:

1. Eat meals at regular times of the day. Don't skip breakfast, and don't eat snacks between meals.

2. Try to choose a variety of different foods from the six basic food groups. That means including ones from the dairy group (e.g. milk, cheese, yoghurt), the meat group (e.g. meat, fish, poultry and eggs, with dried legumes and nuts as alternative sources of protein), fruits, vegetables and the breads and cereals group, and limited amounts of oils and fats. Eat at least five portions of a variety of fruit and vegetables every day. More than five is even better, as actually up to 10 portions per day has recently been shown to be associated with an even lower risk of cardiovascular disease.

3. Limit your intake of red meat (beef, lamb, pork) and processed meat (cured ham, bacon, pepperoni, salami) to no more than 500 g in total per week as larger amounts are associated with an increased risk of bowel cancer.

4. The main source of energy for meals should come from potatoes, bread, rice, pasta or other starchy carbohydrates. However, you should have only small-to-medium

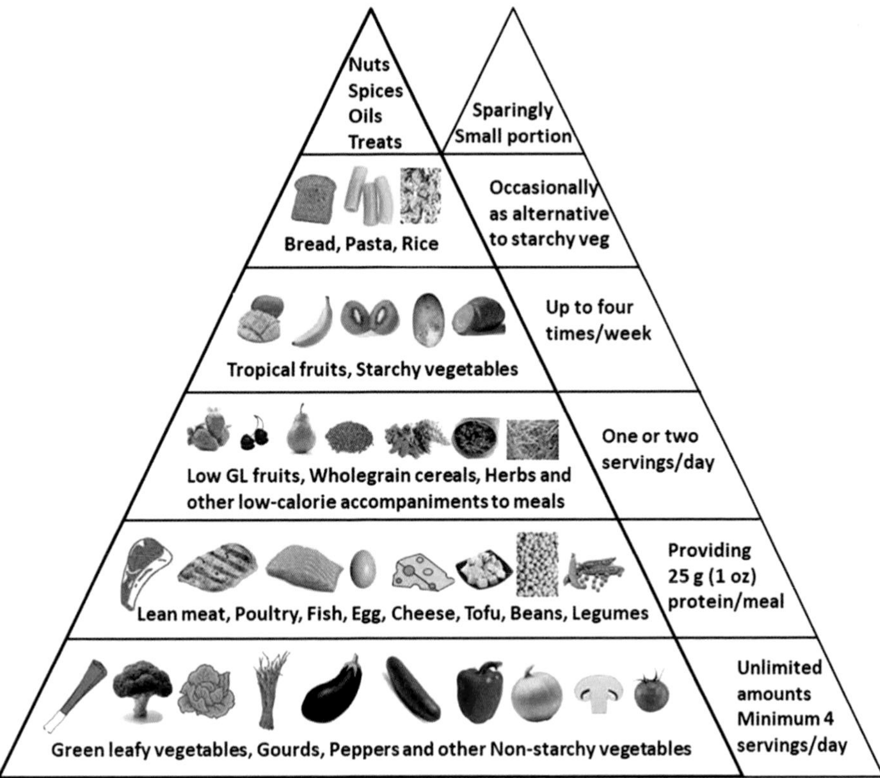

Figure 10.3 A food pyramid that illustrates the principles of healthy eating and provides some guidance on how much of the different food types to consume.

portions of these and choose whole-grain or higher fibre produce where possible. Have starchy vegetables such as potatoes on only up to 4 days of the week and on the other days have bread, rice or pasta instead.

5. Choose lower fat and lower-sugar options where available for things like dairy products, coleslaw, yoghurts etc.

6. Eat some beans, pulses, fish, eggs, meat and other high-protein foods. Aim for two portions of fish every week, one of which should be oily, such as salmon or mackerel. Research studies indicate that consuming 100–120 g of protein per day, spread evenly across three or four meals (i.e. 25–30 g of protein per meal), in combination with some occasional resistance exercise sessions is the most effective way to promote muscle gain and to prevent sarcopenia.

7. Choose unsaturated oils (e.g. rapeseed, olive) and spreads, but only eat them in small amounts.

8. Drink plenty of fluids (6–8 cups or glasses per day are recommended), particularly water (plain, mineral or soda), low-calorie (diet or light) versions of popular beverages (e.g. cola, lemonade and tonic water) and fruit juices with no added sugar. Tea and coffee are also fine in moderation, but if you like them to taste sweet use an artificial sweetener rather than sugar.

9. Limit your intake of alcohol by drinking no more than one 175 mL glass of wine or 350 mL beer with your main meal of the day and on no more than 5 days of the week.

10. Try to limit foods and drinks that are high in fat, salt, and sugar by having these less often and in small amounts. If you feel the need for a snack, choose raw vegetables such as celery or carrot.

NUTRITION FOR MANAGERS, COACHES AND SUPPORT STAFF

Finally, let's not forget the player support staff at the football club. Here, the role of nutrition is to help ensure good health, provide fuel for work and leisure-time physical activity, achieve energy balance and avoid weight gain. For those staff involved in on-pitch or gym-based training such as the strength and conditioning coach, as well as some managers and coaches, the daily physical demands and hence the energy requirements, are higher than those who are not directly involved in player training (other than perhaps observing the activities) or mostly work at a desk such as a football analyst. Essentially, the nutritional advice for support staff is similar to the guidelines previously discussed for the retired player with some adjustments depending on the physical load of the job they do. All staff should be encouraged to engage in at least the minimum volume of exercise needed to support health which, according to Government guidelines, is a minimum of 30 minutes per day of moderate-to-vigorous physical activity on at least 5 days per week.

SPECIAL CONSIDERATIONS

The female player

- Cover same distance in matches as men
- Cover less distance running at high speeds
- Lower body mass than men so overall energy & carbohydrate requirements are proportionally less, but similar expressed per kg BM
- Protein needs are the same (1.6 g/kg BM/day)
- Iron requirement higher than men
- Lower sweat rates than men
- RED(S) and disordered eating more common

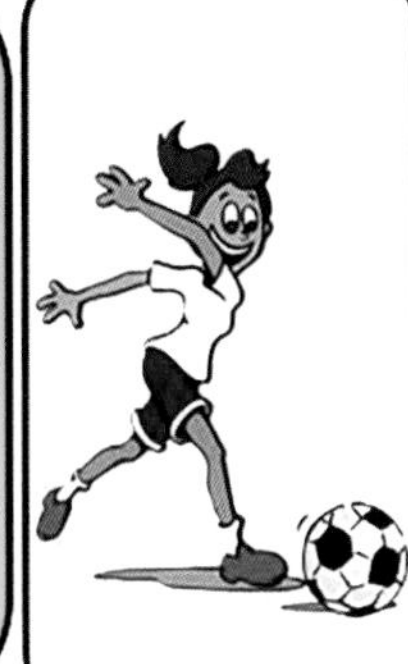

The junior player

- Growth and development of youth players has an impact on their nutritional requirements
- Calcium & phosphorus requirements higher than adults
- Iron requirement of boys higher than men
- Sufficient daily energy & protein intake is a concern with regular evening training sessions on school days
- Daily energy needs can be as high as senior players
- Energy, protein & micronutrient deficits can increase risk of bone fractures & ill health

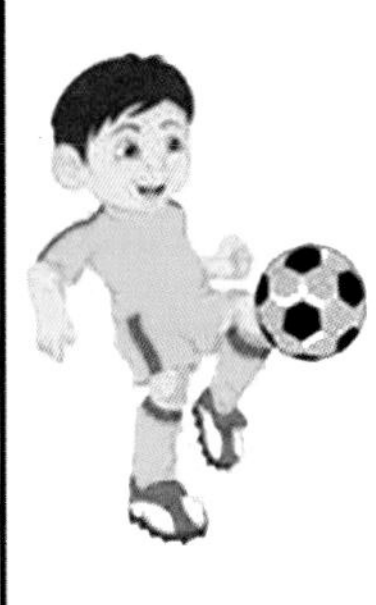

The referee

- Burn ~1200 kcal in a match (~400 kcal less than players)
- Match-day nutrition guidance can be similar to players
- Protein needs are similar (1.2-1.6 g/kg BM/day)
- Training volume generally less than players so daily energy needs are proportionally less
- During training, total energy & carbohydrate intakes should be appropriate to the individual training load & increased only around match days
- Caffeine can be considered as an ergogenic aid

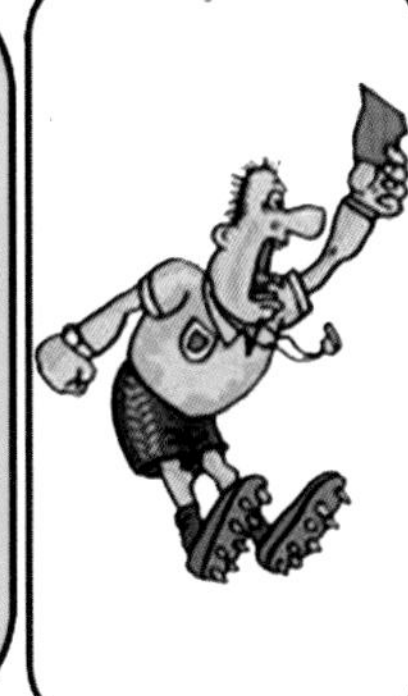

Infographic 10 Special considerations: Nutritional differences for female players, junior players and match officials.

CHAPTER 11

Football for Everyone

- The Health Benefits of Playing Regular Football
- Health Risks of Playing Football
- The Amateur Player
- The Fans

Some people like to play football for fun, or might be doing some football training and some occasional match play (friendly or competitive) because they want to be physically active for health reasons, so in this chapter, I will describe some of the health benefits of playing regular football that have come to light in recent years, as well as acknowledging some of the known potential health risks. I will also explain how the more serious amateur player can use the information in this book about what the professionals eat and drink (or, more accurately, what they are advised to consume) to improve their own match-play performance and subsequent recovery. Finally, I'll consider the fans who usually have to remain seated for 90 minutes or more (other than for a half-time toilet break) while watching a match in a stadium, on the big screen in a pub or at home on the television.

THE HEALTH BENEFITS OF PLAYING REGULAR FOOTBALL

Whether you play competitively or just for fun, football helps keep you fit and brings you the health benefits of other aerobic activities as well as some strengthening and flexibility exercises. Football counts towards your recommended amount of daily physical activity and brings benefits, including reducing your risk of several chronic illnesses such as heart disease, stroke and Type 2 diabetes. It will help improve your overall cardiovascular health, and you should see your fitness and endurance increase over time if you play frequently.

As mentioned in the early chapters of this book, in the professional game players cover typically 8–13 km in a 90-minute match and expend, on average, about 1,600 kcal. For many recreational players, these numbers won't be very different, so playing football regularly can assist with weight loss if dietary energy intake is adjusted accordingly. The combination of running, walking, sprinting, twisting, turning, jumping and kicking in football can bring benefits, including increased stamina, improved cardiovascular health, reduced body fat, improved muscle strength and tone, increased bone density and improved coordination (figure 11.1). In fact, the intensity and range of movements involved in the game provide better overall exercise than just running or weight training, according to a series of published scientific studies. Several of these potential health benefits help to oppose age-related declines in physiological functions. For example, we all lose some muscle mass as we get older (the clinicians refer to this as sarcopenia) but

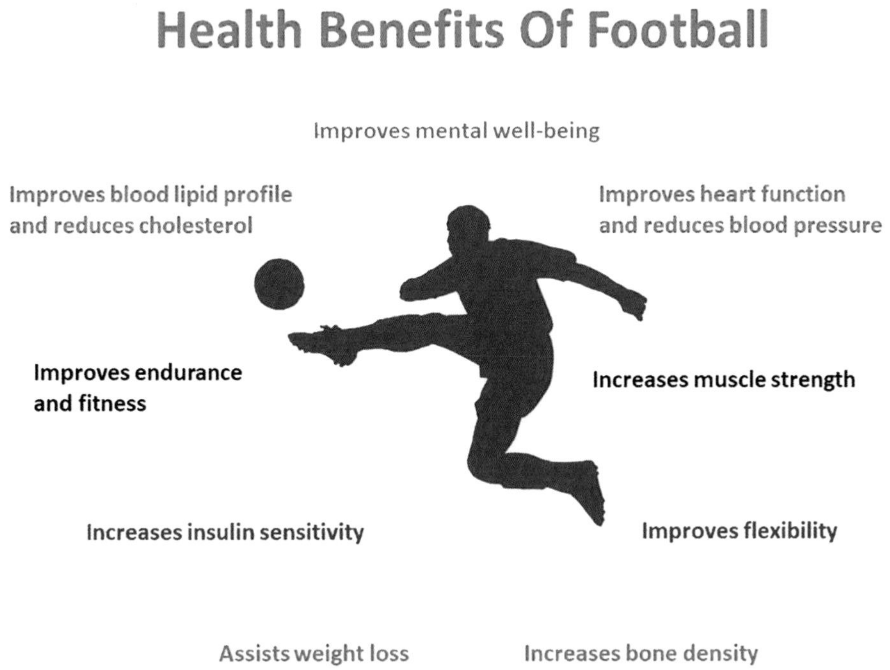

Figure 11.1 Some of the important health benefits of playing regular football.

this can be delayed, minimised, prevented or even reversed by resistance training, which should be a component of training in football. In men, and even more so in women after the menopause, osteoporosis can develop, which makes the bones more brittle and more susceptible to fractures. Participating in weight-bearing exercise such as running helps to prevent this. The risk of coronary heart disease – a major cause of death in the over-50s – can also be significantly reduced by engaging in regular physical activities such as football training and match play.

Playing regular sports such as football is also thought to help improve symptoms of some mental health issues, for example depression and stress. Participation in regular sport can lead to increased confidence and self-esteem and can help to reduce anxiety. Football match play and training provide great workouts and lots of fun. The health and other associated benefits from playing regular sport are as follows:

- Increases aerobic capacity and cardiovascular health.
- Reduces blood pressure in those with hypertension.
- Improves the blood lipid profile and lowers cholesterol.
- Assists with weight loss.
- Lowers body fat.
- Improves muscle tone.
- Increases leg and body core muscle strength.
- Builds strength, endurance and flexibility.
- Increases bone density.
- Teaches coordination.
- Helps with the mental skills of thinking and concentration.
- Encourages determination, persistence and self-discipline.
- Encourages communication, teamwork and sharing responsibility.
- Provides an opportunity to increase confidence and self-esteem, and helps to reduce anxiety and depression.
- Boosts your mood and makes you feel good.
- Boosts immune function and resistance to respiratory infections.
- It is also a great way to meet people and exercise with friends.

The numerous benefits of doing some regular exercise such as football for individuals with insulin-dependent Type 1 diabetes mellitus or noninsulin-dependent Type 2 diabetes include an increase in insulin sensitivity, a reduction of blood-glucose levels, improved immune function, improved blood lipid profiles, reduced adiposity and reduced risk of health problems including hypertension, kidney failure and cardiovascular disease. In order to reverse their condition, individuals with Type 2 diabetes need to lose some weight (refer to my book *Beating Type 2 Diabetes* [Meyer & Meyer Sport, 2020] if this applies to you), and playing football can help with this.

Exercise is one of the three main lifestyle behaviours that people can modify to improve their physical and mental health. The other two are getting good sleep quality and good nutrition (figure 11.2). As you have read about in this book, nutrition has an important impact on our ability to perform exercise, and in chapter 7, I explained how nutrition can also influence how well we sleep. For more detailed explanations about these issues, I suggest that you read my healthy lifestyle guidebook *Eat, Move, Sleep, Repeat* published by Meyer & Meyer Sport in 2020.

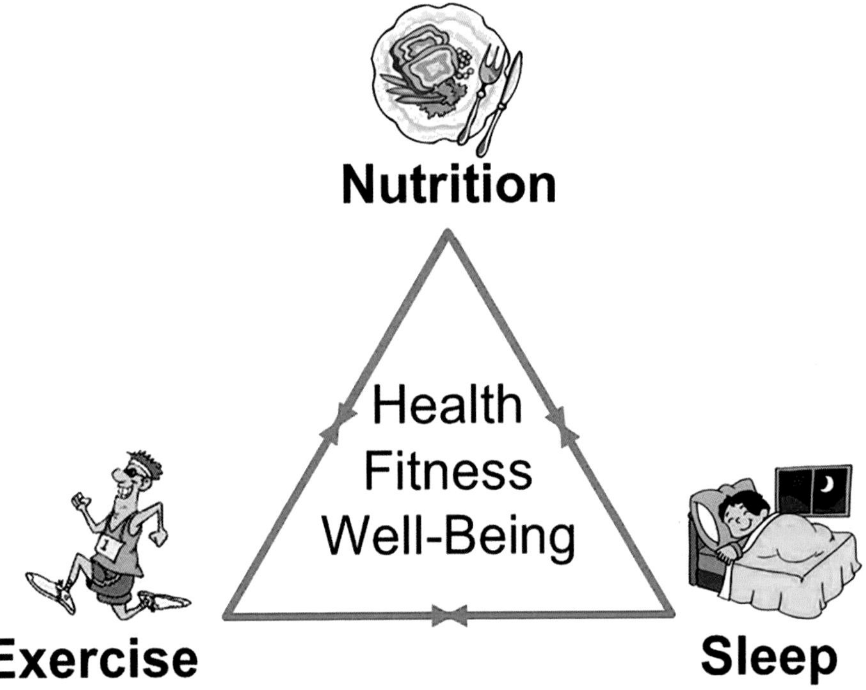

Figure 11.2 Our nutrition, exercise and sleep behaviours have important influences on our health, well-being and longevity. Note the bidirectional arrows in the triangle indicating that (a) nutrition and sleep affect our ability to exercise, (b) nutrition and exercise affect how we sleep and (c) exercise and sleep influence our nutrition (appetite and food choices).

For the older player, instead of the traditional 11-a-side game, participation in other forms of the beautiful game such as 5-a-side (also known as futsal) or walking football can be a good option. These games can be played outdoors or indoors in leisure centres or school gyms in inclement weather. Futsal can be a very high-intensity workout, but in walking football no running or jogging, with or without the ball is allowed, so it is low intensity but great fun to play for older folk. These forms of the game are shorter than the normal 11-a-side football matches, with two halves of exactly 20 minutes playing time, and they are also associated with health benefits. It is good to know that the biggest reduction in risk of chronic diseases such as coronary heart disease occurs when you go from doing no physical activity to doing some activity amounting to about 30 minutes per day on 5 days per week.

HEALTH RISKS OF PLAYING FOOTBALL

While many extol the potential health benefits of regularly playing football, it also needs to mentioned that it comes with some potential health risks, but then so do many other team sports such as rugby, hockey and American football. In soccer, the main danger is the risk of injury, most frequently as a result of bad tackles and accidental collisions during match play. The most common injuries are muscle pulls and tears, knee ligament ruptures, ankle sprains and broken bones. Some facts about the incidence of injury among elite players in the professional game were mentioned in chapter 9, and the potential risk of developing eating disorders, particularly among female and junior players was discussed in chapter 10. Also, in the professional game, there appears to be an increased risk of developing dementia and other neurological problems in later life, and it has been linked to repeated heading of the ball in both training and match play. Since 1937, the dry weight of the ball has been specified by the laws of the game to be 14–16 oz (equivalent to 390–450 g) and the circumference is 68–70 cm (27–28 in). This is known as a size five ball and is used by both male and female players from the age of 13. Balls used to be made of thick leather and they picked up water and mud on wet pitches, which made them considerably heavier in the later stages of a match or an on-pitch training session. In the modern professional game, the standard soccer ball is made of a synthetic leather, called polyurethane, which is stitched around an inflated rubber or rubber-like bladder. It still has a dry weight of 14–16 oz but does not pick up water like the old leather balls used to. Even so, it is probably advisable to limit the amount of heading in training for adult players and not allow heading in games or training for junior players. Young academy players under the age of 13 should also be using smaller, lighter balls in proportion to their smaller body size and strength compared with senior players.

THE AMATEUR PLAYER

Most adult amateur players will either have a full-time day job or be in full-time education at university or college. Team training sessions usually take place in the evening and probably only once or twice per week, with a competitive or friendly game at the weekend (commonly Sunday morning in the UK). Any other training is usually done individually, involving running on the road or in a park or having a workout in the gym. Some coaches may offer some advice about nutrition (although they not be the best qualified people to give it), but often, the timing and composition of meals are largely left to each individual's discretion. Therefore, some appropriate knowledge of what the professionals do (or are advised to do) can potentially go a long way to improving the performance of the amateur player.

Furthermore, although the title of this book emphasises the impact of nutrition clearly in relation to performance, it is not meant to imply that it is all just about what to eat on match day. As mentioned from the start in chapter 1, nutrition is important for many aspects of football that may indirectly influence performance – things like recovery, ability to train hard, adaptation to the training stimulus, body composition, immunity and overall health. Players who train and eat well are generally more resilient to common football injuries and illness making them more likely to be available for selection as they are stronger on the ball, and they can last the full 90 minutes and maintain high-intensity efforts for longer. They can also stay focused, they can react and move more efficiently at high speed, and they can adapt to and recover from training faster. Notice that none of these qualities directly involve use of the ball; they are all things that are under your control and this book provides you with the nutritional knowledge required to achieve them.

NUTRITION FOR DAYS WHEN TRAINING IN THE EVENING

If you are attending a training session in the evening, after a day at work or at an educational institution, you should eat and drink something before travelling, or while on the move if you have to travel some distance by car or public transport. It may be more convenient to ensure you have a good breakfast before your day's work and a good lunch with both meals high in carbohydrate (2 g/kg BM) and protein (0.5–0.6 g/kg BM) so that you then only need a lighter and rapidly digestible meal or snack (e.g. a cereal bar, chicken or tuna sandwich, mixed bean salad followed by some fruit such as banana, apple or grapes) in the early evening after work. Make sure you stay well hydrated throughout the day by drinking water every few hours and take a 500 mL bottle of a sports drink (6–8 g CHO/100 mL) with you to drink during and/or after training. As you may not get home from training until after 10:00pm, have a sandwich (with a chicken, turkey or ham filling and some salad leaves) or a microwavable ready meal (e.g. spaghetti bolognese or carbonara, ham and mushroom tagliatelle, macaroni cheese, chicken and mushroom risotto, chicken curry with rice) in the fridge for when you arrive or ask your partner (nicely!) to prepare something ready for you to eat before you go to bed.

Some people find that eating a large meal shortly before bedtime impairs their ability to sleep well, and if that applies to you it is best to opt for a lighter meal that will still provide some carbohydrate (to restore liver and muscle glycogen) and protein (for muscle repair and adaptation) together with some fluid to replace sweat losses. In addition to the meals listed previously, others can include Greek yoghurt with fruit and granola, scrambled eggs on toast or a bowl of cereal with milk and banana. Alternatively, particularly if your appetite is small, make your own recovery drink such as a homemade smoothie with milk, Greek yoghurt, banana, whey protein and chocolate powder.

NUTRITION FOR THE DAY BEFORE A MATCH

The most important meal on the day before a match, especially if the match kick-off is in the morning, is your evening dinner. This should be a high-carbohydrate (2–3 g/kg BM) meal with 0.4–0.6 g protein/kg BM with around 20–30% of the total energy coming from fat. You may recall from chapter 6 that the main purpose of this meal is to boost your muscle glycogen stores. Suitable meals include any lean meat, fish or poultry with pasta or boiled/mashed potatoes or rice together with some cooked vegetables such as beans, broccoli, asparagus, mushrooms, onion, tomato, peppers etc. to provide fibre and phytonutrients. Suitable meal plans can be very similar to the ones described in chapter 12 for training-day dinners or the post-match main meals and desserts that the professionals commonly have. If you prefer something less complicated for dessert, have some chopped fruit with yoghurt or a bowl of rice pudding, and drink according to your thirst.

NUTRITION ON MATCH DAY

Your nutrition on match day can be as close as possible to what I described in chapter 6 for the professional player. If your match is in the morning – let's say for example it's a 10:00am kick-off – then your pre-match meal is going to be breakfast, with the emphasis on consuming some readily digestible carbohydrate and plenty of fluid (water or a sports drink) 2–3 hours before kick-off. The main purpose of this meal, just as it is for the professionals, is to increase your liver glycogen stores which will be depleted after a night's sleep. This will help to prevent your blood glucose levels dropping in the later stages of a match – important for your brain as well as for your muscles. You can follow

Table 11.1 Match-day nutrition recommendations for a 10:00am kick-off

Timing	Feeding
07:00: Wake up	Individual preparation. Drink 250 mL water
07:30–08:00: Pre-match meal	70–150 g CHO + 20–30 g PRO + fluid + beetroot juice if desired
9:00–9:15	Drink 250 mL cup of strong coffee
9:50: After the warm-up	30 g CHO (e.g. 1 gel or 250 mL sports drink)
10:00: Kick-off	
10:45–11:00: Half-time	30–60 g CHO + 250–500 mL fluid (e.g. sports drink). Chew gum containing 100 mg caffeine if desired
11:45: Full time (to start recovery)	30–60 g CHO + 250–500 mL fluid (e.g. sports drink)
13:00–14:00: Meal	150–200 g CHO + 20–30 g PRO + fluid
17:00:	Fluid as required according to thirst
19:00: Dinner	100–150 g CHO + 20–30 g PRO + fluid
21:00–22:00	30–40 g PRO
23:00: Sleep	

the nutritional strategy shown in table 11.1. If you want to use some dietary ergogenic aids, then have a couple of 70 mL shots of concentrated beetroot juice with your breakfast and a cup of strong coffee (not decaf!) for a suitable dose (up to 3 mg/kg BM) of caffeine one hour before kick-off. Alternatively, do what Leicester City's Jamie Vardy has often done, and drink a caffeinated energy drink such as Red Bull instead of coffee.

Try out things you may be unfamiliar with (e.g. beetroot juice, strong coffee or caffeinated gum) on a normal day or your training day before using them on match day to ensure that you are comfortable with them. If you don't like them, or you think they are not doing anything for you, then ditch them. Dietary ergogenic aids don't work for everyone, although research generally shows that they do tend to be more effective for non-elite sporting people than for top professional games players or other types of elite athlete.

After the match, you are eating to refuel, rehydrate and repair damage to muscles, but the speed of recovery is not quite as critical as it is for the professional player. You will, however, will want to eat enough to ensure that you are ready to go to work the next day and that your physical and mental performance is not going to be impaired by your exertions on match day. Again, the advice is to generally follow what the professional players eat and drink after a match. As soon as possible after the full-time whistle, down a 500 mL sports drink and a carbohydrate gel or a cereal bar and then have a main meal 1–2 hours later. For many, this may be a traditional Sunday lunch at home or in a pub. That is fine if you choose a meal plan similar to the one described in chapter 12. Later in the day, drink fluids according to your thirst but limit your consumption of alcohol. One pint of beer or a glass of wine with your main meal is acceptable, but no more than this if you are looking to optimise your recovery. Fruit juice, tea or a soft drink are better choices. Another lighter meal can be eaten in the evening, and you can consider having a high-protein snack an hour or so before bed.

Finally, in table 11.2 is a list of my top ten tips on how the amateur player can improve their performance and recovery with appropriate nutrition choices.

Table 11.2 Top ten tips on how the amateur player can improve their performance and recovery with appropriate nutrition choices

	Likely Benefit	Nutritional Tip
1	Increased running speed	Attempt to lose any excess weight you may be carrying by eating a high-protein but reduced calorie diet. That will allow you to lose around 0.5 kg of body fat per week while maintaining your muscle mass
2	Improved match play endurance	On the day before a match, consume a high-carbohydrate evening meal containing 150–200 g CHO and 30–40 g protein
3	Improved match play endurance	On match day, consume a pre-match meal 2–4 hours before kick-off containing about 70–150 g CHO and some protein (10–30 g), but low in fibre and fat
4	Improved match play endurance and reduced risk of muscle cramps	Ensure you are well hydrated before a match by consuming 5–7 mL/kg BM of water 2 hours before kick-off
5	Improved match play endurance	Drink two 70 mL shots of concentrated beetroot juice 2 hours before kick-off
6	Improved match play endurance and mental performance	Ingest 100–200 mg caffeine by drinking a strong cup of coffee or caffeine tablets or chewing gum about 1 hour before kick-off
7	Improved match play endurance	Consume 30 g CHO (e.g. 1 gel or 250 mL sports drink) 5–10 minutes before kick-off

	Likely Benefit	Nutritional Tip
8	Improved second-half performance including sprint speed, motor skills and even mood in the final minutes	At half-time and when there are prolonged breaks in play (e.g. due to an injured player receiving treatment on the pitch) mouth rinse and consume some sport drink containing carbohydrate and some sodium
9	Improved recovery	Consume a meal high in carbohydrate and protein within 2 hours after training or match play and rehydrate according to your weight loss after a game
10	Stay healthy	Eat a healthy, well-balanced and diverse diet sufficient to meet your daily energy needs and focus on foods with high nutrient content; try to avoid eating junk food and processed meals; take a daily 1,000–2,000 IU vitamin D3 supplement in the winter months

THE FANS

Nowadays, most football stadia in the professional game are all-seater and fans spend at least 90 minutes mostly sitting on their bottoms while watching a match (maybe apart from when a goal is being celebrated or your team has a strong shout for a penalty, or a referee has done something that you particularly dislike!), and that does not expend much energy – only about 100 kcal for the average adult in fact. So, watching football does not add anything extra to the usual day's energy expenditure. For that reason, it is not a good idea to eat anything during the game, although a cup of tea or coffee or at half-time is fine. Take a bottle of water with you to quench your thirst on warm weather days. Nowadays, many clubs offer excellent catering facilities at their stadia and it is possible (though often rather expensive) to have a meal a few hours before kick-off. That is fine, as long it is a substitute for your normal main meal of the day and not an added extra. As mentioned in chapter 3, in order to be weight stable we have to be in energy balance. In other words, our daily/weekly energy intake should match our daily/weekly energy expenditure.

I remember that back in the 1960s, 70s, 80s and 90s, the only food you could get before kick-off or at half-time in football stadia (when many more people stood to watch a match than were seated) was a meat pie, a burger or a hot dog (figure 11.3). They weren't healthy food choices then and they aren't now, so don't be tempted by these

Traditional Match-Day Nutrition For Fans

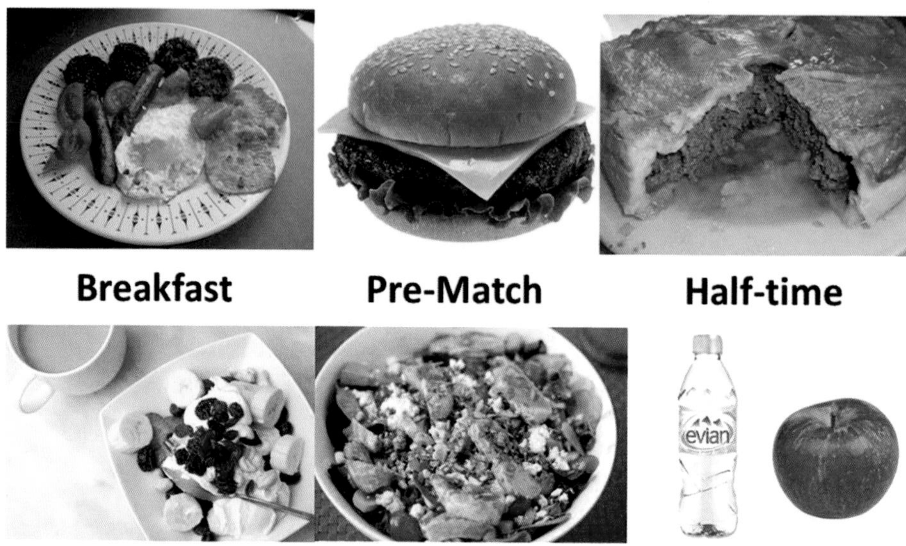

Recommended Match-Day Nutrition For Fans

Figure 11.3 Some traditional foods consumed by football fans on match day (which are not recommended!) and some more appropriate and healthier alternatives.

fatty fast foods! Fans should select healthier options for all meals that they have before watching a match, and at half-time as illustrated in figure 11.3. For additional advice on healthy eating, refer to the information provided in the previous chapter on nutrition for the retired footballer, or get yourself a copy of my healthy lifestyle guidebook *Eat, Move, Sleep, Repeat* published by Meyer & Meyer Sport in 2020.

I know that many avid fans like to have a beer before a game to calm their nerves.

Well OK, we are all allowed a treat once in a while and there is a precedent for this in professional football that I recall from the 1970s. Brian Clough's Nottingham Forest were underdogs for the first ever all-English European Cup fixture, a first-round tie in September 1978 against Liverpool. Forest were the English champions, but Liverpool were in prime form and seeking a third successive European Cup triumph. This was the second leg of the tie (the first ended 2–0 to Forest at the City Ground) and it saw Clough's intuitive man-management at its best. Before the match, he concentrated on relaxing his players as he had detected that many of them appeared nervous. On the team's coach journey to the Anfield stadium, home of the mighty Liverpool, Clough stood up and asked: 'Does anyone fancy a beer?' He duly produced two cans for each player and insisted that they drank them. It seemed that this rare ploy worked, as the second leg finished in a goalless draw so Forest won the tie 2–0 on aggregate. Forest went on to defeat AEK Athens, Grasshopper Club Zürich, Cologne and, in the final, Malmö, to win the European Cup for the first time in their history. The following year, Forest successfully defended the trophy. Two years previously, they had been in the old Second Division. I love those amazing fairy-tale stories in football! In Leicester, we had one of our own when the Foxes, against all the odds, were the surprise winners of the English Premier League title in 2015/16 at pre-season odds of 5,000–1. It's a funny old game and that is one of the reasons that so many people love it. It is still possible, even in these big-money times, for the current bottom club in the league to beat the top team, or for a famous team with a long history of success to get beaten by a lower-league team in a national major cup competition. For example, I was in tears of joy when I watched my beloved Oldham Athletic beat the mighty Liverpool 3–2 in the 4th round of the FA cup in January 2013. I started this book by mentioning my love of football and my lifelong support of 'the Latics', so this seems a very good way to end it. I hope that you have enjoyed reading my book on the importance of nutrition in football. In the final chapter of this book, you will find some suitable meal plans and recipes for what players should be eating on training days and match days.

NUTRITION FOR AMATEUR PLAYER

CARBOHYDRATE
4-6 g/kg BM/day on day prior to match & match day to elevate muscle glycogen stores

ENERGY
Typically consume 3000 kcal to match total energy needs on match days

RECOVERY
Begins immediately post-match with fluid, carbs, protein in sports foods & protein shakes

PRE-MATCH MEAL
High in low-fibre carbohydrate 1-2 g/kg BM to replenish liver glycogen stores

MATCH-DAY

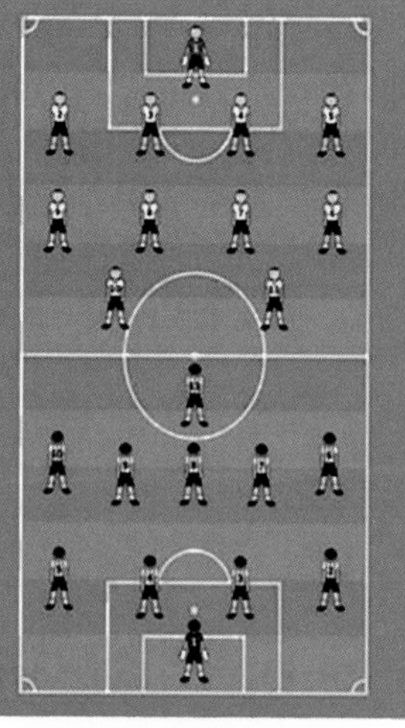

POST-MATCH MEAL
Begin restoration of muscle glycogen & repair by consuming 2 g/kg BM carbohydrate & 40 g high quality protein within 2-3 h post-match

HYDRATION
Start match well-hydrated by drinking 5-7 ml/kg BM fluid 2-4 hours before kick-off

BREAKS IN PLAY
Drink water to avoid dehydration on warm days.
Mouth rinse then swallow sport drink

PRE-MATCH ERGOGENIC AIDS
Beetroot shots with pre-match meal
Caffeine 1-3 mg/kg BM 1 h before KO

WARM-UP JUST BEFORE KICK-OFF
Ingest 30 g carbohydrate as gels or sport drinks

HALF-TIME
Ingest 30-60 g carbohydrate as gels or sport drinks.
Caffeine chewing gum (spit out before returning to pitch)

Infographic 11a Match-day nutrition for the amateur player.

EVENING TRAINING FOR AMATEURS

Carbs 45-65%
Protein 15-20%
Fat 20-35%
Water
Eat a well-balanced & diverse daily diet

ENERGY
Have 2500-3000 kcal to match energy needs on training days but only 2000-2500 kcal on other days or according to occupational demands

ESSENTIAL MICRONUTRIENTS
Vitamins/Minerals
Any deficiency can cause ill health & impair performance
Vit D3 supplement

DAILY CARBS
3-5 g/kg BM
Depending on the specific training scenario & individual player training goals

TRAINING DAY

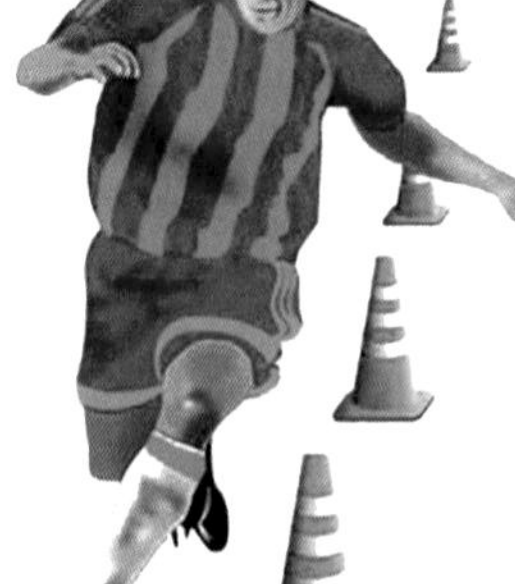

BEFORE TRAINING
Have a substantial high-carb breakfast & lunch & a rapidly digestible snack after finishing daytime work, ideally at least 2 h before training

DAILY PROTEIN
1.4-1.6 g/kg BM

0.3-0.4 g/kg BM high quality protein per meal

DURING TRAINING
Have a sport drink or carb-gel just before the training session begins

DAILY FAT
1.0-1.5 g/kg BM with <0.5 g/kg BM from saturated fats

WATER
>2 L/day
Arrive at training well-hydrated & avoid body mass deficit of >2% during training sessions

AFTER TRAINING
Have a pre-prepared meal ready to heat up & eat when back home. Meal should contain 1-2 g/kg BM carbs & 25-40 g protein

Infographic 11b Nutrition for amateur players having an evening training session.

CHAPTER 12

Meal Plans and Recipes for Footballers

- Training Days
- Match Days

Nutritionists have a tendency to talk about nutrition in terms of requirements for certain amounts of energy in kilocalories, and amounts of macronutrients in grams or grams per kilogram body weight, but the reality is, of course, that players eat real foods and essentially need to know what foods to eat – and how much to eat – to achieve the desired nutritional goals. It is also important that as well as being nutritious meals should be well prepared, attractive to look at and taste delicious. As I mentioned in the first chapter, eating good food is part of the enjoyment of life, and there is no point in preparing a wonderfully nutritious meal if it doesn't look, smell or taste good! Eating should never be a chore, and often it is a social occasion to enjoy with teammates, partners, family or friends. Players should really enjoy their food and eat everything that is served on the plate to achieve the nutrition goals set by the nutritionist. This chapter describes some example meal plans for breakfasts, lunches and evening dinners for footballers. Each of these meal plans indicates the ingredients and the amounts needed to make a meal for one person. If you are preparing meals for two people simply double the amounts. For each meal plan, the total energy content (kcal) and the amount (in grams) of carbohydrate, protein and fat it contains are shown. The meal plans described in this chapter can be varied to some degree to suit your personal food and taste preferences, substituting like-for-like for the meats, green vegetables, legumes, breads, and pasta items that are mentioned below. For example, it is perfectly fine to use turkey instead of chicken; lean pork or non-oily fish such as cod instead of beef; asparagus, spring greens, leeks, cabbage or green beans instead of spinach; sweet potato, corn, or rice instead of potato; peas or butter beans instead of red beans or baked beans; and penne pasta, macaroni, linguine or noodles instead of spaghetti. Just stick to the guideline amounts in grams and the calorie (kcal) amounts will not be very different.

I have not attempted to provide full recipes with cooking times and temperatures for all of the meals listed here, as I don't think I need to teach people how to cook the more basic dishes. The breakfast meals, for example, are all generally quite simple to prepare and I assume that most people will know how to boil eggs, potatoes, rice or pasta; steam vegetables; grill, roast or fry meat; and oven-bake fish, casseroles and curries. Just bear in mind that generally steaming is preferable to boiling for most vegetables that need cooking because more of the essential nutrients are retained, and that grilling is preferable to frying for most meats, as no oil needs to be added. When you do fry food such as steak, use a non-stick frying pan and only enough vegetable oil (no more than two teaspoons, which is 80 kcal and 9 g of fat) to thinly coat the bottom of the pan, and if you are only cooking for one person, use a small diameter pan. Alternatively, brush each side of your steak with one half teaspoon of vegetable oil (rapeseed, sunflower or corn oil are suitable choices) before placing it in a hot non-stick frying pan.

For all meal plans and recipes described in this chapter, I give you the ingredients with their weight or volume and the total energy (kcal) and macronutrient (g) content of the whole meal, rounded up to the nearest 10 kcal and whole gram, respectively. Note that some meal plans specify dry uncooked weights for rice and pasta items while others give the cooked weight. Take care to check which it is, as the energy content of boiled rice or pasta is about 130 kcal per 100 g, but that of uncooked dry rice or pasta is nearly three times that value at 370 kcal per 100 g.

In this chapter, several of the meal plans for the more complex dishes do include recipes with brief instructions on how to prepare and cook them. These have been prepared by my good friends Bruno Cirillo and Rachel Muse. Bruno is Head of Nutrition for the Danish Superliga football club FC Nordsjælland based in Farum in Denmark. Bruno is also an elite performance chef with some great ideas for dishes that resemble some fast food or takeaways that are very popular with footballers (and many other people), but have modified ingredients and/or cooking methods to make them more nutritious and healthier. Rachel is one of the best elite performance chefs in Europe and is the founder of a business called *Talk, Eat, Laugh* and its sister company *Discrete & Delicious*, based in Salisbury in England, which trains and provides performance chefs for high-level clients including many elite athletes and footballers. Rachel has an excellent understanding of the nutritional needs of football players and works in concert with club nutritionists/ dietitians to produce meals with the desired macronutrient content that are also tasty and attractive and cater to the individual preferences of her clients. As you read through the meal plans and recipes in this chapter, she advises the following: 'Read through each recipe before you plan to cook it and ensure you have the ingredients and equipment you need. Aim to cook all meat from room temperature, which means getting individual (defrosted) portions of meat out of the fridge 40 minutes before you plan to cook them and getting a joint of meat or a chicken out of the fridge and hour and a half before you plan to cook it. This is really important for steak and slightly less important for other types of meat. This doesn't include fish. Fish can easily go bad if not kept in the fridge so cook that straight from the fridge. If you need to defrost meats that have been kept in the freezer, keep them in their packaging and place them on a plate in your fridge until they are thawed. How long this takes will depend on the portion size of the meat but for most portions suitable for one person about 24 hours is about right.' Please note that where oven temperatures are indicated in the following recipes they are for a fan-assisted oven. If your oven does not have a fan you should add 10ºC to the suggested temperature setting.

TRAINING DAYS

A typical training day involves a 2-hour morning on-pitch training session followed by a lunch break and then some gym work and testing in the afternoon, before the players travel home. The meal plans and recipes described here that include a breakfast, post-training lunch and evening dinner will provide about 3,000 kcal in total; the amounts can be modified if daily energy expenditure is expected to be lower or higher than this.

BREAKFASTS

These contain 650–750 kcal with at least 50 g CHO, at least 30 g protein and some fat. They are generally quite simple to prepare and easily digestible. They can be accompanied by a drink of water, fruit juice (e.g. cranberry, orange, apple, tomato) with no added sugar, milk or a hot beverage (e.g. green tea, coffee) as desired.

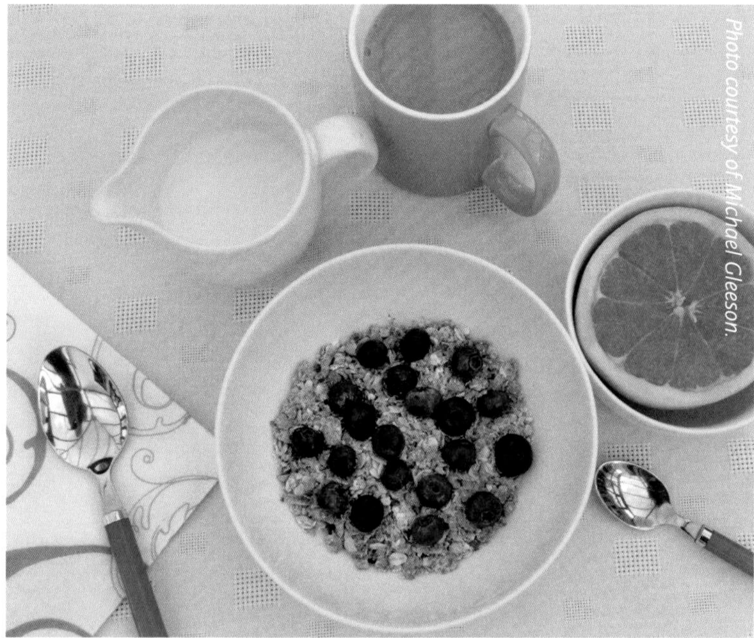

Photo 12.1 Grapefruit half and a blueberry muesli.

Grapefruit half and a blueberry or cherry muesli followed by a vegetable omelette

Half a pink grapefruit and 40 g Swiss style muesli with 75 mL whole milk and 20 blueberries or four pitted chopped red cherries. Followed by a mixed vegetable and olive omelette made with two medium-sized eggs cooked with one tablespoon of rapeseed oil, 60 g fresh spinach, two chopped tomatoes, four sliced mushrooms, one chopped red or green pepper and five pitted olives. Add a pinch of ground pepper and a sprinkling of herbs (e.g. chives, oregano, parsley, sage, or a mixture) to add flavour. Serve with one thick slice of wholemeal bread (730 kcal, 82 g carbohydrate, 34 g protein, 34 g fat).

Fruit and bran cereal followed by scrambled eggs with asparagus and bacon

Half a large orange or a small pink grapefruit, followed by 40 g All-Bran cereal with 75 mL whole milk and half a medium-sized banana, chopped into thin slices. Followed by two scrambled eggs made with 50 mL whole milk and two teaspoons of margarine, with four steamed chopped asparagus spears and two slices of lean bacon. Serve with one slice of toasted whole-grain bread (690 kcal, 77 g carbohydrate, 31 g protein, 31 g fat).

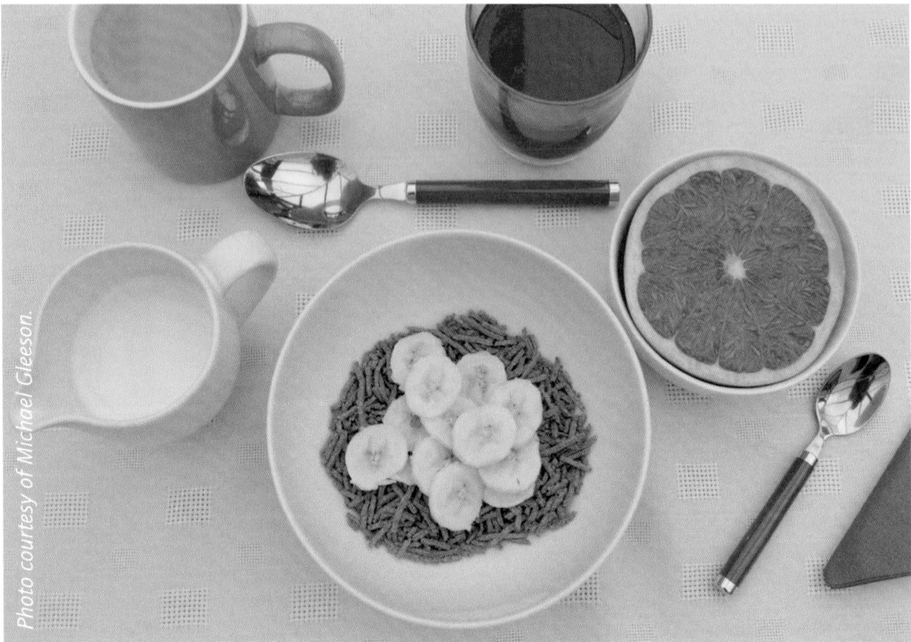

Photo 12.2 Grapefruit and All-Bran cereal with sliced banana.

Whole-wheat cereal with strawberries followed by a bacon sandwich

Two whole-wheat biscuits (such as Shredded Wheat, Weetabix, or Oatibix) with 100 mL whole milk and 12 medium-sized strawberries. Lean bacon sandwich using four slices of lean back bacon, grilled or microwaved. Served between two slices of wholemeal bread or in a toasted bun with one large finely chopped tomato (610 kcal, 77 g carbohydrate, 31 g protein, 21 g fat).

Fruit smoothie followed by smoked salmon and avocado

Fruit smoothie made with one large ripe banana, 300 mL cranberry juice (no added sugar version) and 100 g frozen mixed red berries blended together and served with an English muffin, toasted and spread with a 'light' margarine spread or marmite. Followed by 100 g smoked salmon with half a sliced ripe avocado, sprinkled with black pepper. Serve with one slice of whole-grain bread (750 kcal, 118 g carbohydrate, 32 g protein, 20 g fat).

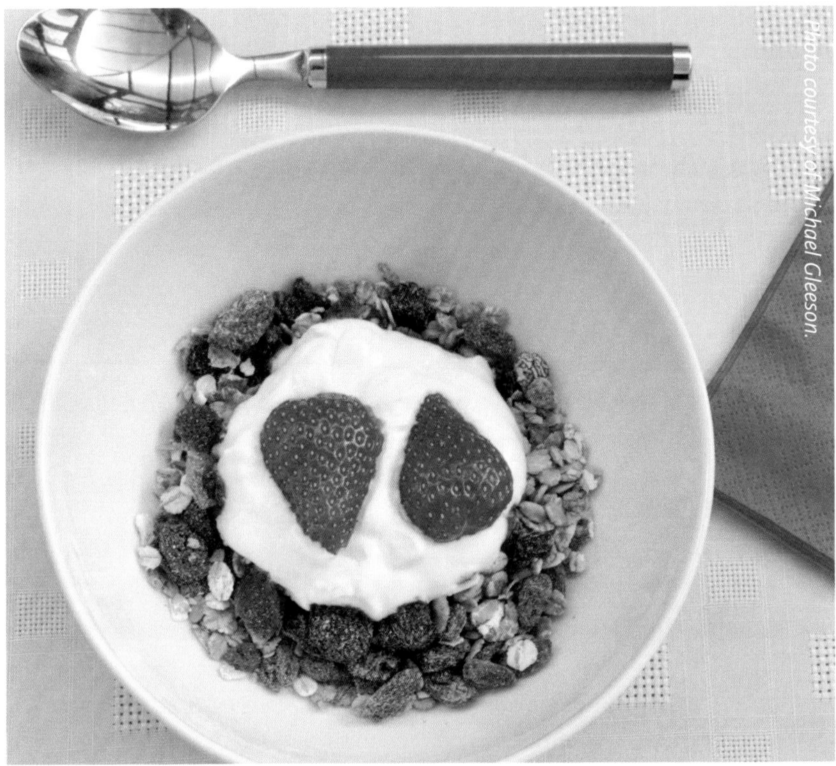

Photo 12.3 Muesli comprising rolled oats, wheat flakes, dried raisins and sultanas, served with low-fat yoghurt and topped with strawberry.

Muesli followed by smoked haddock kedgeree

Muesli (50 g) comprising rolled oats, wheat flakes and 30 g of a variety of dried fruits (e.g. cranberries, raisins, sultanas) served with 100 g Greek yoghurt and topped with a large strawberry. Followed by a kedgeree made from 100 g poached smoked haddock, 100 g boiled brown rice and one tablespoon of curry paste or red pesto, topped with one sliced hard-boiled egg (750 kcal, 93 g carbohydrate, 51 g protein, 22 g fat).

Porridge followed by cheese and red pepper omelette

Porridge oats (40 g) made with 100 mL whole milk and topped with a tablespoon of honey and 30 raisins. Followed by a two-egg omelette cooked with one tablespoon of rapeseed oil oil, 30 g grated cheddar cheese and one whole sliced red pepper (700 kcal, 61 g carbohydrate, 30 g protein, 40 g fat).

Oatmeal with nuts and yoghurt followed by bacon, egg and tomato

One half cup of oatmeal and 100 g Greek yoghurt with 10 chopped pecan nut halves. Followed by three thick slices of grilled lean bacon, one poached egg, one grilled tomato sprinkled with oregano and 50 g sauerkraut. Serve with one slice of wholemeal bread (680 kcal, 53 g carbohydrate, 37 g protein, 36 g fat).

Baked beans on toast followed by a Spanish omelette

Half a can (200 g) of baked beans on two slices of toasted wholemeal bread. Followed by a Spanish omelette made with three eggs, cooked with one tablespoon of rapeseed oil, 30 g cottage cheese, one chopped chilli pepper, five pitted black olives and a tablespoon of tomato salsa (700 kcal, 74 g carbohydrate, 39 g protein, 27 g fat).

Fruit smoothie followed by poached eggs with mushrooms

Fruit smoothie – one large ripe banana, 300 mL cranberry juice (no added sugar version) and 100 g frozen mixed red berries blended together, and served with an English muffin toasted and spread with jam or marmite. Followed by two large poached eggs, with 80 g sliced mushrooms fried in two teaspoons of rapeseed oil and 30 g spinach leaves seasoned with ground black pepper and a pinch of salt. Serve with one thick slice of wholemeal bread (750 kcal, 112 g carbohydrate, 30 g protein, 25 g fat).

Chocolate protein oats followed by beans on toast

Rolled oats (40 g) made with 150 mL whole milk, one sliced medium-sized banana, 40 g of mixed red berries and 20 g of chocolate-flavoured whey protein isolate. Followed by half a can (200 g) of baked beans on a thick slice of toasted wholemeal bread (740 kcal, 119 g carbohydrate, 42 g protein, 10 g fat).

Here are a couple of other breakfast ideas created by elite performance chef Rachel Muse. These are lower calorie meals than the ones previously described, but can be preceded by a bowl of cereal and milk, if desired, to increase the calorie and carbohydrate content.

Egg muffins

This makes three muffins but it usually works better to make it for more (I usually do four times this amount and make 12). They can be eaten hot or stored in the fridge for up to 3 days.

(270 kcal, 3 g carbohydrate, 18 g protein, 18 g fat) per portion (3 muffins).

INGREDIENTS

- One rasher of bacon
- Quarter tablespoon of oil
- Two medium-sized eggs
- One spring onion
- 10 g grated cheese
- Two cherry tomatoes
- 25 mL milk

PREPARATION

1) Pre-heat oven to 180°C; **2)** chop the bacon into small pieces and fry in the oil in the frying pan until they start to go crispy; **3)** grate the cheese and chop the tomatoes and spring onion into small pieces (about 5 mm); **4)** if using silicon muffin cases lay three out on a baking sheet, or alternatively grease three in a muffin tin; divide the bacon, cheese, onion and tomatoes between the three cases; **5)** break the two eggs into a clean jar, add the milk and a pinch of salt and pepper, then shake the jar vigorously until the eggs are well beaten; if you are using a bowl instead, beat the eggs with a fork; **6)** pour the egg mixture into the part-filled cases, leaving a gap at the top for expansion and oven-bake at 180°C for 20 minutes.

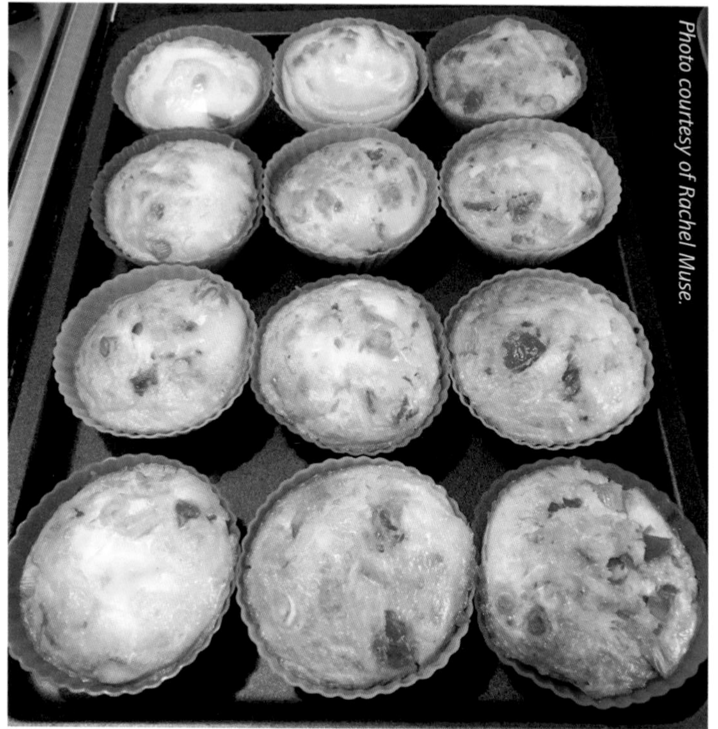

Photo 12.4 Egg muffins.

Cassoulet

(480 kcal, 75 g carbohydrate, 27 g protein, 10 g fat)

INGREDIENTS

- 40 g streaky bacon (or one small sausage)
- Quarter of a large onion, peeled and sliced
- Quarter of a large carrot, peeled and sliced
- Quarter tablespoon oil
- 100 g tinned chopped tomatoes
- 50 g lentils
- 50 g quinoa
- Quarter of a stock cube

PREPARATION

1) In a small bowl, soak the lentils in half a cup of boiling water; **2)** cut the bacon into small bits with scissors or de-skin the sausage and make two mini sausages; **3)** fry the onion in the oil in the frying pan, stirring until soft, then add the bacon or sausages and carrot and continue to stir; **4)** sieve or drain the lentils and add them to the pan, then add just half of the quarter stock cube and the quarter tin of tomatoes, then add 300 mL boiling water; turn the pan down to a low heat and simmer for 20 minutes, stirring occasionally; **5)** put the quinoa and the rest of the stock cube into a small saucepan and add 600 mL of boiling water; stir well then turn to a low heat and simmer for 15 minutes; **6)** serve the quinoa and cassoulet up, next to each other on a plate.

Note: This dish can also be served as a post-training lunch

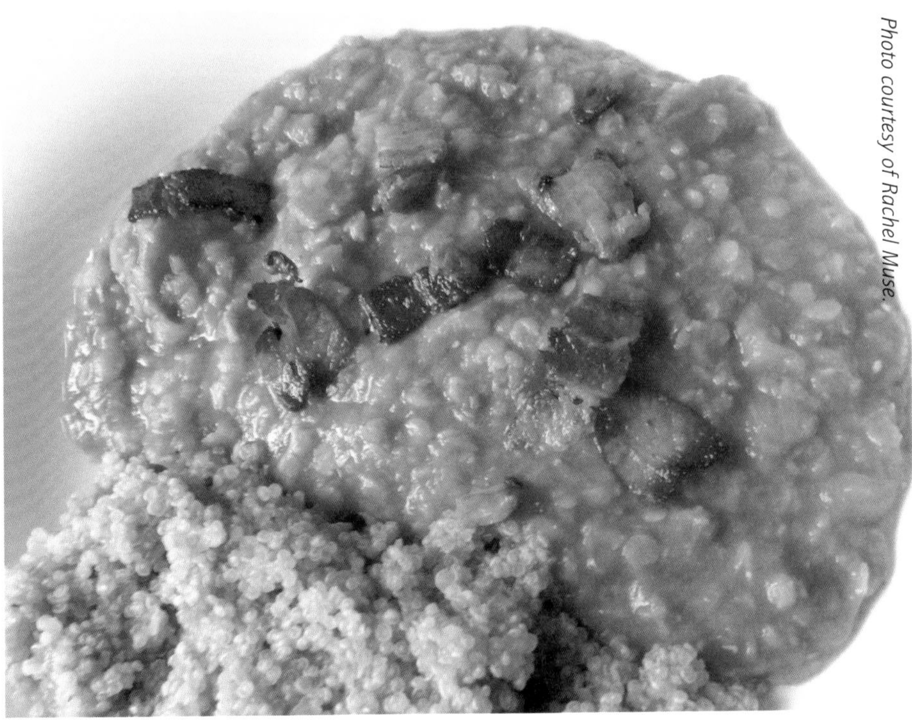

Photo courtesy of Rachel Muse.

Photo 12.5 Cassoulet.

POST-TRAINING LUNCHES

These contain 600–900 kcal with about 50–120 g CHO, at least 30 g protein and about 20–40 g fat. These values indicate a fairly wide range because the actual needs will depend on the duration and intensity of the training session. If the training session last about 2 hours and is intensive, the energy and nutrient needs can be specified in a narrower range (figure 12.1). The lunch recipes listed here can be followed with a selection of fruits (approximately 100–200 kcal) for dessert. They can be accompanied by a drink of water, fruit juice (e.g. orange, apple, grape, tomato – using the no added sugar versions), or a hot beverage (e.g. green tea, coffee) as desired.

The meal recipes that follow have been created by elite performance chef Rachel Muse.

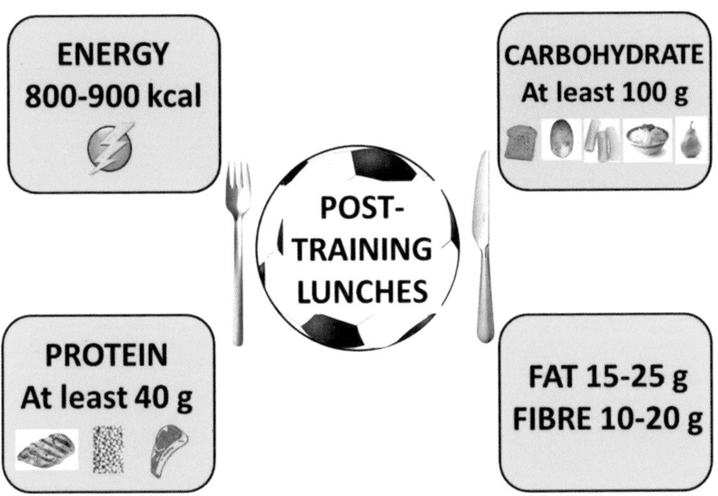

Figure 12.1 Post-training lunch nutrition targets following a 2-hour intensive morning training session. On days with shorter and lighter training sessions, the energy and carbohydrate needs will be correspondingly less.

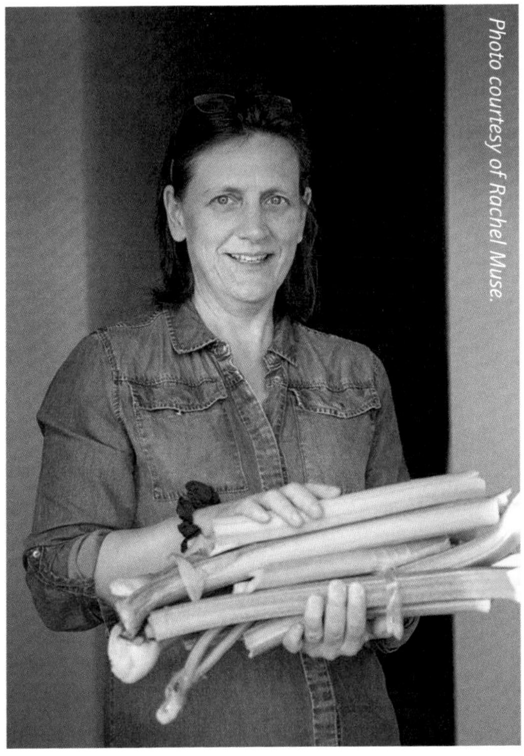
Photo courtesy of Rachel Muse.

Photo 12.6 Elite performance chef Rachel Muse.

Chicken BLT sandwich

(610 kcal, 51 g carbohydrate, 48 g protein, 21 g fat)

INGREDIENTS

- One pre-cooked roast chicken breast (skin removed)
- Two bacon rashers
- Large tomato
- Pinch of sea salt
- Pinch of sugar
- One tablespoon of mustard dill sauce
- Three slices of bread
- Lettuce leaves: two big leaves, or a small handful of small leaves
- Two cocktail sticks

PREPARATION

1) Remove the breast from the chicken carcass and cut into 5 mm slices; **2)** in a hot frying pan dry fry the bacon 2 minutes a side; in cooking the first side of the bacon, fat will be released and when the bacon is turned over the second side will fry in the released oil; **3)** toast the bread; **4)** slice the tomato and sprinkle on the sugar and the salt; **5)** assemble the club sandwich: take a slice of toast, spread with a thin layer of mustard dill sauce, top with sliced tomato and bacon; spread a second slice of toast with mustard dill sauce and place that on the bacon, sauce side down; spread the upper side of the toast with mustard dill sauce, top with sliced chicken and lettuce; spread the final slice of toast with mustard dill sauce and fix everything in place with two cocktail sticks; cut triple-decker sandwich in half and serve.

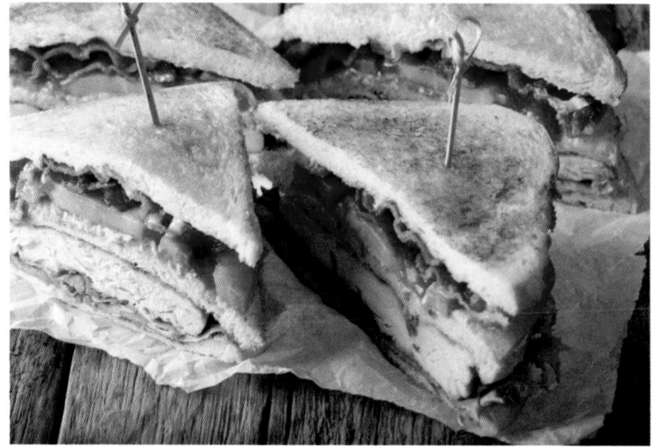

Photo 12.7 Chicken, bacon, lettuce and tomato sandwich.

Thai green chicken curry with brown rice and stir-fried vegetables

(900 kcal, 75 g carbohydrate, 60 g protein, 40 g fat)

INGREDIENTS

- Two pre-cooked chicken thighs (skin removed)
- One teaspoon of Thai green curry paste
- Two tablespoons of coconut milk
- One lime
- One spring onion
- 70 g brown rice
- Four baby sweetcorn cobs
- 30 g sugar snap peas
- One tablespoon of rapeseed fry oil (or toasted sesame oil)
- One garlic clove
- One red pepper
- One orange pepper
- Two teaspoons of soya sauce

PREPARATION

1) Strip the meat from the bone of the chicken thighs, place in a small bowl and mix with the Thai green curry paste, coconut milk and juice from half a lime; slice the spring onion and set aside; **2)** place the rice in a saucepan and rinse in cold water, drain through a sieve and add 150 mL of cold water and cook on a medium heat; **3)** in a small pan on a low heat warm the chicken and curry paste mixture; **4)** cut the sweetcorn and the sugar snap peas in half lengthwise and cut the peppers into thin strips; **5)** in a large frying pan or a wok, heat the oil then add the sweetcorn and stir, the heat should be high enough that there is a bit of sizzle but not so hot that there is smoke; add the garlic and the strips of peppers and stir twice in the course of 1 minute; add the sugar snaps and stir twice in the course of 1 minute and then take the vegetable mixture off the heat; **6)** as soon as the rice has absorbed all the water, test and see if the rice is cooked; brown rice is naturally firmer when cooked than white rice, but if it's still starchy add a splash more water and cook for a few more minutes; **7)** once the rice is cooked, spoon it on to a plate, make a little dip in the top of the rice; top the rice with the chicken mixture and then top with the spring onion and the juice from the remaining half of the lime; **8)** put the vegetables back on the heat for a moment, add the soy sauce and stir; spoon on to the plate beside the chicken and rice.

Spiced smoked salmon kedgeree

(560 kcal, 67 g carbohydrate, 29 g protein, 23 g fat)

INGREDIENTS

- Half an onion
- One tablespoon of vegetable oil
- One tablespoon of curry powder
- One egg
- 65 g white rice
- Half a teaspoon of turmeric
- 80 g frozen peas
- 50 g smoked salmon
- 10 g butter
- One teaspoon of parsley
- Salt
- Pepper

PREPARATION

1) Wash, rinse and drain the rice, then transfer to a pan and add 150 mL of cold water, the turmeric and a pinch of salt; cook for 12 minutes then stir in the frozen peas and cook for a further 2 minutes, until the water has evaporated; **2)** in another pan of water, boil the egg until just hard (about 5 minutes); remove from the heat, drain and run under cold water; once cooled, peel the egg and chop into quarters lengthwise; **3)** peel and finely slice the onion and warm the oil in a large frying pan, add the sliced onion and curry powder and fry over a low heat for 5 minutes; **4)** now add the butter and the rice/pea mixture; taste a bit, and add salt, pepper and more curry powder (if desired) to taste; **5)** mix in half the smoked salmon, then add the remaining salmon, eggs and parsley and garnish with a sprinkle of curry powder.

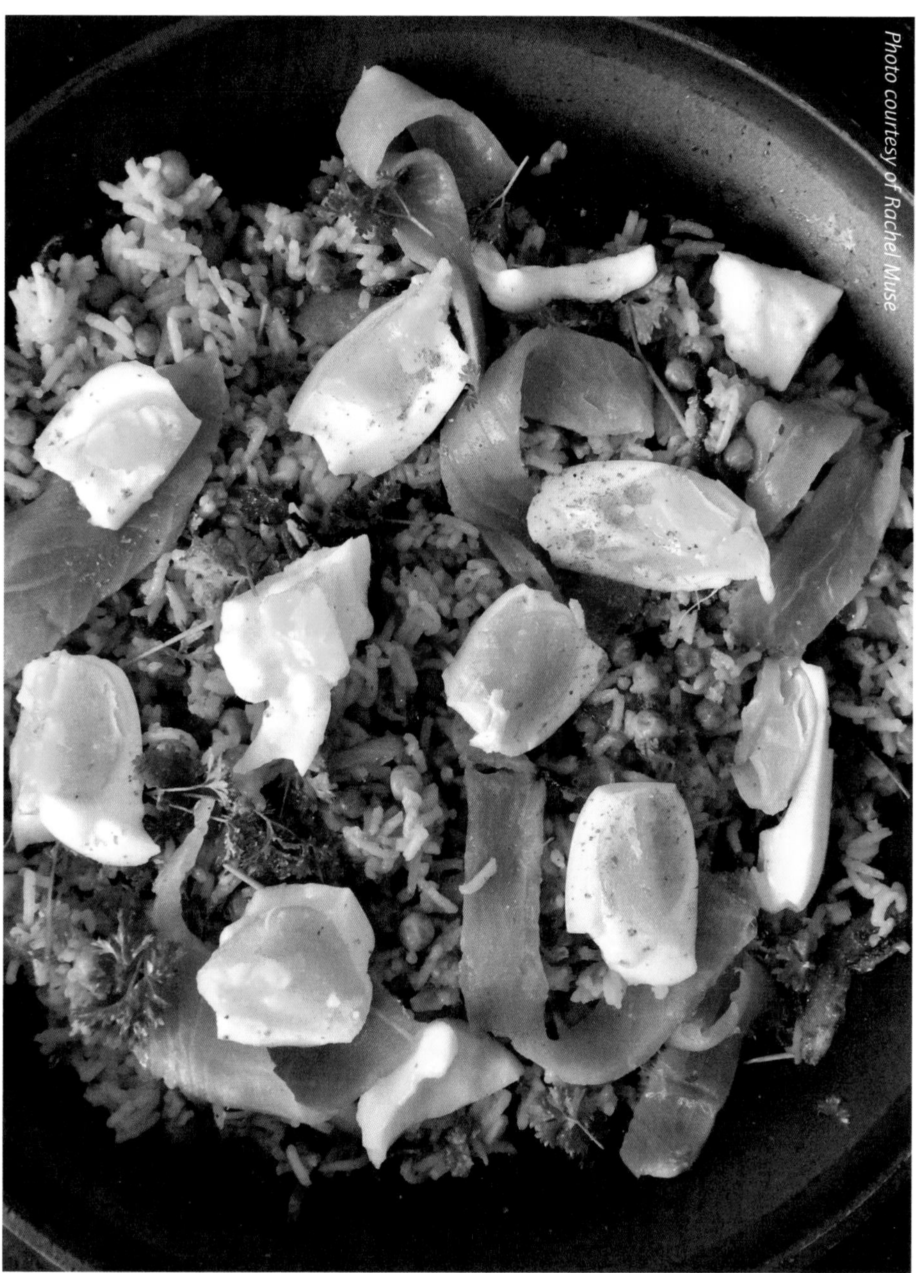
Photo courtesy of Rachel Muse

Photo 12.8 Spiced smoked salmon kedgeree.

Ginger beef and noodles

(640 kcal, 52 g carbohydrate, 59 g protein, 25 g fat)

INGREDIENTS

- 125 g rump steak
- 100 g mushrooms
- 150 g fresh egg noodles (not dried ones)
- Half a large onion
- Three spring onions
- Half a tablespoon of chilli sauce
- Half a tablespoon of ginger paste
- 15 mL sesame oil
- 20 mL soy sauce
- 50 g kale

PREPARATION

1) Mix half a teaspoon of oil and half a tablespoon of soy sauce and rub it into the steak on the plate; **2)** put the heat on low under the empty pan/wok, then chop the mushrooms and add to the pan with half a tablespoon of oil; fry for 1 minute then transfer to the serving bowl; fry the steak in the same pan; slice the onion and add it to the pan, with an

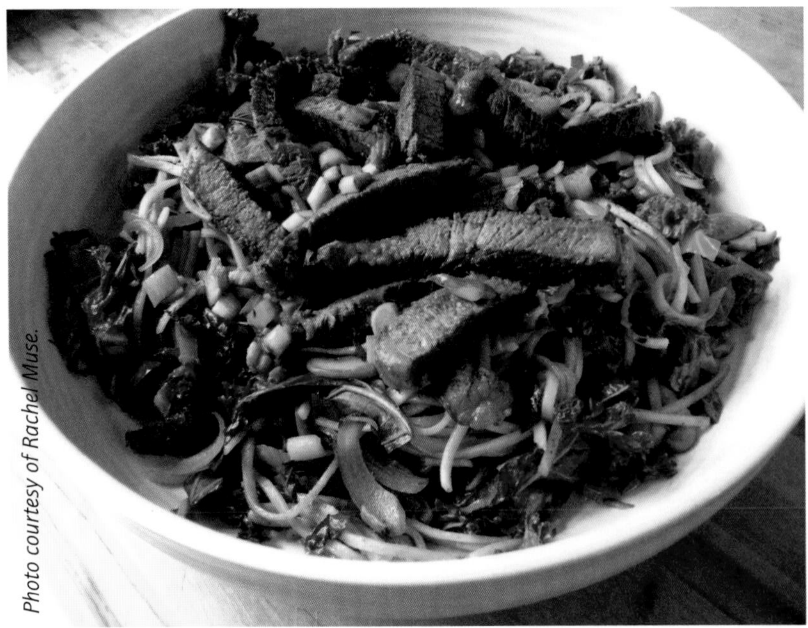
Photo courtesy of Rachel Muse.

Photo 12.9 Ginger beef and noodles.

extra half a teaspoon of oil, when you turn the steak; stir fry the onions around the steak; when cooked remove the steak and put on a chopping board; **3)** add the kale to the pan with the onion and stir until it wilts, then transfer to the serving bowl; **4)** add the noodles to the pan with half a teaspoon of oil, half a tablespoon of soy sauce, half a teaspoon of ginger paste and half a tablespoon of chilli sauce and stir well; add the kale, onions and mushrooms to the noodles, mix well and transfer to the serving bowl; **5)** slice the steak and chop the spring onions. add both to the pan with 1 teaspoon of oil and 1 tablespoon of soy sauce; fry for 1 minute then tip onto the noodles.

Vegan burgers with kidney bean salad

(810 kcal, 105 g carbohydrate, 32 g protein, 28 g fat)

INGREDIENTS FOR THE BURGER

- Half a can of red kidney beans, drained and liquid reserved
- 15 g nut butter of your choice
- 40 g oats
- Half a grated courgette (no need to peel)
- Pinch of salt
- One teaspoon of a spice of your choice (e.g. cumin, paprika, harissa etc)
- One finely sliced garlic clove
- Liquid from the beans (90 mL)
- One tablespoon of rapeseed oil

INGREDIENTS FOR THE SALAD

- Remaining red kidney beans from the can
- One teaspoon of chives
- Juice from half a lemon juice
- One tablespoon of olive oil
- Pinch of salt
- Pinch of sugar
- One small grated carrot (no need to peel)
- 80 g salad leaves
- One teaspoon of nuts or seeds

(continued)

(continued)

PREPARATION

1) In a large, flat-bottomed bowl, mash the beans for the burgers with a potato masher or with a fork but don't mash until all the beans are mashed – a few kidney beans should remain whole; add all the remaining burger ingredients to the mashed kidney beans except for the oil; mix together by hand until the liquid is absorbed by the oats; **2)** add the oil to a heavy-based frying pan on a medium heat, form the burger mixture into two patties and fry the patties in the pan for 5 minutes on each side; **3)** whilst the patties are frying, assemble the salad; place all the ingredients, except for the seeds and nuts, in a large bowl and mix together with your hands; **4)** place on the serving plate and top with seeds and nuts; as soon as the burgers are fried place next to the salad.

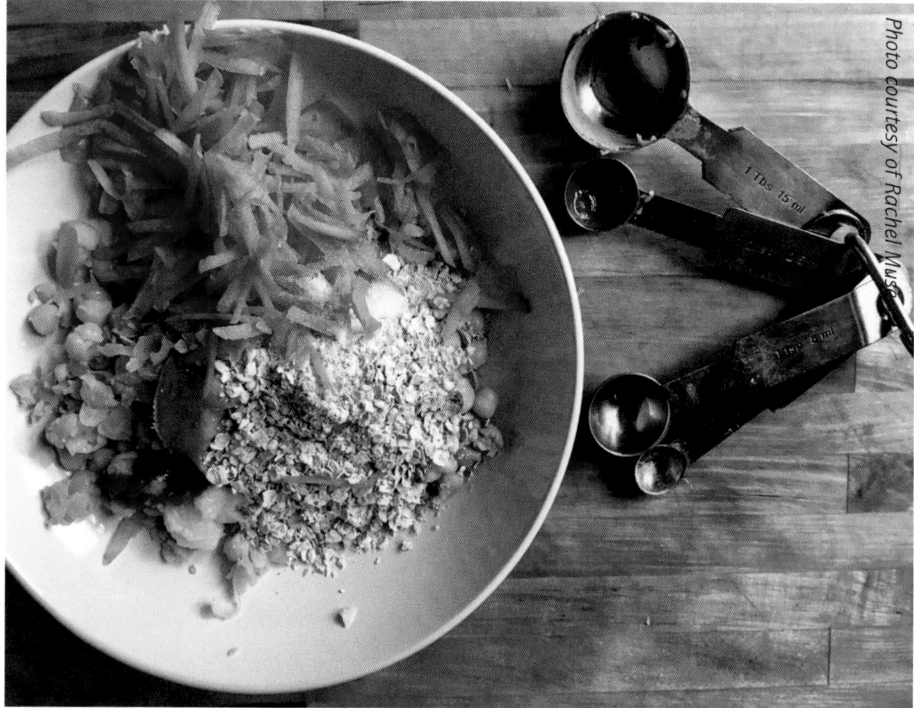

Photo 12.10 Vegan burger ingredients.

Here are some additional meal plans of my own.

Beef stifado stew with new potatoes

(820 kcal, 113 g carbohydrate, 51 g protein, 21 g fat)

INGREDIENTS

- 150 g lean beef, cubed
- 100 g shallots
- One large chopped onion
- One medium-sized tomato cut into wedges
- One clove of garlic
- One vegetable stock cube
- One tablespoon of rapeseed oil
- One tablespoon of red wine vinegar
- One tablespoon of tomato puree
- One bay leaf
- One teaspoon of dried rosemary
- Pinch of nutmeg
- Pinch of salt and black pepper.
- 50 g mixed salad leaves
- 250 g new potatoes
- One thick slice of whole-grain crusty bread

(continued)

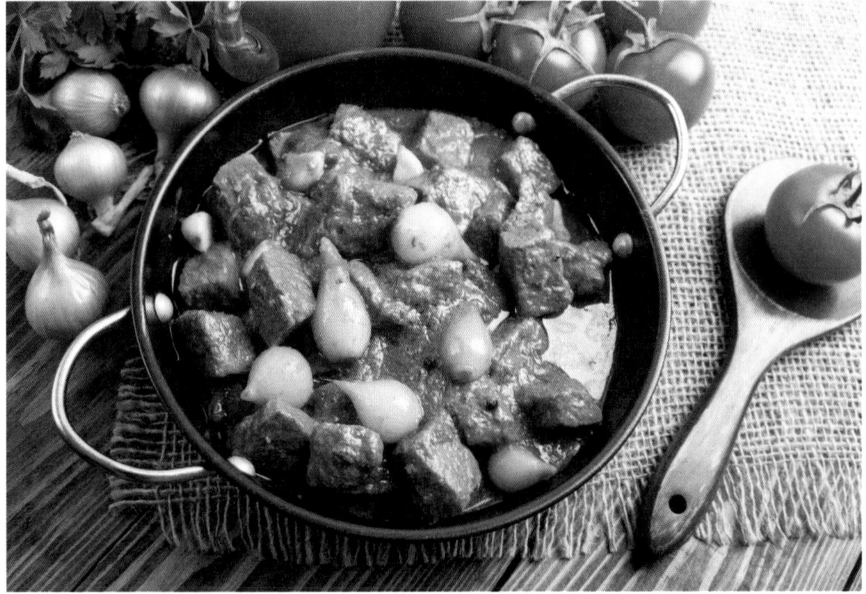

Photo 12.11 Beef stifado stew with onions and tomatoes.

(continued)

PREPARATION

1) Season the cubed beef with salt and pepper and fry in rapeseed oil until sealed; **2)** place the beef in a casserole dish and add chopped shallots, onion, tomato wedges, crushed clove of garlic, vegetable stock cube, red wine vinegar, tomato puree, bay leaf, dried rosemary and a pinch of nutmeg; **3)** serve with 50 g mixed salad leaves, 250 g steamed new potatoes and a thick slice of whole-grain crusty bread.

Seafood and chicken paella

(810 kcal, 104 g carbohydrate, 50 g protein, 22 g fat)

INGREDIENTS

- 100 g chopped chicken breast (skin removed)
- 70 g peeled prawns
- One tablespoon of rapeseed oil
- 50 g garden peas
- One chopped large red pepper
- One chopped medium-sized onion
- One vegetable stock cube dissolved in 200 mL water
- 100 g (uncooked weight) brown rice
- One teaspoon of parsley

PREPARATION

1) Slice the chicken breast into eight pieces and fry in the oil until cooked; **2)** add the prawns, peas, chopped pepper and onion and cook for an additional 10 minutes; **3)** in a separate pan, boil the brown rice for 15 minutes in the water containing the crushed vegetable stock cube and then add the meat and vegetables and simmer for 10 minutes; **4)** serve on a plate and sprinkle with parsley.

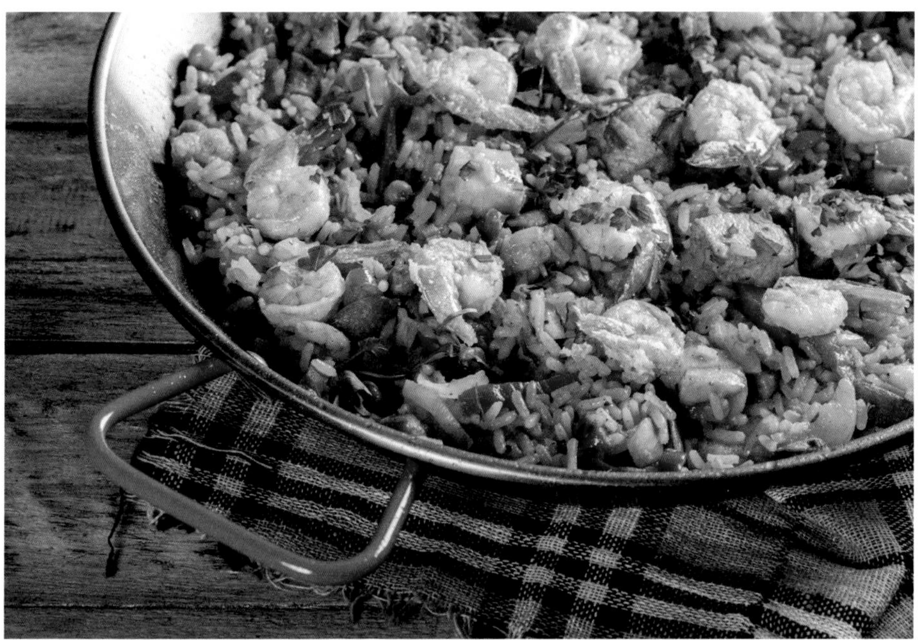

Photo 12.12 Traditional seafood paella with shrimp, fish, chicken and brown rice.

Chicken and mixed vegetable rice risotto

(800 kcal, 113 g carbohydrate, 48 g protein, 17 g fat)

INGREDIENTS

- 150 g diced chicken breast (skin removed)
- 20 g margarine
- One finely chopped garlic clove
- Half a cup of dry Arborio rice
- One vegetable stock cube dissolved in 150 mL boiling water
- 50 g canned chickpeas, drained and rinsed
- 100 g mixed fresh vegetables, such as asparagus, diced red pepper, baby corn, onion, sliced button mushroom

(continued)

(continued)

- Pinch of salt and black pepper
- One tablespoon of chopped fresh herbs, such as parsley or thyme
- One tablespoon of grated hard Italian cheese

PREPARATION

1) Slice the chicken breast into 12 small cubes, season with salt and pepper and fry in the margarine until sealed; **2)** add the chopped garlic and chickpeas followed by the boiled water containing the vegetable stock cube and simmer for 5 minutes; **3)** add the Arborio rice and the vegetables, add one tablespoon of chopped fresh herbs and simmer until the rice is cooked; **4)** after cooking, sprinkle on one tablespoon of grated hard Italian cheese.

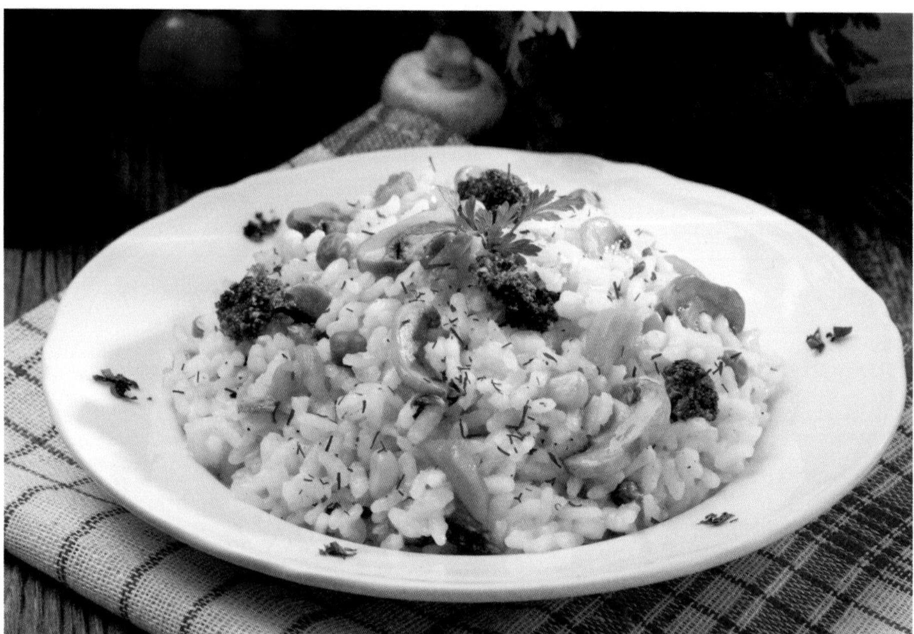

Photo 12.13 Mixed vegetable rice risotto.

Meat and vegetable skewer with egg noodles

(800 kcal, 105 g carbohydrate, 61 g protein, 16 g fat)

INGREDIENTS

- 200 g diced large cubes of lean lamb, pork, beef or chicken
- Three 25 cm (10 in) metal skewers
- Six medium-sized tomatoes
- One courgette (zucchini), cut into six pieces
- One large onion
- One aubergine (eggplant) cut into cubes
- One red, green or yellow pepper
- 300 g (cooked weight) of boiled or microwavable egg noodles

PREPARATION

1) Place the cubes of meat alternated with the tomato, courgette, aubergine, onion and peppers on three skewers and grill for 10–15 minutes turning the skewers occasionally until the meat is thoroughly cooked; **2)** serve with 300 g (cooked weight) of boiled or microwavable egg noodles.

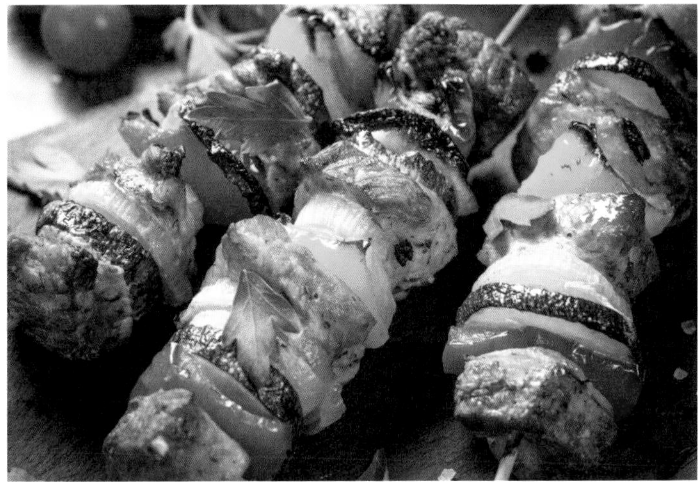

Photo 12.14 Grilled pork on skewers with tomato, zucchini, onion and peppers.

Fruity desserts

(All about 100–200 kcal, mostly from carbohydrate)

Cup of mixed chopped fruits (e.g. apple, grapes, persimmon, nectarine, melon, cherries, blueberries, raspberries, strawberries) with one tablespoon of Greek yoghurt and four crushed walnut halves.

- 12 strawberries with one tablespoon of low-fat crème fraîche, Greek yoghurt or vanilla ice cream.
- 120 g chopped watermelon with a dozen grapes.
- 120 g slice of Honeydew or Piel de Sapo (frog skin) melon sprinkled with ginger powder.
- Peeled segments from one medium-sized orange or large satsuma with 20 blueberries.
- One 50 g piece of chocolate ice cream with 10 strawberries sprinkled with one tablespoon of shredded coconut.

DINNERS

The main meals contain 600–1,000 kcal with 40–120 g CHO, at least 40 g protein and some fat. They can be followed by a dessert (approximately 200 kcal). The lower energy meals (600–800 kcal) can be preceded by a soup or salad starter like the ones shown below. This allows the inclusion of more of the nonessential but health-promoting nutrients fibre and phytonutrients, which are needed for optimal health – something everyone should be aspiring to attain. The meals can be accompanied by a drink of water, fruit juice (e.g. orange, apple, grape, tomato – using the no added sugar versions), non-alcoholic beer or wine, or a hot beverage (e.g. green tea, coffee) as desired. Several of these meals (chicken teriyaki, chilli con carne and mixed bean salad followed by cod loin in tomato sauce with macaroni) are suitable for the important evening dinner on the day before a match, and these courses can be followed by any one of the desserts.

Soup or salad starters

Beef and vegetable, chicken noodle, lentil and bacon, pea and ham, broccoli and stilton soups etc (400 mL – a full can) and a crusty whole-grain bread roll (340 kcal, 48 g carbohydrate, 18 g protein, 7 g fat).

Mixed green leaf salad

60 g mixed green salad leaves (e.g. lettuce, rocket, watercress, spinach) with two stalks of chopped celery, one medium-sized tomato, five spring onions, five pitted green olives and one diced 25 g thin slice of roast ham, drizzled with juice from half a squeezed lime or lemon. Serve with one slice of toasted wholemeal bread (260 kcal, 30 g carbohydrate, 13 g protein, 12 g fat).

Greek salad

Greek salad made with five olives, two large vine tomatoes cut into wedges, half a chopped red onion, 50 g cubed peeled cucumber and 30 g feta cheese cut into chunks. Drizzled with one teaspoon of extra virgin olive oil, juice from half a lemon and sprinkled with dried oregano. Serve with one slice of crusty whole-grain bread (310 kcal, 32 g carbohydrate, 12 g protein, 16 g fat).

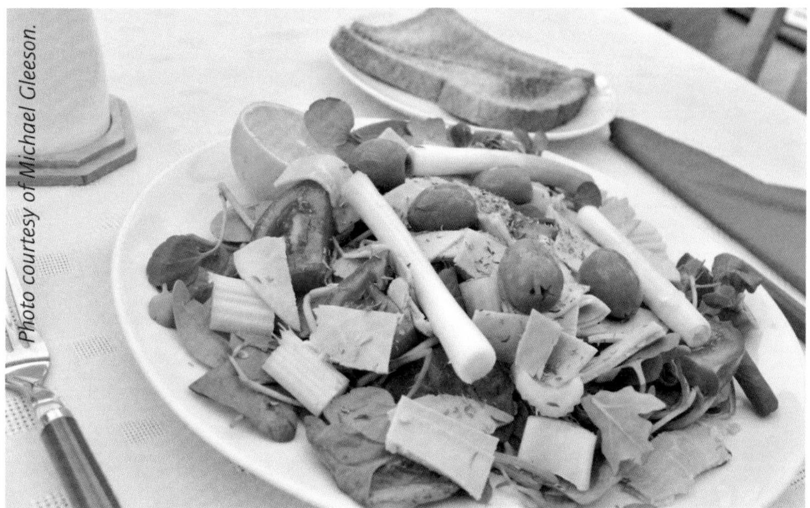

Photo 12.15 Mixed leaf salad with spring onion, green olives and diced roast ham with a slice of toasted wholemeal bread.

Mixed bean salad

Mixed bean salad made with half a can (200g) of mixed beans (e.g. red kidney, black eye, barlotti, green lima, pea navy, cannelloni beans) and 50 g beansprouts with one slice of crusty whole-grain bread (320 kcal, 55 g carbohydrate, 18 g protein, 4 g fat).

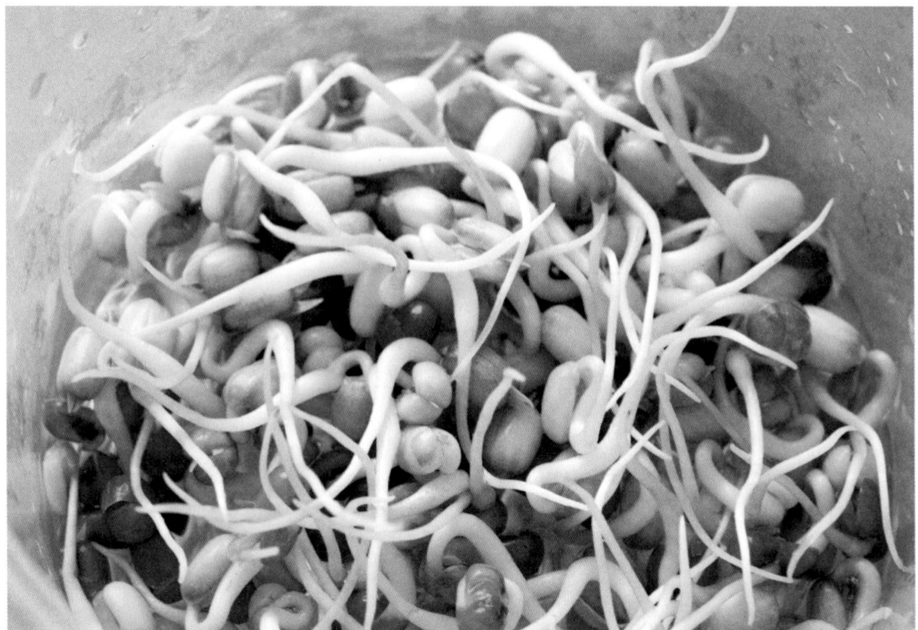

Photo 12.16 Mixed bean salad.

Main meals

Baked cod loin in tomato sauce with macaroni

(730 kcal, 120 g carbohydrate, 57 g protein, 4 g fat)

INGREDIENTS

- 200 g cod loin
- Half a can of chopped tomatoes
- A few slices of aubergine (eggplant) and courgette (zucchini)
- One chopped red pepper
- One chopped medium-sized onion
- 50 g mixed salad leaves
- 100 g (uncooked weight) macaroni

PREPARATION

1) Oven-bake the cod loin in a casserole dish with the chopped tomato and mixed vegetables for 40 minutes at 180°C; **2)** boil the macaroni as per instructions until soft and place on a plate; **3)** placed the cooked cod in tomato over the top of the macaroni and serve with the mixed salad leaves.

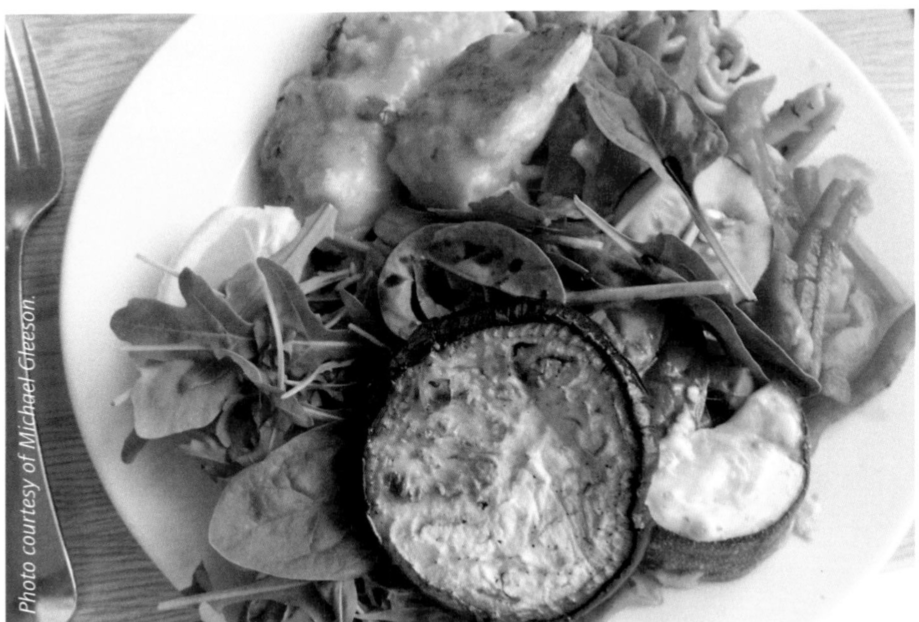

Photo 12.17 Oven-baked cod loin in tomato sauce with macaroni, mixed vegetables and salad leaves.

Beef stir-fry

(900 kcal, 109 g carbohydrate, 74 g protein, 25 g fat)

INGREDIENTS

- 200 g beef rump steak strips
- 100 g beansprouts
- Five sliced mushrooms
- One sliced red or green pepper
- One medium-sized, chopped onion or 30 g water chestnuts
- Two teaspoons of rapeseed oil
- Two tablespoons of dark soya sauce
- Two cups of boiled whole-wheat pasta

PREPARATION

1) Fry the beef rump steak strips in the rapeseed oil for 5 minutes; **2)** add the sliced mushrooms, pepper and onion (or water chestnuts) and fry for an additional 5 minutes; **3)** add the beansprouts and dark soya sauce and cook for 2 minutes more; **4)** serve with two cups of boiled whole-wheat pasta.

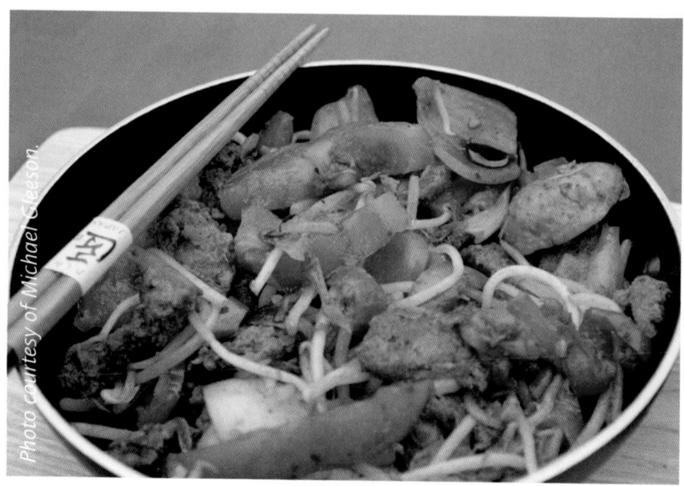

Photo 12.18 Beef stir-fry made with beef rump steak strips, beansprouts, mushrooms, pepper, onions and soya sauce.

Chicken teriyaki

(820 kcal, 98 g carbohydrate, 54 g protein, 23 g fat)

INGREDIENTS

- 200 g sliced chicken breast (skin removed)
- One tablespoon of Japanese soy sauce
- One tablespoon of sake
- Two tablespoons of mirin (or a sweet white wine)
- One tablespoon of honey
- One teaspoon of grated ginger
- One crushed garlic clove
- One tablespoon of rapeseed oil
- One teaspoon of ground black pepper
- One finely chopped small green chilli
- 200 g boiled white rice
- 80 g broccoli florets

PREPARATION

1) Fry the sliced chicken breast in the rapeseed oil until thoroughly cooked; **2)** prepare the teriyaki sauce in a pan by combining the Japanese soy sauce, sake, mirin, honey, grated ginger, crushed garlic, ground black pepper and chopped green chilli and bringing it to the boil and simmering for 2 minutes; **3)** boil the rice until soft; **4)** steam the broccoli for 15 minutes; **5)** plate out the rice and mix in the broccoli, place the chicken on top and pour over the teriyaki sauce.

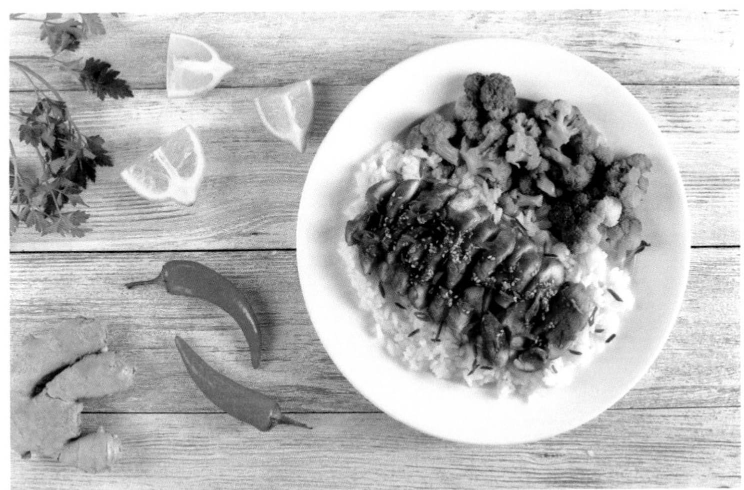

Photo 12.19 Teriyaki chicken breast with boiled white rice and broccoli.

Chilli con carne

(880 kcal, 111 g carbohydrate, 62 g protein, 21 g fat)

INGREDIENTS

» 200 g beef cubes or lean mince (5% fat)
» Two teaspoons of rapeseed oil
» One chopped large onion
» 100 g red kidney beans
» Half a can of chopped tomatoes
» One tablespoon of hot red chilli powder
» 200 g boiled white or brown rice

PREPARATION

1) Sear the beef or mince for a few minutes in a frying pan with the rapeseed oil; **2)** add the meat to a casserole dish with the chopped onion, red kidney beans, chopped tomatoes and chilli powder and cook in an oven for 60 minutes at 180°C; **3)** serve with 200 g boiled white or brown rice.

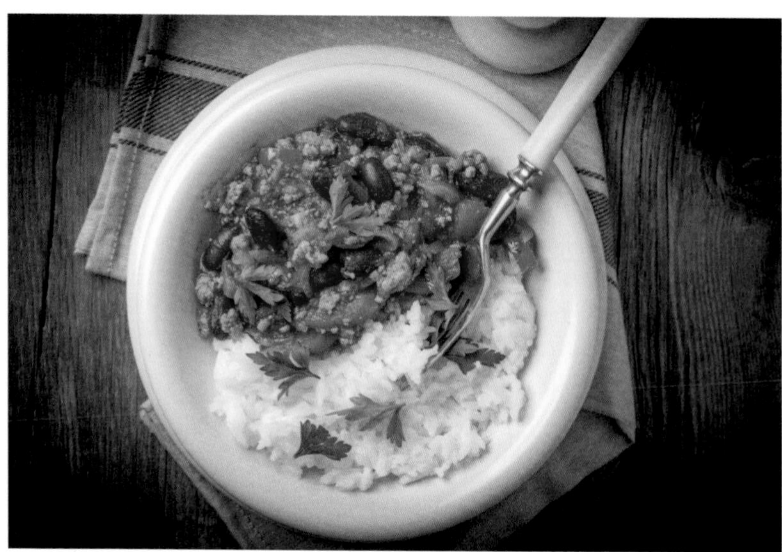

Photo 12.20 Chilli con carne made with lean minced beef, accompanied by boiled white rice.

The meal recipes for the main courses, sauces and desserts that follow have been created by elite performance chef Rachel Muse.

Roast chicken with spice, roast Mediterranean vegetables and couscous

(820 kcal, 58 g carbohydrate, 44 g protein, 40 g fat)

The recipe described here involves cooking a whole 1.2 kg chicken providing two breasts, two drumsticks and two thighs, which can be used in other lunches or dinners on subsequent days.

INGREDIENTS FOR THE CHICKEN

- One roast chicken breast (skin removed)
- One tablespoon of rapeseed oil
- One tablespoon of Soy sauce (or Worcestershire sauce)
- One large brown onion
- Two teaspoons of your preferred spice (e.g. cumin, paprika, curry powder, chilli powder etc.)

PREPARATION

1) Pre-heat the oven to 180ºC; line a roasting tray with aluminium foil and pour the oil and the soy sauce onto the centre of the foil; roll the chicken around in the oil and sauce and sprinkle on your choice of spice; finish with the chicken on its front (breast side), with the back facing up and place the peeled and quartered onion under the chicken so the chicken is balanced on top of the onion sections; **2)** roast the chicken in the oven for 50 minutes, then turn it over and roast for a further 15 minutes to brown the breast; **3)** remove from oven and allow to rest for 10 minutes, which allows the juices in the meat to remain in the flesh when the chicken is cut into, meaning that it will be juicy rather than dry when it's eaten; **4)** once rested, cut the legs off and then cut down the middle of the breast, either side of the breastbone; allow the rest of the bird to cool until it is at room temperature, then put on a plate, cover and put in the fridge; the chicken must be eaten within four days; **5)** use the juice from the bottom of the roasting tray to pour over the chicken as a 'gravy'.

INGREDIENTS FOR THE MEDITERRANEAN VEGETABLES

- Choose three of the five following vegetables:
- Courgette, medium-sized
- Pepper (colour of your choice)
- Brown onion, medium-sized
- Aubergine, small
- Tomato, large
- Two tablespoons of rapeseed oil
- Half a teaspoon of sea salt
- Half a teaspoon of granulated sugar
- Sprig of fresh rosemary, or half a teaspoon of dried rosemary

PREPARATION

1) If using onion, top and tail it with a sharp knife and then peel it; all other vegetables just wash and don't peel; cut the vegetables into slightly larger-than-bite-sized chunks (they will shrink slightly during cooking); once each vegetable is cut into chunks put it in a section of a baking tray – the idea is to keep each vegetable in a separate section because one type of vegetable may cook slightly quicker than the others and if they aren't all mixed together one of the types of the vegetable can removed from the oven before the others; **2)** if using fresh rosemary, pull the leaves off the stalk and roughly chop, then drizzle the oil, salt, rosemary and sugar over the vegetables; **3)** cook for 35–40 minutes at 180ºC until your preferred level of 'doneness'; if one of the groups of vegetables is done ahead of time, remove it with a fish slice.

INGREDIENTS FOR THE COUSCOUS

- 60 g couscous (whole-grain, ideally)
- Half a stock cube (chicken or vegetable)
- Boiling water (90 mL)
- 100 g spinach (or rocket)
- Half a lemon

PREPARATION

1) In a cup or jug, make up the stock with the stock cube and the boiling water, stir until the stock cube dissolves; **2)** place the couscous in a bowl and pour the stock on the couscous and stir; cover with a plate, leave for 10 minutes then take off the plate and stir; the couscous will have absorbed the majority of the water; replace the plate and leave another 5 minutes; **3)** stir in the spinach or rocket, replace the plate and let stand until you are ready to serve; just before you want to serve, squeeze on the juice of half a lemon; **4)** finally, assemble the roast chicken portion, roast vegetables and couscous on a plate and season with a mill of black pepper.

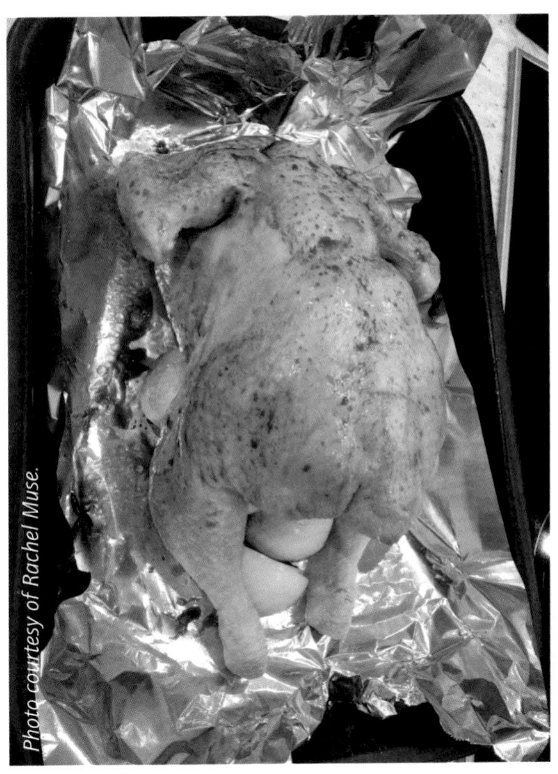

Photo 12.21 Roasting a whole chicken.

Steak and sweet potato wedges with salad

(870 kcal, 50 g carbohydrate, 48 g protein, 59 g fat)

INGREDIENTS

- Steak of choice 200 g (4 or 5 cm thick); tuna can be used instead of beef
- One large sweet potato
- Two tablespoons of rapeseed oil
- Sea salt and pepper
- 80 g salad leaves of choice
- Quarter of a red onion
- Six cherry tomatoes
- Juice from half a lemon
- Two teaspoons of olive oil
- Two tablespoons of low-fat crème fraîche
- Two teaspoons of mustard (or 20 g blue cheese, or one teaspoon of green peppercorns) for the steak sauce

PREPARATION

1) Take the steak out of the fridge and pre-heat the oven to 180ºC; **2)** wash the sweet potatoes and, with a sharp knife, top and tail but don't peel the sweet potato; cut them in half widthways, then, with the potato cut side on the board, cut in half and then in half again, each potato will be cut into eight wedges; **3)** take a baking tray and add one tablespoon of rapeseed oil; using your hands, roll the wedges in the oil, add a pinch of salt and roll about again; spread the wedges out on the tray and put in the oven for 20 minutes; **4)** meanwhile, make the sauce: in a small bowl place the crème fraîche, if using blue cheese, crumble it in and mix, taste, and add salt and pepper to taste; if using mustard or green peppercorns, mix into the crème fraîche and add a pinch of salt if needed; **5)** now assemble the salad: wash the leaves and the tomatoes and pat dry with kitchen paper; cut the tomatoes in half and, on the chopping board, season with a pinch of sugar and a pinch of salt; put the leaves and the tomatoes in the bowl you will use to serve the salad; peel the red onion, slice thinly and add to the salad; at the last moment before serving, add the olive oil and lemon juice to the salad; **6)** remove the wedges from the oven and turn the wedges, using two forks or tongs, so the surface that was in contact with the tray is now facing upwards; sprinkle on a little more salt; from this point the wedges will need another 15 or 20 minutes to finish cooking, depending on thickness; when the wedges are browning they are done; **7)** pour a tablespoon of rapeseed oil on a saucer or small plate; to fry the steak, take a thick-bottomed frying pan and put, empty, on a medium heat; season the steak with sea salt and black pepper then lay it flat in the saucer of oil on both sides then fry the steak in the hot pan for one minute on each side using a fork or tongs to turn; if the pan is smoking, turn the heat down slightly; for cooking, cook each side for one minute at a time following the guide below for the desired level of 'doneness'(for a 5 cm thick steak), then rest on a clean chopping board for 5 minutes, covered with a plate.

- Blue 2 minutes a side.
- Rare 2 minutes 30 seconds a side.
- Medium rare 3 minutes 45 seconds a side.
- Medium 5 minutes a side.
- Medium well 6 minutes 30 seconds a side.
- Well done 7 minutes 30 seconds a side.

8) Once the steak is out of the pan, assemble the other elements of the dish: take the sweet potato fries out of the oven, squeeze the lemon juice onto the salad, add the olive oil and a bit of salt, pepper and a small pinch of sugar; toss to combine; **9)** put the sauce in a jug ready to serve, and place the steak and the sweet potato fries on the serving plate.

Note: you can use this exact recipe for making tuna steaks, although, for a sauce, I would suggest crème fraîche with the juice of half a lemon, a pinch of salt and some finely chopped spring onions all mixed together.

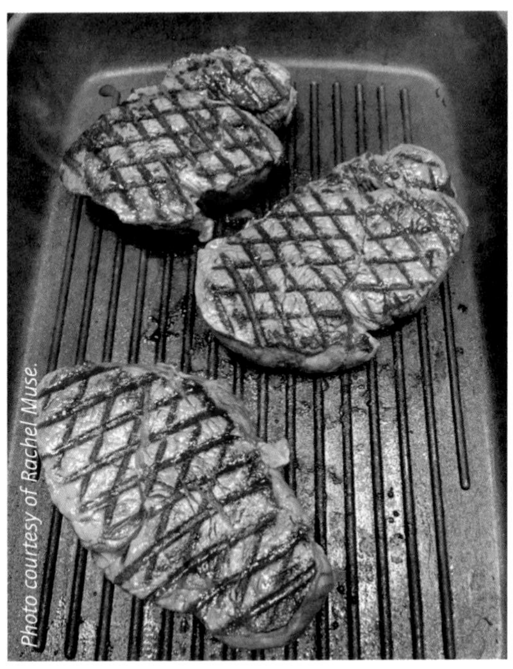

Photo 12.22 Frying beef steaks.

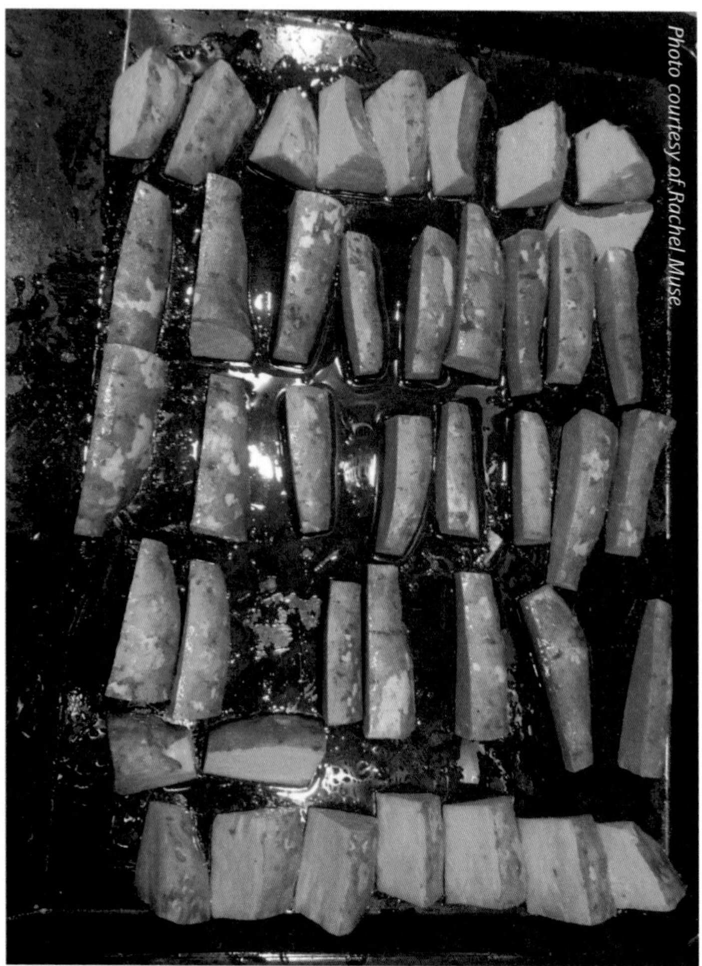

Photo 12.23 Sweet potato wedges ready to roast.

Salmon with spinach pesto and new potatoes

(970 kcal, 45 g carbohydrate, 66 g protein, 60 g fat)

INGREDIENTS

» 250 g salmon

» One tablespoon of rapeseed oil

- 100 g cherry tomatoes (about six)
- 40 g green pesto
- 50 g spinach (a handful)
- 200 g new potatoes
- 70 g frozen or fresh peas (three tablespoons)
- 100 g asparagus or tenderstem broccoli
- Salt and pepper

PREPARATION

1) Pre-heat oven to 180ºC; if you have a large frying pan with a handle that can go in the oven (i.e. not plastic) this recipe is an ideal chance to use it; **2)** boil the new potatoes in a pan that's a bit too big, with a bit too much water, since this pan will also be used to briefly boil the asparagus or tenderstem broccoli; **3)** cut the salmon in half; heat the frying pan with the oil and when the oil is hot place the salmon in, skin side up, and cook until just browned (about 2–3 minutes); turn over and cook skin side for 2–3 minutes; add the cherry tomatoes and roll around in the oil; season with salt and pepper; if the frying pan can go in the oven, then put it in the oven, otherwise place the salmon and the tomatoes on a baking sheet covered in aluminium foil; **4)** put the pesto and spinach in a food processor or NutriBullet with a pinch of salt and blend until smooth; **5)** once the potatoes have been boiling for 10 minutes and are half done, add the asparagus or tenderstem broccoli to the pan, leave for a minute then take the asparagus or broccoli out of the pan with a fork and put in a bowl; **6)** put the asparagus or tenderstem broccoli into the oven in with the salmon and the tomatoes; add the peas to the potatoes and cook a further 5 minutes, then drain the potatoes and peas; **7)** carefully remove the salmon from the oven (if you have been using a frying pan make sure you remove the pan from the oven with an oven glove as it will be very hot); **8)** plate up the salmon, the tomatoes and the asparagus (or broccoli), add a tablespoon of the pesto mix to the potatoes and peas and plate up; use the remaining pesto to drizzle over the salmon.

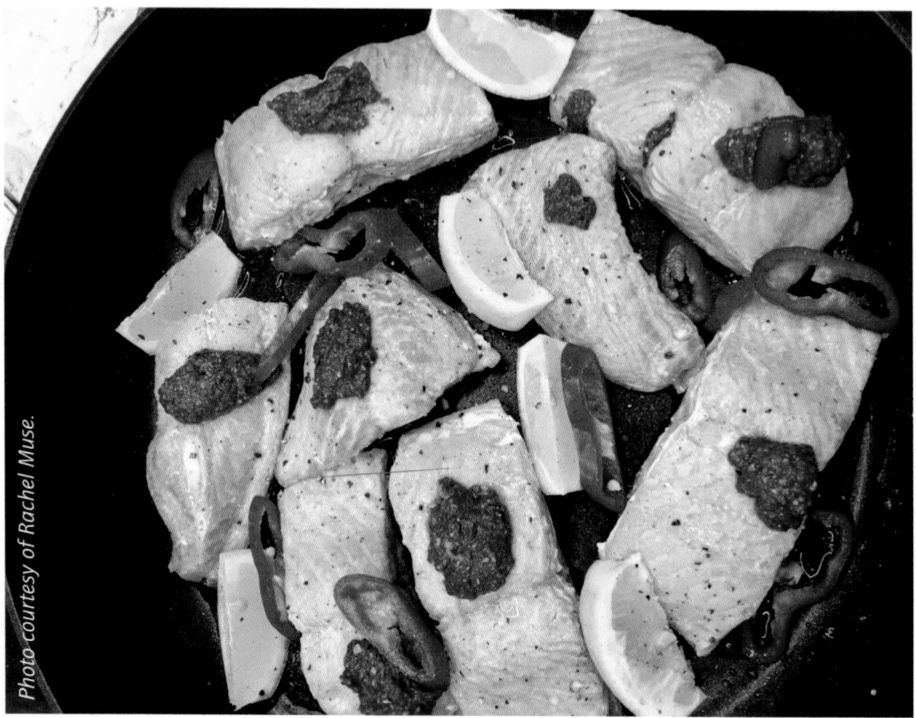

Photo 12.24 Salmon with spinach pesto.

Chicken drumsticks with mustard potato salad and boiled eggs

(840 kcal, 39 g carbohydrate, 40 g protein, 48 g fat)

INGREDIENTS

- Two pre-cooked roast chicken drumsticks (skin on)
- 200 g new potatoes
- Two eggs

- One teaspoon of mustard
- One tablespoon of yoghurt
- Three pinches of sea salt
- Pinch of sugar
- Juice from half a lemon
- Two teaspoons of olive oil
- 80 g salad leaves
- Black pepper

PREPARATION

1) Remove the drumsticks from the roast chicken and place on a dinner plate; **2)** boil the new potatoes in a pan that's a bit too big, using one pinch of salt; **3)** in a medium-sized bowl mix sugar, lemon juice, a small pinch of salt and olive oil; **4)** after 10 minutes when the potatoes are half cooked add the two eggs to the boiling water; after cooking for 20 minutes remove the potatoes and eggs from the heat; drain, put the potatoes and eggs back in the pan and refill it with cool water; **5)** mix the salad leaves into the lemon juice and olive oil mixture and place on the plate with the drumsticks; peel the eggs and slice onto the salad leaves; **6)** drain the cold water from the potatoes and cut in half and place in a little bowl; add the yoghurt, a mini pinch of salt and the mustard to the potatoes and stir to combine; add potato salad to the serving plate and add a few twists of pepper from the pepper mill.

Lamb (or beef) kebabs with cauliflower rice and tomato salsa

(880 kcal, 43 g carbohydrate, 62 g protein, 52 g fat)

INGREDIENTS

- 200 g diced lean lamb (or beef) rump
- One medium-sized red onion

(continued)

(continued)

- Two teaspoons of cumin or spice of choice
- Two teaspoons of chopped herb of choice (chives, parsley, basil)
- Sea salt and pepper
- Pinch of sugar
- One tablespoon of rapeseed oil
- One medium-sized cauliflower head
- Two medium-sized tomatoes
- Two tablespoons of crème fraîche or yoghurt
- One clove of garlic

PREPARATION

1) You'll also need two metal skewers or wooden skewers that have been soaked in water; pre-heat the oven to 180ºC; **2)** put the lamb in a plastic or china bowl; peel and halve the onion; in a food blender or NutriBullet put half the onion and the spice of choice, process until smooth, pour onto the lamb and stir so that the lamb is covered; **3)** line a baking tray with aluminium foil and pour on the oil; with a sharp knife, cut the florets from the cauliflower and place half the florets into the food processor and process until the cauliflower looks like grains of rice; remove from the processor and put on the sheet of foil on the baking tray, then repeat with the other half of the cauliflower; add two pinches of salt to the cauliflower and mix with your hands; pat the cauliflower down to an even layer of about 1 cm and place in the oven; **4)** roughly chop the herb and place in a small bowl, then cut the tomatoes in half and then into cubes and add to the herb; season with a pinch of salt and a pinch of sugar; **5)** put the yoghurt or crème fraîche in a small bowl; peel then chop the garlic clove as finely as possible and mix the garlic into the yoghurt with a pinch of salt; **6)** cut the remaining onion half into four pieces, take the lamb and thread on to the two skewers, at some point on each skewer, place two sections of onion; once the lamb is on the kebabs season with salt and pepper; **7)** take the cauliflower out of the oven and, with a fish slice, carefully pick it up and turn it over without ripping the foil underneath; **8)** cover a second baking tray with foil and a drizzle of oil, then place the lamb skewers on the tray and cook for 5 minutes a side; remove kebabs from the oven, place on a clean chopping board and cover with a plate; **9)** while the lamb is resting, assemble the dish: place the cauliflower rice on a plate; pour any liquid that has come off the kebabs onto the cauliflower; place the kebabs on top of the rice, top the kebabs with the garlic yoghurt and serve with the tomato salsa on the side.

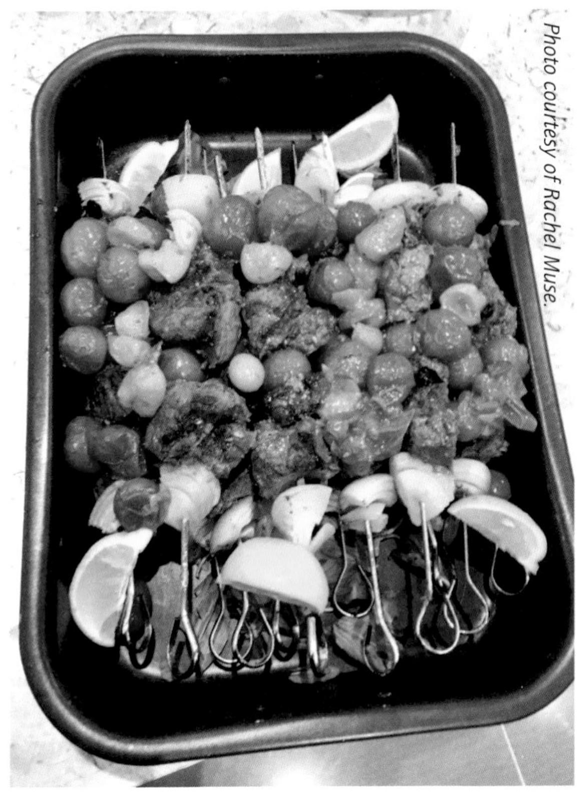

Photo courtesy of Rachel Muse.

Photo 12.25 Meat kebabs.

Sauces

Mustard dill sauce with crème fraîche

This sauce works really well to add a bit of excitement to meat, fish, or in a sandwich instead of mayonnaise; or as a dip for raw vegetables. It's more than one portion, but it keeps well in the fridge. If you can't find crème fraîche, low-fat sour cream works just as well. It's important that everything is super clean for this recipe because then the sauce will keep for a week in the fridge; otherwise, it will only keep for a day or two.

(120 kcal, 10 g carbohydrate, 1 g protein, 8 g fat) per portion (two tablespoons)

INGREDIENTS (TO MAKE SIX PORTIONS)

- Half a tub of low-fat crème fraîche (150 mL)
- Two teaspoons of mustard

(continued)

(continued)

- One sprig of dill (ideally fresh, but if not use half a teaspoon of dried dill)
- Half a teaspoon of sea salt
- Pinch of granulated sugar

PREPARATION

1) In a super clean lidded container (e.g. old jam jar or Tupperware) mix crème fraîche, mustard, salt and sugar together; **2)** if using fresh dill, wash it and dry it on kitchen paper and use scissors to cut dill into 5 mm lengths, straight into the crème fraîche; stir to combine, with a completely clean spoon; taste and add more mustard and salt (if desired) to suit your own taste.

Fake cream

This is the sweet version of the mustard/dill sauce and also a great way to use up the other half of the tub of crème fraîche. Use a dollop of it to make banana cakes into a pudding then garnish with berries, or serve with any sliced fruit. The recipe is more than one portion and it keeps well in the fridge so it can be used over the course of a week, provided that everything you use is super clean.

(90 kcal, 1 g carbohydrate, 1 g protein, 9 g fat) per portion (two tablespoons)

INGREDIENTS (TO MAKE FIVE PORTIONS)

- Half a tub of low-fat crème fraîche (150 mL)
- Half a teaspoon of vanilla essence (the best quality you can afford)

PREPARATION

1) In a clean lidded container (e.g. old jam jar or Tupperware) mix the crème fraîche with the vanilla with a super clean spoon; **2)** and that's it, as somehow the vanilla tricks our brains into thinking the crème fraîche tastes much sweeter!

Mango and avocado salsa

This makes enough for four portions as it is pretty much impossible to do it for one, and it is best eaten immediately or the avocado will go brown.

(150 kcal, 22 g carbohydrate, 2 g protein, 8 g fat) per portion (two tablespoons)

INGREDIENTS (TO MAKE FOUR PORTIONS)

- Small bunch of fresh coriander
- Half a small red onion
- One mango
- One avocado
- One orange
- Pinch of salt

PREPARATION

1) Top and tail the mango and slice the peel off with a sharp knife; then carve the flesh from round the stone and finely dice it; **2)** top and tail the orange and slice the peel off with a sharp knife; holding the peeled orange in one hand, use the knife to slice into the middle and remove the segments, leaving the membranes behind; chop into pieces the same size as the mango; **3)** finely dice the onion, halve the avocado and use the knife to remove the stone; cut into quarters and peel the skin off, then dice into pieces the same size as the mango and orange; **4)** finely chop the coriander, stalks included, then add everything to a bowl with a pinch of salt and mix well.

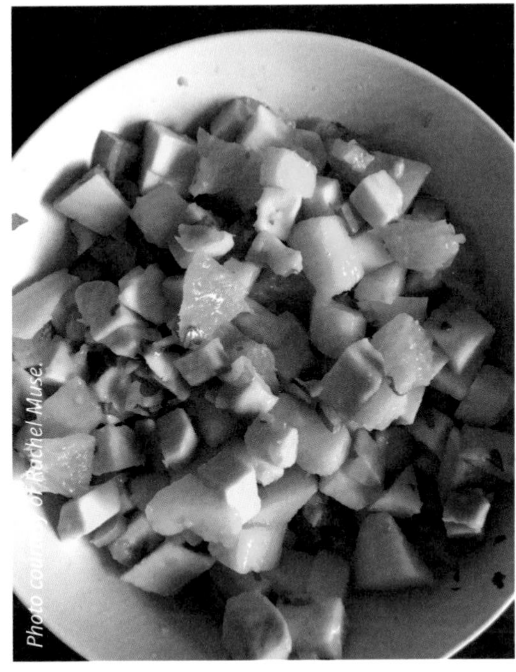

Photo 12.26 Mango and avocado salsa.

Desserts

Chocolate banana muffins

This will make eight muffins. Best eaten straight out of the oven, or can be allowed to cool to room temperature then put in an airtight container and eaten the following day. Keeps for up to three days.

(440 kcal, 60 g carbohydrate, 10 g protein, 18 g fat) per portion (two muffins)

INGREDIENTS (TO MAKE EIGHT MUFFINS)

» 140 g self-raising flour

» Pinch of sea salt

» Three tablespoons of vegetable oil

» 75 g light brown sugar (ideally but granulated sugar is fine)

» One egg

» Three medium-sized ripe bananas

» 50 g chocolate chips or chopped nuts

» Half a teaspoon of vanilla extract (optional)

PREPARATION

1) Pre-heat the oven to 180ºC; **2)** in large flat-bottomed bowl, mash the bananas with a potato masher and place all other ingredients on top of the mashed bananas; mix together with a wooden spoon (but not too much: very slightly under mixed with tiny pockets of white flour still visible is better than overmixed as it starts to go too elastic; **3)** set eight paper muffin cases in a muffin tin and divide the mixture into the paper cases with a wooden spoon; bake for 13–15 minutes, or until risen and the tops are just starting to 'crack'.

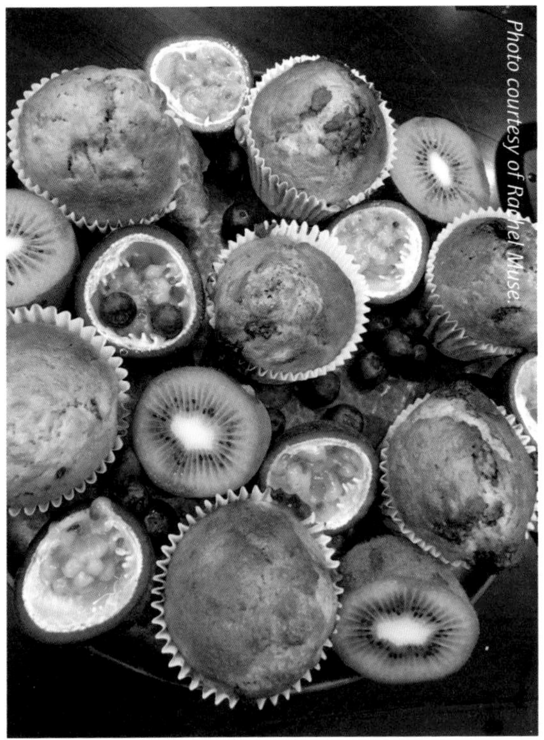

Photo 12.27 Chocolate banana muffins.

Strawberries dipped in chocolate

(370 kcal, 50 g carbohydrate, 5 g protein, 17 g fat)

INGREDIENTS

- 250 g strawberries
- 50 g dark chocolate
- Two teaspoons of vegetable oil
- Pinch of sea salt

PREPARATION

1) Wash and dry the strawberries; I leave the green leaves on the strawberries because I like the clash of colour, but feel free to cut off the very top of the strawberry and remove

(continued)

(continued)

the leaves; **2)** put the chocolate and oil and the smallest amount of salt that's visible to the naked eye into a non-metallic bowl; either microwave for 40 seconds initially, then in batches of 20 seconds on high until melted, stirring with a teaspoon between each 20 seconds to assess the melting process, or set the bowl above a little saucepan of boiling water over a low heat and stir on and off until melted; **3)** take a dinner plate and cover it with cling film; put the bowl of melted chocolate half on and half off a scrunched-up tea towel so that the bowl is at an angle and then take each strawberry and dip it in the deep end of the liquid chocolate; the chocolate will stick to the bottom of the strawberry so each strawberry will be half covered in chocolate; if you have cut off the leaves you may need to use a fork to help with the dipping process; if the strawberries are cold, then the chocolate may cool down a bit and start to thicken up, if so gently reheat until just liquid again; **4)** now put the dipped strawberries on the cling-filmed plate, placing the strawberries close together on the plate otherwise you will run out of space on the plate; **5)** if you have any leftover chocolate, dip a teaspoon into the chocolate and use it to make a drizzle over the top of the strawberries; place in the fridge for 20 minutes until the chocolate is set and then gently peel the strawberries off the cling film.

Bananas dipped in chocolate and chopped nuts

(520 kcal, 75 g carbohydrate, 8 g protein, 24 g fat)

INGREDIENTS

» Two medium-sized ripe bananas

» 40 g chocolate of choice

» One teaspoon of vegetable oil

» Pinch of sea salt

» Two tablespoons of mixed seeds (flax, sunflower etc) or chopped nuts

» Cocktail sticks

PREPARATION

1) Peel the bananas and cut into 1.5 cm slices; stick a cocktail stick into each slice so that they look like mini lollipops; **2)** put the chocolate and oil and the smallest amount of salt that's visible to the naked eye into a non-metallic bowl; either microwave for 40 seconds initially, then in batches of 20 seconds on high until melted, stirring with

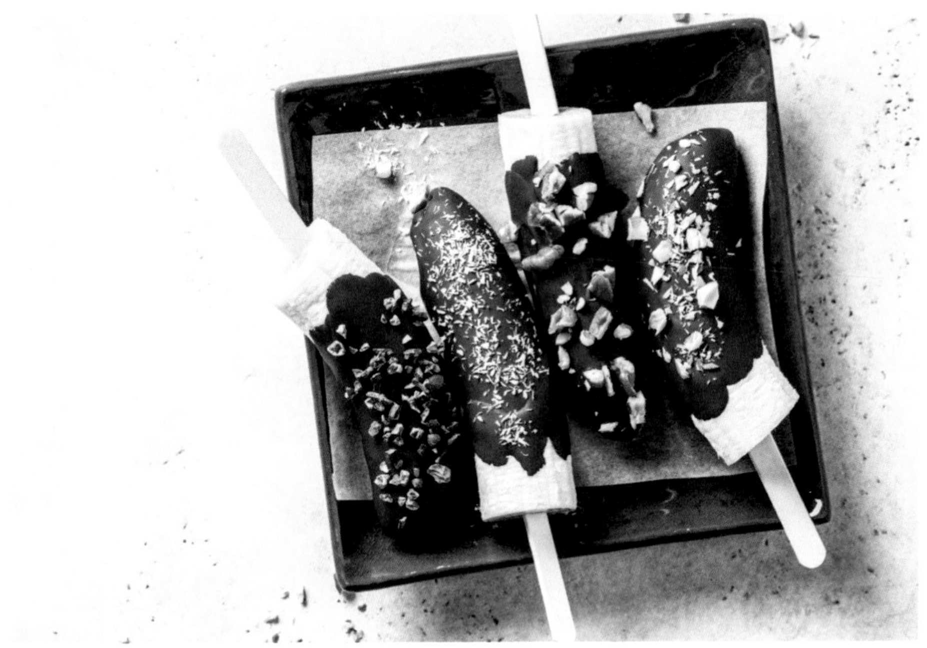

Photo 12.28 Bananas dipped in chocolate and chopped nuts.

a teaspoon between each 20 seconds to assess the melting process, or set the bowl above a little saucepan of boiling water over a low heat and stir on and off until melted; **3)** take a dinner plate and cover it with cling film; put the bowl of melted chocolate half on and half off a scrunched-up tea towel so that the bowl is at an angle; put the nuts or seeds in a different bowl and also set half on, half off the tea towel, so the bowl is at an angle; **4)** take each banana 'lollipop' and dip it in the deep end of the liquid chocolate covering just the bottom half of the banana slice and then dip the chocolate into the seeds or chopped nuts; the chocolate may cool down a bit and start to thicken up, if so, gently reheat until just liquid again; **5)** set the dipped bananas on the cling-filmed plate, placing the banana slices close together on the plate otherwise you will run out of space on the plate; **6)** if you have any leftover chocolate, dip a teaspoon into the chocolate and use it to make a drizzle over the undipped part of the banana; place in the fridge for 20 minutes until the chocolate is set and then gently peel the bananas off the cling film.

Chocolate and mango mousse

This makes two small portions. One for today and one for tomorrow.

(410 kcal, 59 g carbohydrate, 5 g protein, 21 g fat) per portion

INGREDIENTS (TO MAKE TWO PORTIONS)

- One ripe avocado
- One ripe mango
- 40 g milk or dark chocolate of choice
- One teaspoon of cocoa powder
- Four dates (with stone removed)
- Pinch of sea salt
- 60 g mixed berries (e.g. raspberries, blueberries, strawberries)

PREPARATION

1) The mango and avocado need to be really ripe, but not over ripe, so you may have to wait a day or two after purchasing until the avocado and mango are at peak ripeness; **2)** melt the chocolate in a non-metallic bowl in the microwave on full for 40 seconds, then in batches of 20 seconds stirring between 20 seconds until just melted; add a very small pinch of salt and the cocoa powder and stir to combine; **3)** in a NutriBullet or food processor, process the avocado and mango until no little green pieces of avocado remain and then add all remaining ingredients and process until the mixture turns a shade lighter (this shows that air has been incorporated into the mix); **4)** using a spatula, scrape the mixture into two little glasses and serve with a mixture of berries.

Lemon mousse

(125 kcal, 11 g carbohydrate, 15 g protein, 3 g fat) per portion

INGREDIENTS (TO MAKE TWO PORTIONS)

» 250 g fat free (or low-fat) Quark soft cheese
» One tablespoon of lemon curd (ideally one with butter in the ingredient list)
» Juice of one lemon juice
» Two tablespoons of low-fat crème fraîche or sour cream
» One passion fruit

PREPARATION

1) Combine all ingredients except the passion fruit in a NutriBullet or food processor and process for 30 seconds or until everything is well combined; **2)** using a spatula divide into two glasses and allow to set in the fridge for 30 minutes; **3)** serve with half a passion fruit; if leaving a mousse until the following day, cover the glass with cling film and keep in the fridge.

Sweet potato and orange cheesecake

» (590 kcal, 42 g carbohydrate, 8 g protein, 44 g fat) per portion (1/8th whole cheesecake)

INGREDIENTS FOR ENOUGH TO MAKE A CHEESECAKE THAT WILL PROVIDE EIGHT PORTIONS

» Three medium-sized sweet potatoes
» Three oranges
» 200 g butter
» 280 g cream cheese
» 80 g almond butter
» 240 g digestive biscuits

(continued)

(continued)

- 25 g almonds
- Two passion fruits (for decoration, not essential)
- Half a pomegranate (for decoration, not essential)

PREPARATION

1) In a medium-sized saucepan, boil the sweet potatoes whole and unpeeled; cover with a lid but allow some of the steam to escape; check water level and top up if needed; **2)** in the meantime, make the base of the cheesecake: put the butter in a pan on a low heat until melted; in a NutriBullet or a food processor weigh the almonds, digestive biscuits, almond butter and blitz; add 75 g of melted butter and blitz for a few seconds; **3)** use the mixture to make a 1–1.5 cm thick base in a loose-based tin 22–25 cm in diameter; smooth out flat and compact slightly with the back of a dessert spoon, then put the tin in the fridge to firm up; if you have too much base mixture, put in a small bowl to be used later; **4)** wash the oranges and use a potato peeler to peel the oranges; finely slice the peel and put in a small saucepan; juice the oranges and add to the pan, making sure there are no pips in the juice; bring the juice to the boil and simmer for 10–12 minutes to reduce the volume of liquid and intensify the flavour; **5)** once the sweet potato is fully cooked (45–60 minutes, try not to test the potatoes by piercing with a fork, the idea is to keep all the nutrition of the potato within the skin), remove from the heat, pour off the hot water and refresh in cold water; change the water as the potatoes cool; **6)** when cool enough, peel the potatoes by hand, then break into thirds and put in

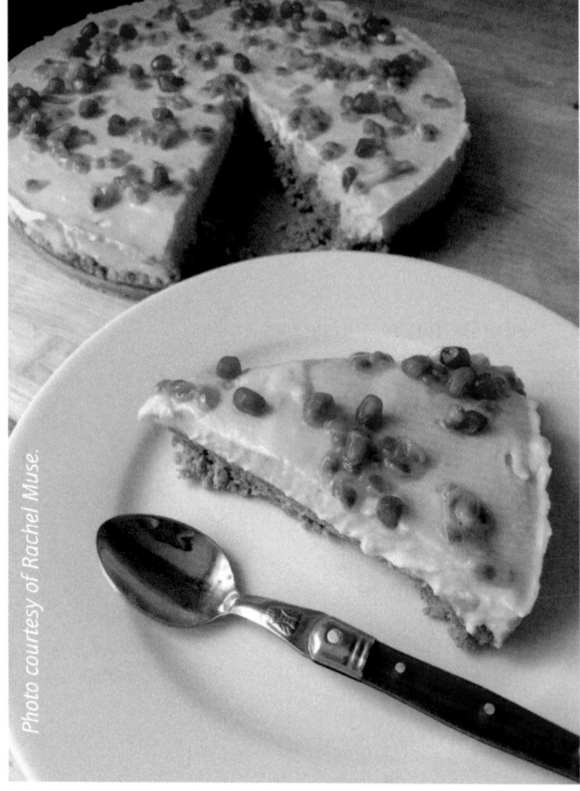

Photo 12.29 Sweet potato and orange cheesecake.

the food processor; add the cream cheese, the remaining melted butter (doesn't matter if it's starting to firm up, just as long as it is not rock hard) and the orange juice/peel mixture; blitz the mixture, scrape down with a spatula and blitz again until uniform; **7)** pour into the tin (the thickness should be 3–3.5cm) and place into the fridge to firm up for 2 hours.

Banana brownie American-style pancakes

(635 kcal, 80 g carbohydrate, 15 g protein, 30 g fat) per portion (three pancakes)

INGREDIENTS (TO MAKE NINE PANCAKES)

- 200 g oats
- 40 g unflavoured protein powder or 40 g more oats
- One tablespoon of baking powder
- Two tablespoons of cocoa powder
- Three medium-sized ripe bananas
- 60 g Nutella
- One large egg
- Pinch of salt
- Two tablespoons of rapeseed oil
- 20 g berries of choice to garnish

PREPARATION

1) Put all dry ingredients (oats, protein powder, baking powder, cocoa powder and salt) into a food processor or NutriBullet and process until smooth; **2)** peel the bananas then add these to the blender with the egg and Nutella and blend again until all ingredients are combined; **3)** heat a heavy-based frying pan on a medium–low heat, add two tablespoons of oil (the oil shouldn't smoke, if it does turn the heat down); for each pancake, place two tablespoons of mixture on top of each other in the pan (the mixture should sizzle when it hits the surface of the pan); the mixture will rise up, cook for two minutes then turn over with a fish slice, cook the second side for one and a half minutes; **4)** garnish and eat one portion (3 pancakes); place the remaining pancakes on a plate and cover with cling film; they will keep in the fridge for four days; to reheat place in the toaster and toast for one minute.

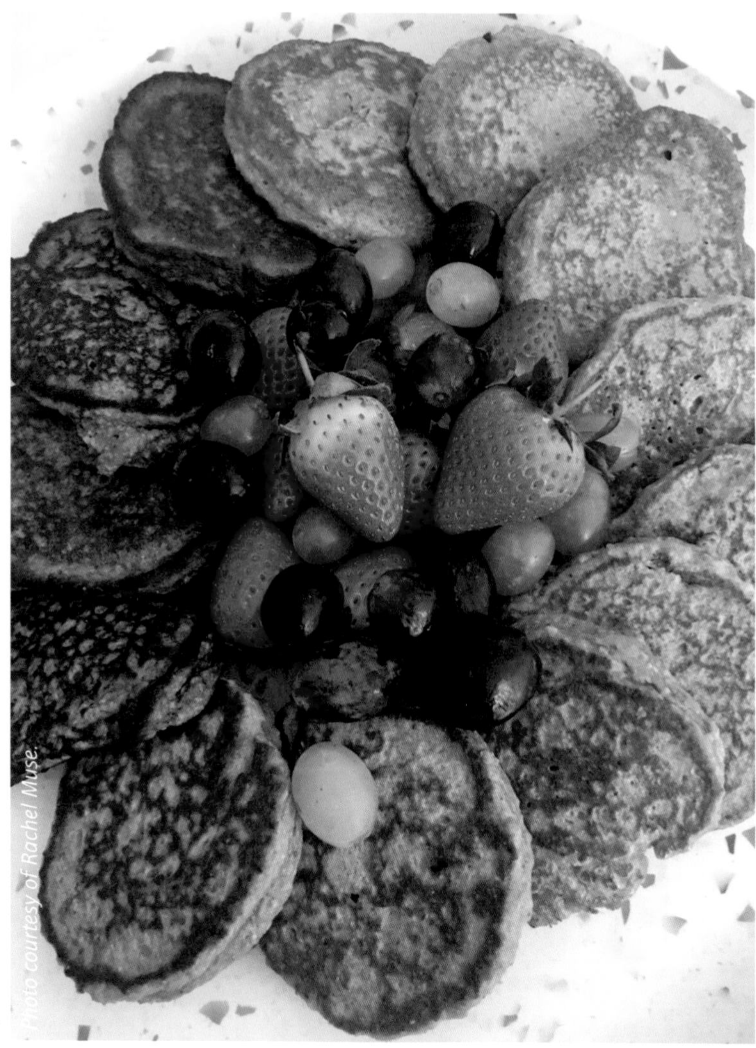

Photo 12.30 Banana brownie American-style pancakes.

SNACKS

In general, snacking is not encouraged in football due to concerns with weight gain and to avoid players consuming foods with a low nutrient content. When players are eating three or four meals per day, between-meal snacks are unnecessary. However, on intensive training days if a player has to wait a longer time than usual between meals and is feeling hungry, then a low-calorie vegetarian snack is acceptable. Here are some suitable examples.

Vegetarian fruit snacks

(All less than 100 kcal, mostly from carbohydrate)

- One medium-sized apple
- One medium-sized pear
- One large peach
- Three small plums
- One cup of grapes, strawberries or cherries
- Five sticks of celery
- Six cherry tomatoes.

One cup of chopped fruit (e.g. apple, grapes, orange, persimmon, plums, melon or strawberries) or a cup containing a mixture of two or three different fruits topped with a tablespoon of low-fat yoghurt

MATCH DAYS

On most match days, there will be an opportunity for breakfast and at least one other pre-match meal where the emphasis will be on providing carbohydrate and fluid with some protein. However, for morning or lunchtime kick-offs, the pre-match meal will be breakfast usually. Sports drinks or carbohydrate gels may be provided to players just before kick-off, at half-time, and often a carbohydrate/protein recovery shake and/or some finger food will be available in the dressing room after the match. For the post-match meal, the emphasis is on providing carbohydrate for restoring muscle glycogen and protein for muscle repair and recovery. Typical match-day energy expenditure for a player who completes a full 90-minute match will be about 3,500 kcal. The meal plans described here will provide about 3,000 kcal per day (as players typically get an additional 500 kcal or so from sports drinks, gels and recovery shakes); the amounts can be modified if daily energy expenditure is expected to be lower (e.g. if a player does not play the full 90 minutes) or higher (if extra-time is played as in many cup competitions if the scores are level after normal time).

BREAKFASTS

These contain 450–500 kcal with at least 70 g CHO, at least 10 g protein and only a small amount of fat. They are generally quite simple to prepare and easily digestible. They can be accompanied by a drink of water, fruit juice (e.g. orange, apple, tomato), milk or a hot beverage (e.g. green tea, coffee) as desired.

Fruit and a strawberry or cherry muesli followed by a toast and honey

Half a large orange or a small pink grapefruit, followed by 40 g swiss style muesli with 75 mL whole milk and 10 strawberries or pitted chopped red cherries. Followed by two slices of wholemeal toast each smeared with a tablespoon of honey (470 kcal, 89 g carbohydrate, 13 g protein, 10 g fat).

Fruit and bran cereal followed by wholemeal bread and jam

Half a large orange or a small pink grapefruit, followed by 40 g All-Bran cereal with 75 mL whole milk and a medium-sized banana, chopped into thin slices. Followed by a thick slice of wholemeal bread smeared with a pat of butter and one tablespoon of raspberry jam (480 kcal, 105 g carbohydrate, 13 g protein, 6 g fat).

Whole-wheat cereal with strawberries followed by a hard-boiled egg

Two whole-wheat biscuits (e.g., Shredded Wheat, Weetabix, or Oatibix) with 100 mL whole milk and 10 medium-sized strawberries. Followed by a runny (3-minute) hard-boiled egg and two slices of toasted wholemeal bread (470 kcal, 72 g carbohydrate, 21 g protein, 12 g fat).

Fruit smoothie with a toasted muffin

Fruit smoothie made with one large ripe banana, 250 mL cranberry juice (no added sugar version) and 100 g frozen mixed red berries blended together and served with an English muffin, toasted and spread with creamed cheese (500 kcal, 100 g carbohydrate, 11 g protein, 11 g fat).

Muesli with dried fruit and walnut with yoghurt

Muesli (50 g) comprising rolled oats, wheat flakes and 30 g of a variety of dried fruits (e.g. cranberries, raisins, sultanas) served with 100 g Greek yoghurt and topped with a large strawberry and six crushed walnut halves (450 kcal, 70 g carbohydrate, 18 g protein, 15 g fat).

Banana and yoghurt followed by baked beans on toast

One small banana, sliced with 50 g Greek yoghurt followed by half a can (200 g) of baked beans on two slices of toasted wholemeal bread (500 kcal, 94 g carbohydrate, 26 g protein, 4 g fat).

PRE-MATCH MEALS

The pre-match meal will be consumed about 3 hours before kick-off and should be easily and rapidly digestible, which means limiting the amounts of fibre and fat and using lighter forms of meat such as chicken and non-oily fish. These meals contain about 600–800 kcal with 70–150 g carbohydrate and about 20–40 g protein (figure 12.2).

The meal recipes that follow have been created by elite performance chef Bruno Cirillo.

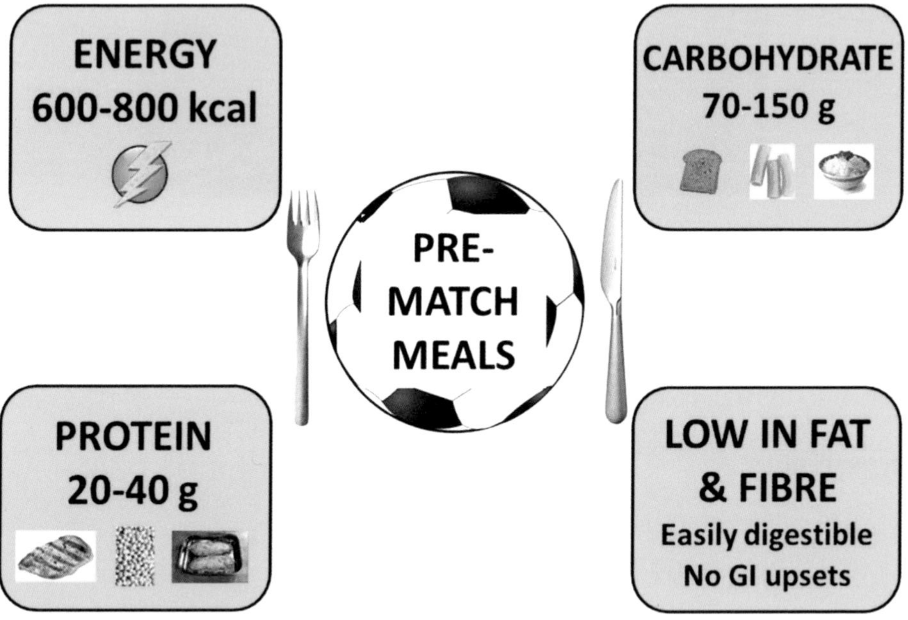

Figure 12.2 Pre-match meal nutrition targets.

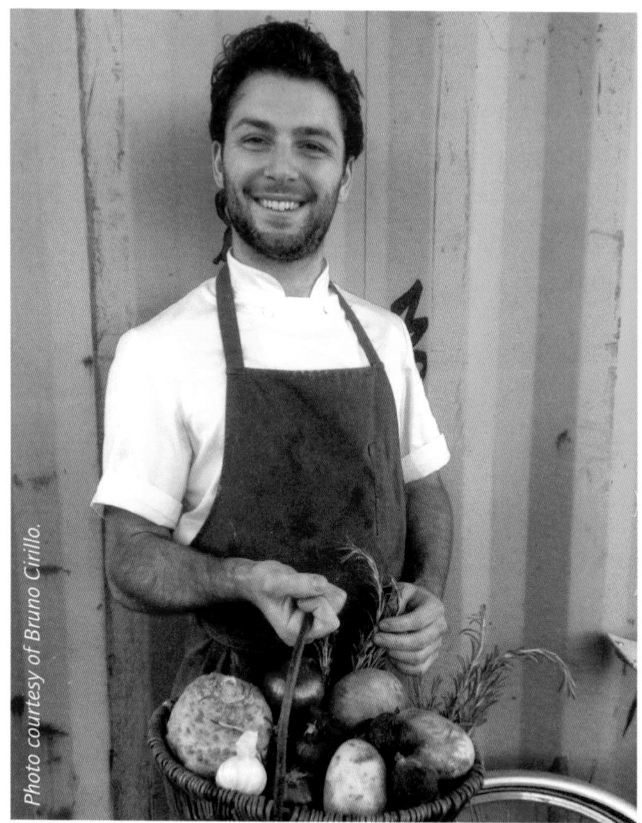

Photo 12.31 Elite performance chef Bruno Cirillo.

Pasta al pomodoro with Parmigiano-Reggiano cheese

(640 kcal, 105 g carbohydrate, 24 g protein, 17 g fat)

INGREDIENTS

- 130 g dry pasta (penne or fusilli style)
- 150 g tomato sauce
- 12 g extra virgin olive oil
- 10 g Parmigiano-Reggiano cheese
- Basil to garnish
- Pinch of salt and black pepper to season

PREPARATION

1) Cook pasta as per instructions; **2)** heat tomato sauce in a pan and season with salt and pepper; **3)** when pasta is cooked, drain and stir in the tomato sauce; **4)** garnish with basil, olive oil and Parmigiano-Reggiano cheese.

Pasta with pumpkin cream and chickpeas

(670 kcal, 107 g carbohydrate, 25 g protein, 18 g fat)

INGREDIENTS

» 120 g dry pasta (penne or fusilli style)
» 150 g pumpkin/winter squash
» 70 g canned chickpeas
» 15 g extra virgin olive oil
» 7 g nutritional yeast
» Pinch of salt and black pepper to season

PREPARATION

1) Cook pasta as per instructions; **2)** dice and steam until the pumpkin becomes very soft; blend it and season with olive oil, salt and pepper; **3)** when the pasta is cooked, drain and stir in the pumpkin sauce adding the chickpeas; **4)** sprinkle nutritional yeast to season and serve.

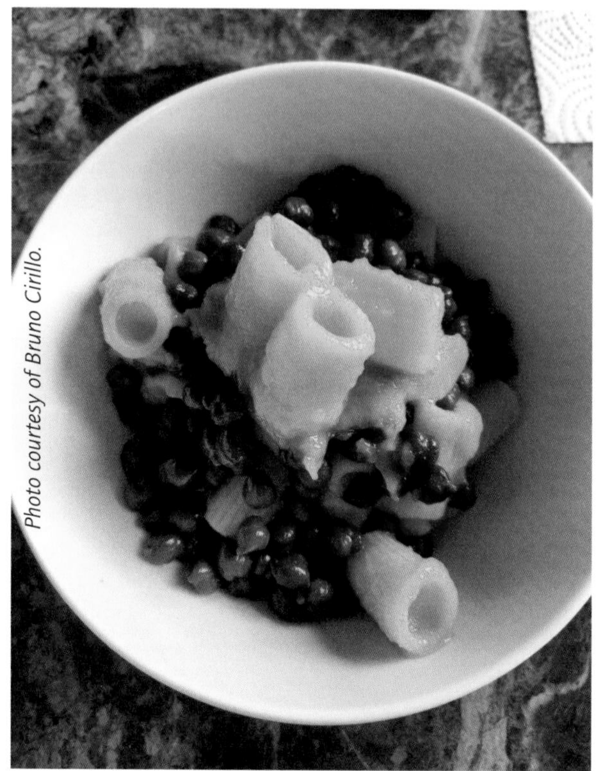

Photo 12.32 Pasta with pumpkin cream and chickpeas.

Fruity porridge

(730 kcal, 130 g carbohydrate, 23 g protein, 10 g fat)

INGREDIENTS

- 150 g rice milk
- 110 g dry rolled oats
- One medium-sized banana
- 100 g frozen mixed berries
- 50 g egg (1 large egg)
- 21 g honey
- Cinnamon

PREPARATION

1) Finely cut the banana and place all the ingredients in a small pot; **2)** bring to a simmer and stir continuously until a soft consistency is achieved (about 10 minutes).

Rice with sticky chicken and fried vegetables

(620 kcal, 90 g carbohydrate, 24 g protein, 17 g fat)

INGREDIENTS

- 150 g courgette (zucchini)
- 80 g dry white rice (basmati/jasmine)
- 70 g carrots
- 60 g bell pepper
- 60 g diced chicken breast (skin removed)
- 50 mL chicken stock
- 15 g brown sugar
- 12 g extra-virgin olive oil
- 10 g soy sauce
- Lime and spring onions to garnish
- Pinch of salt and black pepper to season

PREPARATION

1) Cook rice as per instructions; **2)** in a pan, add chicken stock, sugar and soy sauce and bring to a simmer; **3)** pan-fry the chicken in the sauce; **4)** in another pan, stir fry the vegetables with the olive oil; **5)** serve with lime and spring onions.

Rice and vegetable burritos

(740 kcal, 111g carbohydrate, 26 g protein, 10 g fat)

INGREDIENTS

- 130 g tortilla wraps (two wraps, but depending on size)
- 150 g cooked white rice
- 150 g canned black beans
- 70 g finely chopped lettuce
- 60 g diced bell pepper
- 60 g diced tomatoes
- Coriander to garnish
- Lime juice to moisten
- Pinch of salt and black pepper to season

PREPARATION

1) Combine ingredients (already prepared) inside the wraps as desired; **2)** can be prepared in bulk in advance and be stored in the freezer.

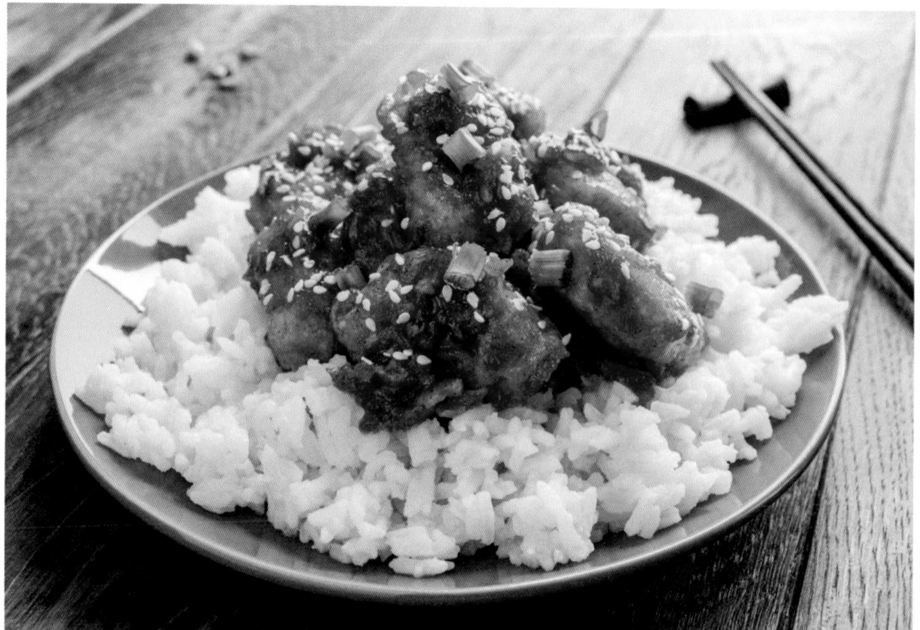

Photo 12.33 Rice with sticky chicken and fried vegetables.

Jacket sweet potato with smoked salmon and sour cream dressing served with hummus toast

(540 kcal, 76 g carbohydrate, 20 g protein, 12 g fat)

INGREDIENTS

- 350 g sweet potato (one or two sweet potatoes, depending on size)
- 50 g sour cream (reduced fat)
- 30 g smoked salmon
- Finely cut chives to garnish
- 30 g wholemeal bread slice
- 30 g hummus

PREPARATION

1) Give the potatoes a scrub and prick evenly with a fork. Heat the oven to 200°C, when warm, place the potatoes to cook until soft inside (about 60 minutes); **2)** split open and top as desired with sour cream, salmon and chives; **3)** on the side prepare the toast with hummus.

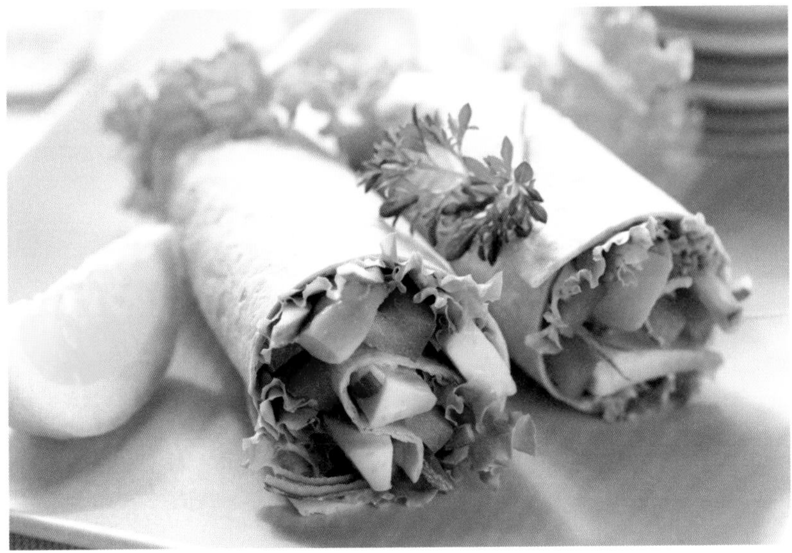

Photo 12.34 Rice and vegetable burritos.

Here are some additional meal plans of my own.

Chicken and tomato pasta bake

(580 kcal, 85 g carbohydrate, 43 g protein, 7 g fat)

INGREDIENTS

» 120 g chicken breast (skin removed)

» 200 g tomato and garlic sauce

» 100 g dry penne pasta

» One teaspoon of oregano

PREPARATION

1) Cut the chicken breast cut into chunks and oven-bake in 200 g tomato and garlic sauce for 60 minutes at 180ºC; **2)** layer over boiled pasta made with 100 g dry penne pasta: **3)** sprinkle with one teaspoon of oregano.

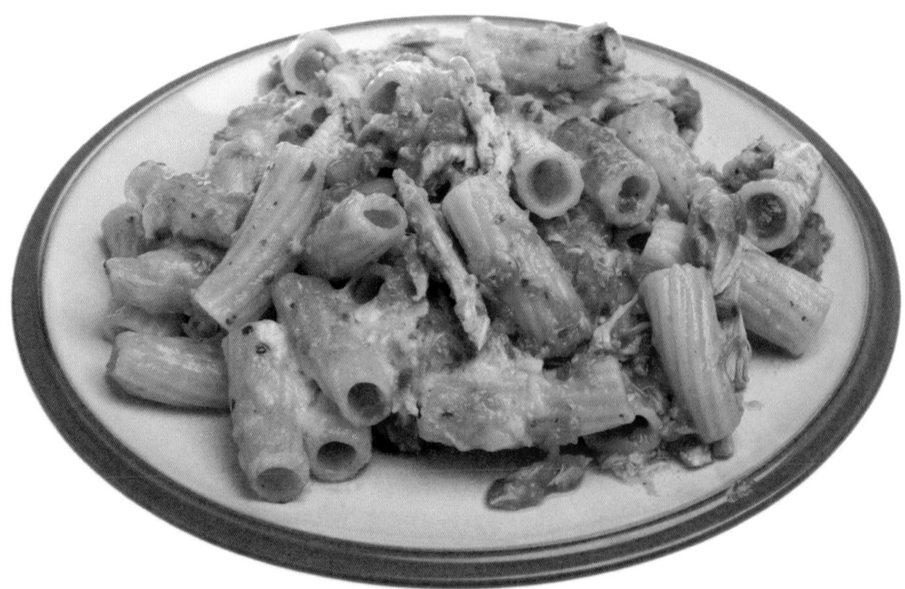

Photo 12.35 Chicken and tomato pasta bake.

Chicken with rice and butter beans

(600 kcal, 88 g carbohydrate, 43 g protein, 7 g fat)

INGREDIENTS

- 120 g chicken breast (skin removed)
- 50 g canned butter beans
- 200 g boiled white rice

PREPARATION

1) Grill or roast the chicken breast and cut it into chunks; **2)** serve with 50 g of pan-cooked butter beans and 200 g boiled white rice.

Chicken and egg-fried rice

(575 kcal, 75 g carbohydrate, 42 g protein, 11 g fat)

INGREDIENTS

- 120 g chicken breast (skin removed)
- 200 g Chinese egg-fried rice (microwavable bag)
- 50 g frozen garden peas
- Two tablespoons of soy sauce

PREPARATION

1) Grill or roast the chicken breast and cut it into chunks; **2)** add to microwaved Chinese egg-fried rice; **3)** add 50 g of pan-cooked garden peas and pour the soy sauce over the meal.

Cod loin with mashed potato and peas

(540 kcal, 65 g carbohydrate, 38 g protein, 14 g fat)

INGREDIENTS

- 150 g cod loin
- One lemon
- One teaspoon of chopped parsley
- 100 g frozen garden peas
- 300 g potato
- 50 mL milk
- One teaspoon of butter

PREPARATION

1) Wrap the cod loin in baking foil with sliced lemon and chopped parsley on top and oven-bake for 30 minutes at 180 ºC; **2)** boil 300 g potatoes in water in a pan then drain the water, mash the potato and add the butter and milk in the hot pan; **3)** serve with serve with 100 g of pan-cooked garden peas.

POST-MATCH MEALS

The post-match meal will normally be eaten within a couple of hours after the final whistle. These meals contain 800–1,000 kcal with 100–150 g CHO, at least 40 g protein and about 20 g fat (figure 12.3). If this is to be the last main meal of the day, these amounts can be increased by 20–30% and accompanied by a starter and/or a dessert such as the ones devised here by Bruno Cirillo, or those already described in this chapter. After a match many professional and amateur players like to eat some sort of comfort food, which if made well, and with appropriate ingredients, is a good solution to satisfy their desire. Pizza, for instance, can be made to deliver adequate amounts of carbohydrate and protein, and the fat content can be reduced by limiting the use of oils and using a little less cheese. Several of these meals (salmon or veal with rice, chicken and ramen noodles, spaghetti bolognese and prawn linguine carbonara) are suitable for the important evening dinner on the day before a match, and these courses can be followed by any one of the desserts.

The meal recipes that follow have been created by elite performance chef Bruno Cirillo.

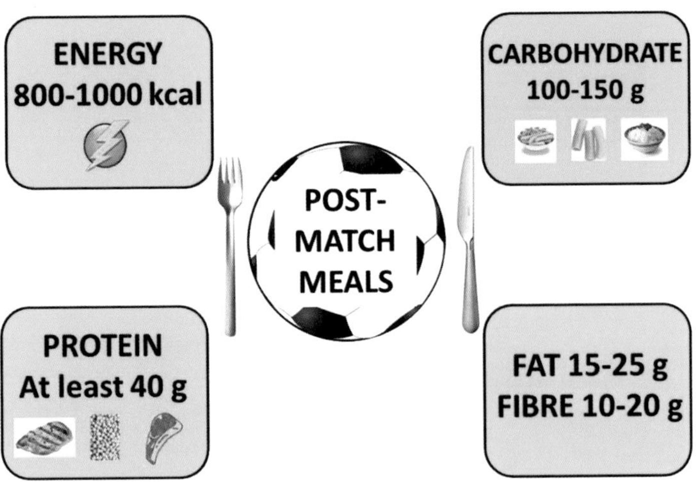

Figure 12.3 Post-match meal nutrition targets.

Cheeseburger with sweet potato 'fries' (preferably home-made) and a bottle of pop

(780 kcal, 88 g carbohydrate, 44 g protein, 22 g fat)

INGREDIENTS

- 300 g oven-baked sweet potato 'fries'
- 120 g lean minced beef patty (7–10% fat)
- 60 g burger bun
- 30 g lettuce leaves
- 30 g sliced tomato
- 20 g cheese slice
- 20 g ketchup
- 330 mL standard soft drink

PREPARATION

1) Grill the minced beef patty for 5 minutes each side until cooked through; **2)** cut the sweet potato into wedges and oven-bake on a baking tray for 30 minutes (these contain far less fat than deep fried); **3)** place the cooked burger in the bun and place the cheese on top of the burger; **4)** serve with the lettuce, tomato and sweet potato.

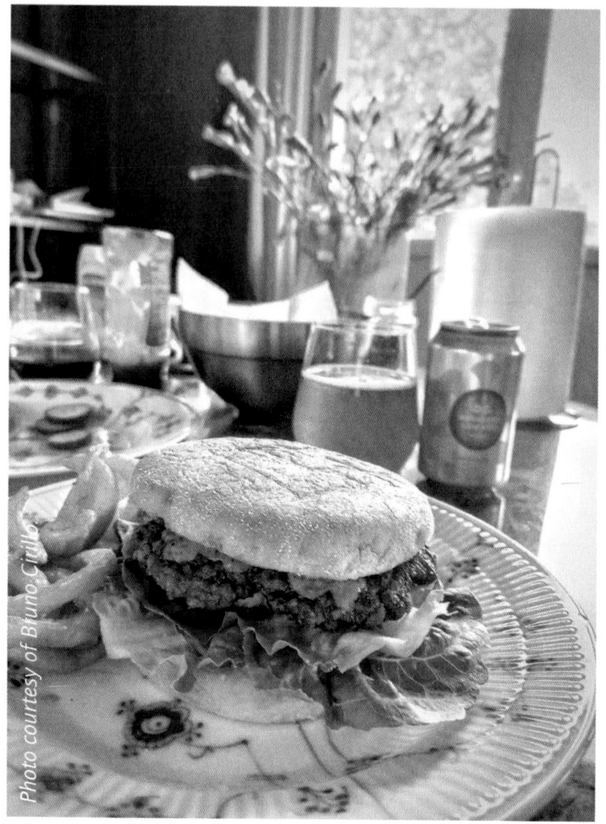

Photo 12.36 Cheeseburger with sweet potato 'fries'.

Pizza rossa con prosciutto crudo

(810 kcal, 107 g carbohydrate, 38 g protein, 24 g fat)

INGREDIENTS

- 180 g dough base (a supermarket own brand sourdough base is a good choice)
- 120 g tomato sauce
- 50 g Prosciutto di Parma (or similar)
- 40 g cherry tomatoes
- 40 g rocket salad (Rucola)
- 14 g extra virgin olive oil

PREPARATION

The vast majority of calories and fat in a pizza come from the oil and cheese. This recipe is for a 'pizza rossa' (a pizza without cheese). Prepare as follows: **1)** Smear the tomato sauce with a drop of olive oil over a ready-made sourdough base (a bit of olive oil on the tomato sauce helps to prevent the dough from going too dry whilst cooking; especially important when there's no cheese); **2)** cook in oven at 250ºC for 5–8 minutes (steady heat, not ventilated); **3)** after cooking add the rocket salad, cherry tomatoes and the ham cut into slices as toppings and drizzle with olive oil.

Rice with salmon fillet in poppy seed crust

(840 kcal, 96 g carbohydrate, 43 g protein, 28 g fat)

INGREDIENTS

- 150 g broccoli
- 120 g salmon fillet
- 90 g dry white rice (jasmine or basmati)
- 40 g cherry tomatoes
- 40 g mixed salad
- 30 g raisins
- 10 g poppy seeds
- 13 g olive oil
- Coriander to garnish
- Lime juice to moisten
- Pinch of salt and black pepper to season

PREPARATION

1) Cook rice as per instructions; **2)** heat the oven to 160ºC and in the meantime roll the salmon fillet on the poppy seeds to cover it entirely. Once the oven is warm, bake for 35 minutes; **3)** steam broccoli and cool down aside; **4)** once chilled, mix with mixed salad, raisins and cherry tomatoes.

Crunchy pork cotoletta with boiled potatoes

(810 kcal, 107 g carbohydrate, 38 g protein, 24 g fat)

INGREDIENTS

» 250 g white potatoes

» 150 g lean pork chop

» 40 g cherry tomatoes

» 40 g mixed salad

» 20 g olive oil

For the crust:

» 1 beaten egg with 30 g whole milk

» 30 g all-purpose flour

» 30 g crushed rye cracker (or rye flour)

PREPARATION

1) Boil the potatoes; **2)** beat down the pork chop until thin as desired (about 3 mm); **3)** coat with breading (prepared by mixing the flour, beaten egg, milk and rye crust); **4)** firstly, pan-fry the breaded pork chop until it has a golden crust and then bake it in the oven at 180ºC for 20 minutes; **5)** serve all together with fresh salad and a light dressing.

Home-made quick and easy ramen

(860 kcal, 94 g carbohydrate, 45 g protein, 24 g fat)

INGREDIENTS

» 400 g chicken/pork bone broth

» 120 g fresh ramen noodles (not dry packaged)

» 70 g pork loin/chicken breast (visible fat and skin removed) or tofu

» 40 g bell pepper

» 40 g oyster mushrooms or similar

- 12 g sesame oil
- 15 g miso paste
- 10 g soy sauce
- Toppings such as coriander, lime and chilli

PREPARATION

1) Oven-bake the mushrooms and a lean cut of meat (if using pork loin first cut off any visible fat) or prepare tofu as desired; **2)** heat the bone broth in a pan and gently stir in it the soy sauce and miso paste; **3)** cook the noodles separately as per instructions; **4)** combine all the ingredients and serve with preferred garnish/toppings.

Creamy veal stew with white rice

(800 kcal, 89 g carbohydrate, 42 g protein, 24 g fat)

INGREDIENTS

- 120 g veal loin strips
- 100 g dry white rice
- 100 bone broth (chicken/pork)
- 40 g carrot
- 40 g white onion
- 40 g white mushrooms
- 20 g cream
- 15 g olive oil
- Flour (enough to coat the veal)

PREPARATION

1) Cook the rice as per instructions; **2)** coat the veal in flour and pan-fry until golden and then set aside; **3)** on the bottom of a pan gently cook (until soft) the finely chopped onion and carrot; **4)** once done, add the mushrooms and bone broth and bring to a simmer; now add the cooked veal and cream and cook for a further 10 minutes and serve on top of the rice.

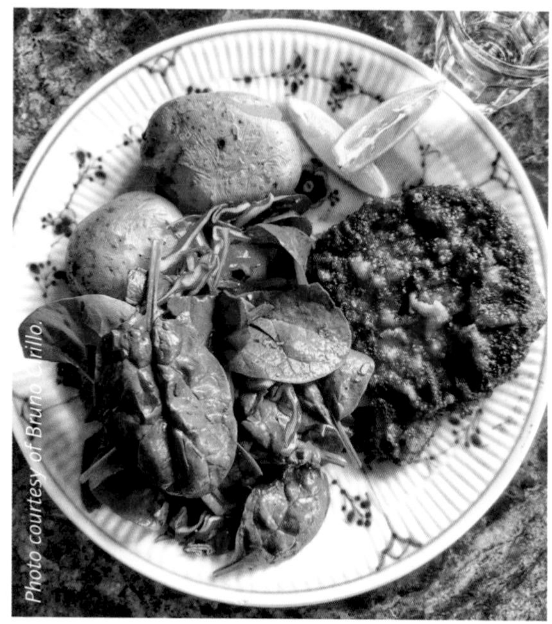

Photo 12.37 Crunchy pork cotoletta with boiled potatoes.

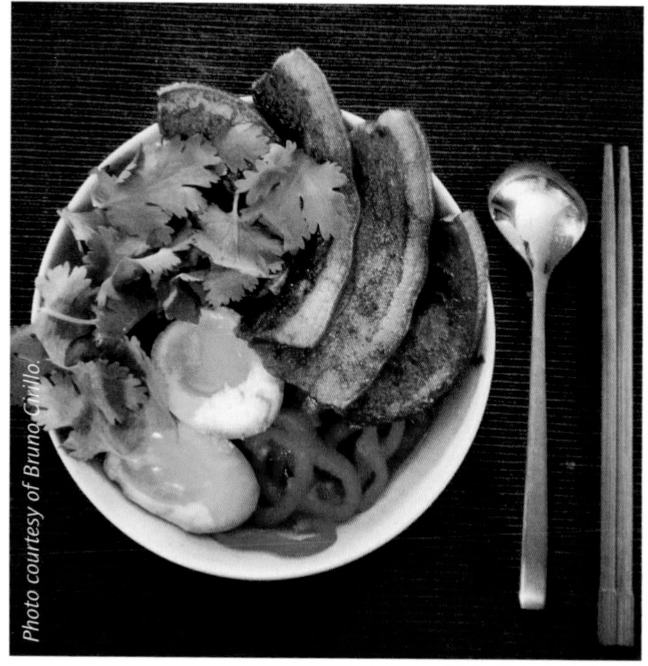

Photo 12.38 Ramen with pork loin and coriander topping.

Here are some additional main post-match meal plans of my own.

Classic spaghetti bolognese

(1,000 kcal, 120 g carbohydrate, 70 g protein, 26 g fat)

INGREDIENTS

- 200 g lean beef mince (5% fat)
- Two teaspoons of rapeseed oil
- 200 g bolognese sauce
- 60 g cannellini beans
- Half a can of chopped tomatoes
- One teaspoon of chopped garlic
- Pinch of chilli flakes
- 200 g boiled whole-wheat spaghetti
- Two 3 cm slices of a baguette
- One teaspoon of garlic paste

PREPARATION

1) Pan-fry the mince in the rapeseed oil for 3 minutes and place it in a casserole dish; **2)** add the bolognese sauce, chopped tomatoes, chopped garlic, chilli bits and cannellini beans and mix thoroughly before baking in an oven for 60 minutes at 180°C; **3)** pour over the boiled whole-wheat spaghetti; **4)** serve with 2 slices of a toasted baguette smeared with garlic paste.

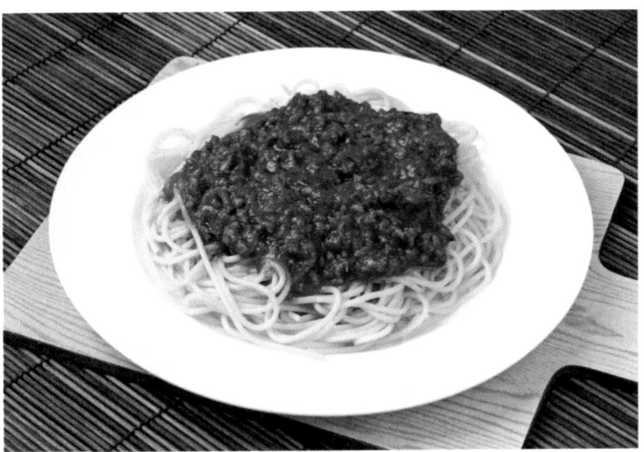

Photo 12.39 Spaghetti bolognese.

Spicy prawn linguine carbonara

(980 kcal, 110 g carbohydrate, 78 g protein, 28 g fat)

INGREDIENTS

- 200 g cooked peeled prawns
- 200 g carbonara sauce (contains egg and milk)
- 100 g chopped courgette (zucchini)
- 100 g cannellini beans
- 60 g chopped shallots
- Two chopped garlic cloves
- Pinch of chilli flakes
- 250 g boiled linguine pasta
- One tablespoon of grated hard Italian cheese

PREPARATION

1) Place the prawns and the carbonara sauce in a casserole dish; **2)** add the cannellini beans and chopped courgette, shallots, garlic cloves and a sprinkle of chilli bits and mix thoroughly; **3)** cook in an oven for 60 minutes at 180ºC; **4)** pour over 250 g boiled linguine pasta and sprinkle on one tablespoon of grated hard Italian cheese.

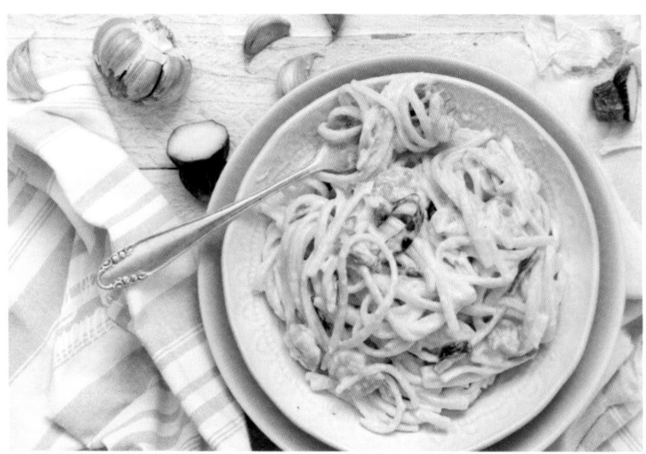

Photo 12.40 Spicy prawn linguine carbonara.

Beefsteak with baked jacket potato, corn and mixed green leaf salad

(900 kcal, 145 g carbohydrate, 55 g protein, 13 g fat)

INGREDIENTS

180 g lean beef steak (e.g. fillet, rump, sirloin or a lamb leg steak or pork loin steak can be used as an alternative to beef if desired)

- One large jacket potato
- 8 cm piece of corn on the cob
- One small sweet potato
- 60 g mixed green salad leaves (e.g., watercress, rocket, spinach)
- Three cherry tomatoes

PREPARATION

1) Grill the steak on both sides and remove any visible fat after cooking; **2)** oven-bake one large jacket potato and a small sweet potato; **3)** serve with a steamed corn on the cob accompanied by the mixed green leaf salad and cherry tomatoes.

Traditional Sunday roast beef dinner

(990 kcal, 118 g carbohydrate, 59 g protein, 30 g fat)

INGREDIENTS

- 180 g topside of beef
- 150 g roast parsnips
- One tablespoon of olive oil
- One teaspoon of chopped garlic
- 300 g new potatoes
- 100 g carrots
- 100 g savoy cabbage leaves (about half a small cabbage with the stalk removed)
- One large onion
- One small pre-baked Yorkshire pudding
- Three tablespoons of beef stock gravy
- One teaspoon of horseradish sauce

PREPARATION

1) Wrap the beef in foil and roast on a baking tray in an oven for 40 minutes at 180ºC; **2)** at the same time, roast the peeled parsnips and half the onion drizzled with a tablespoon of olive oil and a teaspoon of chopped garlic, all wrapped in foil; **3)** steam the new potatoes and carrots for 20 minutes; **4)** chop up the savoy cabbage and the other half of the onion and steam together for 20 minutes; **5)** heat a small pre-baked Yorkshire pudding in the oven for 5 minutes and prepare a beef stock gravy (adding the juices from the cooked meat at the end); **6)** serve with a teaspoon of horseradish sauce.

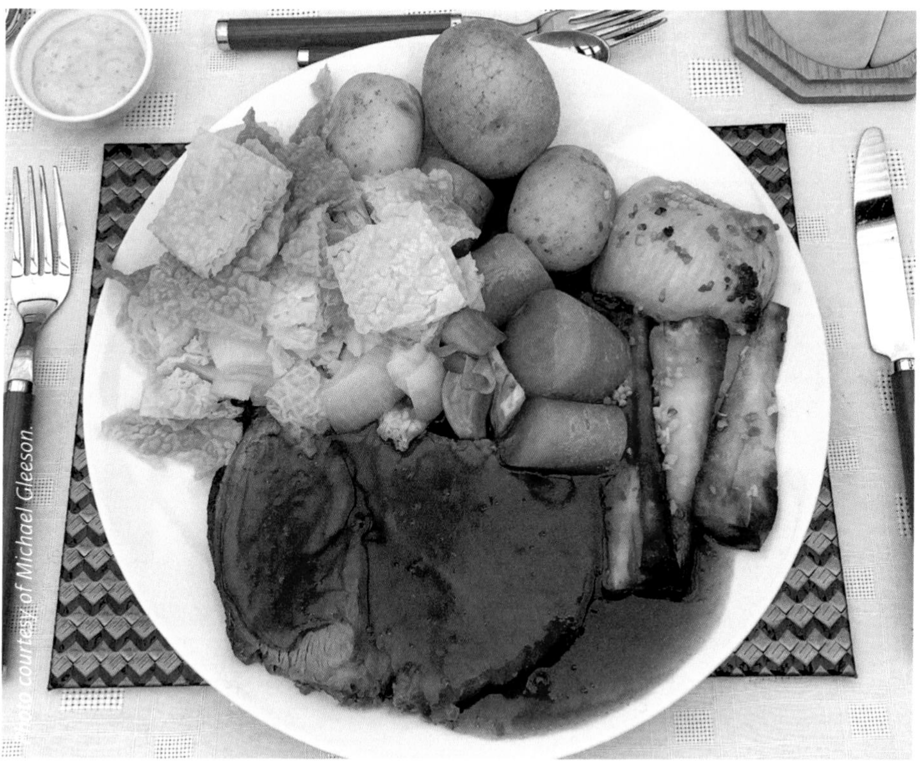

Photo 12.41 Traditional Sunday roast beef dinner.

The post-match dessert recipes that follow have been created by elite performance chef Bruno Cirillo.

Quick and easy tiramisù

(970 kcal, 114 g carbohydrate, 59 g protein, 30 g fat)

INGREDIENTS

- 40 g egg whites (the amount you get from one large egg)
- 33 g Ladyfingers (three pieces)
- 25 g granulated sugar
- 25 g condensed milk
- Espresso coffee to dip Ladyfingers in
- Pinch of salt for whipping the egg white

PREPARATION

1) Whip the egg white, with pinch of salt (first) and granulated sugar (adding slowly); **2)** when whipped to firm, add condensed milk, and stir gently; **3)** dip Ladyfingers in espresso coffee; **4)** make layers of the mixture and the coffee-dipped Ladyfingers in a single glass and refrigerate for at least one hour before serving.

Chocolate mousse

(300 kcal, 50 g carbohydrate, 4 g protein, 9 g fat)

INGREDIENTS

- 60 g sweet potato
- 35 g banana
- 21 g honey
- 16 g coconut milk
- 13 g dark chocolate
- 10 g brown sugar
- Pinch of salt

PREPARATION

1) Dice and steam the sweet potato until it becomes very soft; **2)** soften the dark chocolate in a bain marie (hot water bath); **3)** add all the ingredients into a blender and blend until smooth; **4)** pour into a glass and refrigerate for at least one hour before serving.

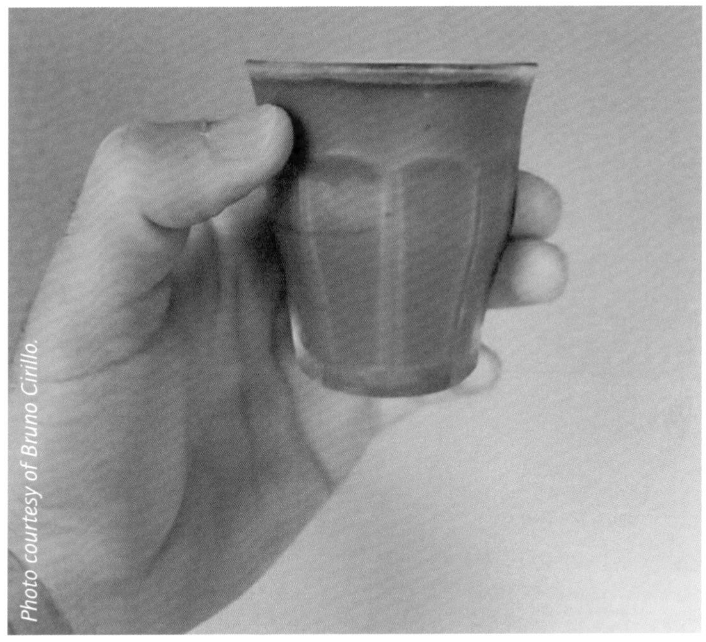

Photo courtesy of Bruno Cirillo.

Photo 12.42 Chocolate mousse.

Fruit salad with ice cream

(320 kcal, 58 g carbohydrate, 10 g protein, 5 g fat)

INGREDIENTS

- 150 g white grapes
- 100 g mixed berries sorbet (a low-fat form of ice cream)
- One medium-sized banana
- 50 g pear
- 21 g honey
- 1 teaspoon of anise seeds

PREPARATION

1) Dice the fruit and place in a bowl; **2)** melt the honey in a saucepan gently with the anise seeds; **3)** add the honey to the diced fruit and serve in a cup with fruit-based ice cream (e.g. mixed berries sorbet).

Crunchy apple trifle

(280 kcal, 58 g carbohydrate, 4 g protein, 4 g fat)

INGREDIENTS

» 150 g skinless and seedless apple

» 30 g crunchy granola (low fat)

» 20 g granulated sugar

» 2 g vanilla sugar

» Pinch of cinnamon or cardamom

PREPARATION

1) Dice the apple and place in a cooking pot with the sugar; simmer until very soft (about 10 minutes); **2)** set aside to cool down or in the fridge; **3)** for serving: in a glass add the apple compôte and crunchy granola as alternating layers; **4)** sprinkle cinnamon or cardamom on top according to personal preference.

Chocolate milkshake

(380 kcal, 68 g carbohydrate, 11 g protein, 7 g fat)

INGREDIENTS

» 250 mL low-fat chocolate milk

» 110 g frozen diced banana

» 70 g ice cream (reduced fat chocolate flavour)

» Pinch of cocoa powder or cinnamon for topping

PREPARATION

1) In a blender, add all the ingredients except the topping and blend until smooth;
2) serve cold with cocoa powder or cinnamon as topping.

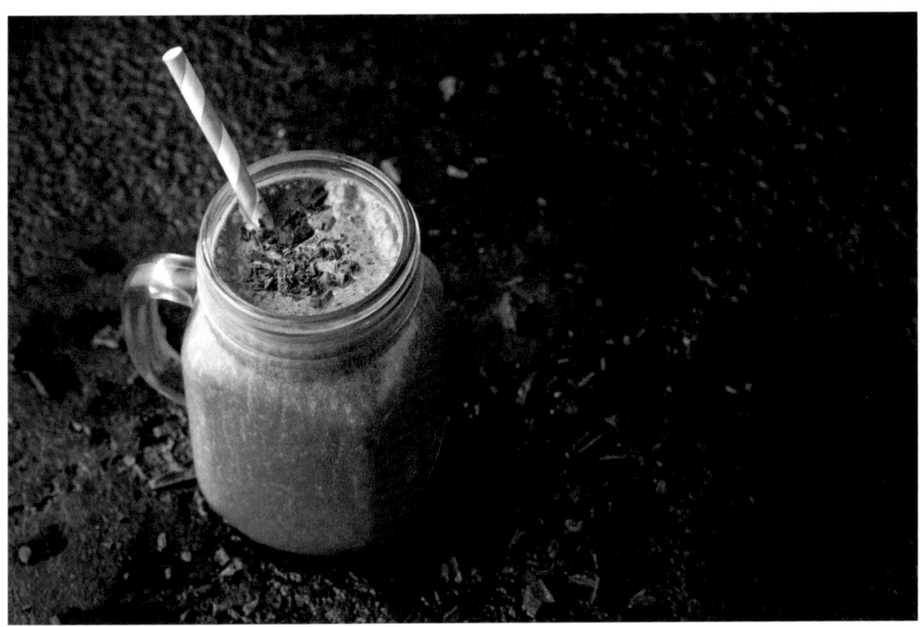

Photo 12.43 Chocolate milkshake.

Energy balls

(290 kcal, 58 g carbohydrate, 7 g protein, 5 g fat)

INGREDIENTS

- 40 g Medjool dates
- 35 g rolled oats
- 6 g tahini (toasted ground hulled sesame)
- 6 g honey
- Pinch of salt to enhance taste
- Two tablespoons of cocoa powder to roll once made

PREPARATION

1) In a blender, add all the ingredients, except the cocoa powder, and blend until a compact dough is formed; if too hard, soften by adding some water; **2)** divide into uniform parts and roll in your own hands to create balls; **3)** once finished, roll on top of cocoa powder and chill in the fridge before serving; **4)** can be prepared in bulk and stored in the fridge for up to a week in an airtight container.

EXAMPLE MEALS FOR PLAYERS

Training Day Breakfast

~700 kcal, >50 g carb & >30 g protein

Fruit smoothie + poached egg
Muesli + smoked haddock kedgeree
Porridge + cheese & red pepper omelette
Oatmeal, nuts & yoghurt + bacon & egg
Baked beans on toast + Spanish omelette
Fruit & bran cereal + scrambled eggs
Chocolate protein oats + beans on toast
Grapefruit, muesli + vegetable omelette
Macaroni cheese & toast

Pre-match Meal

~600 kcal, >70g carb & >40 g protein

Chicken & tomato pasta bake
Chicken, rice & beans
Chicken/prawn & egg fried rice
Cod loin, mashed potato & peas
Pasta with pumpkin cream & chickpeas
Rice with sticky chicken & fried vegetables
Jacket sweet potato with smoked salmon
Rice & vegetable Burritos
Fruity porridge

Post-training lunch

~850 kcal, >100 g carb, >40 g protein & ~20 g fat

Beef stifado stew & potato
Seafood & chicken paella
Chicken & vegetable rice risotto
Meat casserole & mashed potato
Meat & veg skewer & egg noodle
Thai chicken curry & brown rice
Mixed veg & fish rice risotto
Chicken BLT sandwich
Spiced smoked salmon kedgeree
Vegan burger

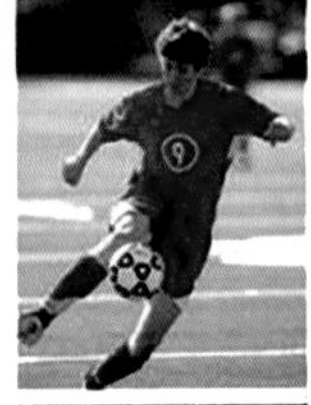

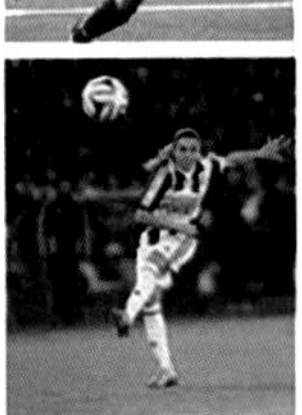

Finger Foods

High carb suitable for travel

Celery, cherry tomatoes & apple
Cup of chopped mixed fruit
Banana & grapes
Fruit yoghurt
Chicken/ham/tuna sandwich
Oven-baked sweet potato wedges
Chicken/ham/tuna Paninis,
Chicken & rice tortilla wraps
Cereal bar
Chocolate milk shake
Sports foods & drinks

Training Day Dinner

~900 kcal, >90 g carb & >40 g protein

Salmon/cod, new potatoes & spinach
Beef/pork stir-fry & egg noodle
Meat & mixed veg with pasta or rice
Lamb/chicken curry, beansprouts & rice
Chicken/beef teriyaki, white rice & broccoli
Beef burger on bun, chips & salad
Chilli con carne & brown rice
Roast chicken, vegetables & couscous
Beef/tuna steak, sweet potato & salad

Post-match Meal

~1,000 kcal, >100 g carb, >40 g protein & ~20 g fat

Spaghetti Bolognese
Spicy prawn linguine Carbonara
Beefsteak, jacket potato, corn & salad
Seafood & chicken paella
Chicken & vegetable rice risotto
Cheeseburger with sweet potato fries
Rice with salmon fillet in poppy seed crust
Ramen noodles with pork

Infographic 12 Examples of meals and snacks for football players.

RECOMMENDED READING AND REFERENCE SOURCES

This is a list of reference sources I have used in putting together this book. You can find the journal articles on the PubMed website (https://www.ncbi.nlm.nih.gov/pubmed). PubMed is a search engine that comprises more than 27 million papers and review articles from the biomedical literature, life science journals and online books. Just type in the title of the article or the lead author surname and initials to bring up a 250-word abstract of the article; for many articles you can click on a link to get the full article for free. The other reference sources in the list are books and websites where you will find helpful information on particular topics.

LIST OF REFERENCE SOURCES

Abaidia A-E et al. (2020). Effects of Ramadan fasting on physical performance: A systematic review with meta-analysis. *Sports Med* 50(5):1009–1026.

Abbott W et al. (2018). Presleep casein protein ingestion: acceleration of functional recovery in professional soccer players. *Int J Sports Physiol Perform* 14(3):1–24.

Abbott W et al. (2020). Tart cherry juice: no effect on muscle function loss or muscle soreness in professional soccer players after a match. *Int J Sports Physiol Perform* 15(2):249–254.

Ackland TR et al. (2012). Current status of body composition assessment in sport. *Sports Med* 42:227–249.

Aerospace Medical Association, Air Transport Medicine Committee. (1996). Medical guidelines for air travel. *Aviat Space Environ Med* 67(10 suppl):1–6.

Afshar M et al. (2015). Acute immunomodulatory effects of binge alcohol consumption. *Alcohol* 49:57–64.

Akenhead R et al. (2016). Examining the external training load of an English premier league football team with special reference to acceleration. *J Strength Cond Res* 30: 2424–2432.

Ali A & Williams C. (2009). Carbohydrate ingestion and soccer skill performance during prolonged intermittent exercise. *J Sports Sci* 27(14): 1499–1508.

Aljaloud SO & Ibrahim SA. (2013). Use of dietary supplements among professional athletes in Saudi Arabia. *J Nutr Metab* 245349:1–7.

American Academy of Pediatrics (2011). Policy statement. Climatic heat stress and exercising children and adolescents. *Pediatrics* 128:1–7.

Anderson L et al. (2015). Quantification of training load during one-, two- and three-game week schedules in professional football players from the English Premier League: Implications for carbohydrate periodization. *J Sports Sci* 4:1–10.

Anderson L et al. (2017). Daily distribution of macronutrient intakes of professional soccer players from the English Premier League. *Int J Sport Nutr Exerc Metab* 27(6):491–498.

Anderson L et al. (2017). Energy intake and expenditure of professional soccer players of the English Premier League: Evidence of carbohydrate periodization. *Int J Sport Nutr Exerc Metab* 27(3):228–38.

Anderson L et al. (2019). Case study: muscle atrophy, hypertrophy, and energy expenditure of a premier league soccer player during rehabilitation from anterior cruciate ligament injury. *Int J Sport Nutr Exerc Metab* 29(5):559–566.

Anonymous. (2006). Consensus statement: nutrition for football: the FIFA/F-MARC consensus conference. *J Sports Sci* 24:663–664.

Ardern CL et al. (2016). Consensus statement on return to sport from the First World Congress in Sports Physical Therapy, Bern. *Br J Sports Med* 50:853–864.

Areta J et al. (2013). Timing and distribution of protein ingestion during prolonged recovery from resistance exercise alters myofibrillar protein synthesis. *J Physiol* 591:2319–2331.

Armstrong LE. (2006). Nutritional strategies for football (soccer): Counteracting heat, cold, high altitude and jet lag. *J Sport Sci* 24(7):723–740.

Armstrong LE et al. (2010). Human hydration indices: acute and longitudinal reference values. *Int J Sport Nutr Exerc Metab* 20(2):145–153.

Armstrong LE et al. (1998). Urinary indices during dehydration, exercise, and rehydration. *Int J Sport Nutr* 8(4):345–355.

Armstrong LE et al. (2014). Novel hydration assessment techniques employing thirst and a water intake challenge in healthy men. *Appl Physiol Nutr Metab* 39(2):138–144.

Babraj J et al. (2005). Human bone collagen synthesis is a rapid, nutritionally modulated process. *J Bone Miner Res* 20(6):930–937.

Baker LB et al. (2014). Acute effects of dietary constituents on motor skill and cognitive performance in athletes. *Nutr Rev* 72(12):790–802.

Baker LB et al. (2015). Acute effects of carbohydrate supplementation on intermittent sports performance. *Nutrients* 7(7):5733–5763.

Baker LB et al. (2016). Normative data for regional sweat sodium concentration and whole-body sweating rate in athletes. *J Sports Sci* 34(4):358–368.

Bangsbo J. (2014). Physiological demands of football. *Sports Sci Exch* 27(125):1–6.

Bangsbo J et al. (1991). Activity profile of competition soccer. *Can J Sport Sci* 16(2):110–116.

Bangsbo J et al. (2006). Physical and metabolic demands of training and match play in the elite football player. *J Sports Sci* 24(7):665–674.

Bangsbo J et al. (2015). Recreational football for disease prevention and treatment in untrained men: a narrative review examining cardiovascular health, lipid profile, body composition, muscle strength and functional capacity. *Br J Sports Med* 49:568–576.

Barbosa A et al. (2012). A leucine-rich diet and exercise affect the biomechanical characteristics of the digital flexor tendon in rats after nutritional recovery. *Amino Acids* 42(1):329–336.

Barnes C et al. (2014). The evolution of physical and technical performance parameters in the English Premier League. *Int J Sports Med* 35:1095–1100.

Barry DW & Kohrt WM. (2007). Acute effects of 2 hours of moderate-intensity cycling on serum parathyroid hormone and calcium. *Calcif Tissue Int* 80:359–365.

Barry DW et al. (2011). Acute calcium ingestion attenuates exercise-induced disruption of calcium homeostasis. *Med Sci Sports Exerc* 43:617–623.

Bell P et al. (2014). The role of cherries in exercise and health. *Scand J Med Sci Sports* 24(3):477–490.

Bell PG et al. (2014). Montmorency cherries reduce the oxidative stress and inflammatory responses to repeated days high-intensity stochastic cycling. *Nutrients* 6(2):829–843.

Bengtsson H et al. (2013). Muscle injury rates in professional football increase with fixture congestion: an 11-year follow-up of the UEFA Champions League injury study. *Br J Sports Med* 47:743–747.

Berglund B & Hemmingsson P. (1982). Effects of caffeine ingestion on exercise performance at low and high altitudes in cross-country skiers. *Int J Sports Med* 3(4):234–236.

Bergman P et al. (2013). Vitamin D and respiratory tract infections: A systemic review and meta-analysis of randomised controlled trials. *PLoS One* 8(6):e65835.

Bergstrom J & Hultman E. (1967). A study of glycogen metabolism during exercise in man. *Scand J Clin Invest* 19:218–228.

Bergstrom J et al. (1967). Diet, muscle glycogen and physical performance. *Acta Physiol Scand* 71:140–150.

Bermon S et al. (2017). Consensus Statement Immunonutrition and Exercise. *Exerc Immunol Rev* 23:8–50.

Berry DJ et al. (2011). Vitamin D status has a linear association with seasonal infections and lung function in British adults, *Br J Nutr* 106:1433–1440.

Best G. (2002). *Blessed – The Autobiography*. Ebury Press, London.

Bjørneboe J et al. (2016). Role of illness in male professional football: not a major contributor to time loss. *Br J Sports Med* 50(11):699–702.

Bradley PS et al. (2009). High-intensity running in English FA Premier League football matches. *J Sports Sci* 27:159–168.

Briggs MA et al. (2015). Assessment of energy intake and energy expenditure of male adolescent academy-level soccer players during a competitive week. *Nutrients* 7(10):8392–8401.

Briggs MA et al. (2017). The effects of an increased calorie breakfast consumed prior to simulated match play in Academy soccer players. *Eur J Sport Sci* 17(7):858–866.

Briggs MA et al. (2015). Agreement between two methods of dietary data collection in male adolescent academy-level soccer players. *Nutrients* 7(7):5948–5960.

Bruno Cirillo Performance Nutrition website: https://www.brunocirillo.com

Burdon et al. (2012). Influence of beverage temperature on palatability and fluid ingestion during endurance exercise: a systematic review. *Int J Sport Nutr Exerc Metab* 22(3):199–211.

Burke LM. (2008). Caffeine and sports performance. *Appl Physiol Nutr Metab* 33(6):1319–1334.

Burke LM. (2010). Fasting and recovery from exercise. *Br J Sports Med* 44:502–508.

Burke LM. (2015). Re-examining high-fat diets for sports performance: Did we call the 'nail in the coffin' too soon? *Sports Med* 45(Suppl 1):S33–S49.

Burke LM et al. (2017). Postexercise muscle glycogen resynthesis in humans. *J Appl Physiol* 122(5):1055–1067.

Burke LM et al. (2017). Low carbohydrate, high fat diet impairs exercise economy and negates the performance benefit from intensified training in elite race walkers. *J Physiol* 595(9):2785–2807.

Bush M et al. (2015). Evolution of match performance parameters for various playing positions in the English Premier League. *Hum Mov Sci* 39:1–11.

Cancela P et al. (2008). Creatine supplementation does not affect clinical health markers in football players. *Br J Sports Med* 42:731–735.

Cardinali DP et al. (2002). A multifactorial approach employing melatonin to accelerate resynchronization of sleep-wake cycle after a 12 time zone westerly transmeridian flight in elite soccer athletes. *J Pineal Rsch* 32(1):41–46.

Carling C & Orhant E. (2010). Variation in body composition in professional soccer players: interseasonal and intraseasonal changes and the effects of exposure time and player position. *J Strength Cond Res / National Strength & Conditioning Association.* (5):1332–1339.

Carter JM et al. (2004). The effect of carbohydrate mouth rinse on 1-h cycle time trial performance. *Med Sci Sports Exerc* 2004:2107–2111.

Castagna C et al. (2007). Physiological aspects of soccer refereeing performance and training. *Sports Med* 37(7):625–646.

Centre for Integrative Sports Nutrition website: https://www.intsportsnutrition.com

Cheuvront SN et al. (2010). Biological variation and diagnostic accuracy of dehydration assessment markers. *Am J Clin Nutr* 92(3):565–573.

Churchward-Venne TA et al. (2020). Dose-response effects of dietary protein on muscle protein synthesis during recovery from endurance exercise in young men: a double-blind randomized trial. *Am J Clin Nutr* 112(2):303–317.

Clark M et al. (2003). Pre- and post-season dietary intake, body composition, and performance indices of NCAA division I female soccer players. *Int J Sport Nutr Exerc Metab* 13(3):303–319.

Clark M et al. (2003). Pre- and post-season dietary intake, body composition, and performance indices of NCAA division I female soccer players. *Int J Sport Nutr Exerc Metab* 13(3):303–319.

Claudino JG et al. (2014) Creatine monohydrate supplementation on lower-limb muscle power in Brazilian elite soccer players. *J Int Soc Sport Nutr* 11(32):1–6

Close GL et al. (2013). Assessment of vitamin D concentration in non-supplemented professional athletes and healthy adults during the winter months in the UK: implications for skeletal muscle function. *J Sports Sci* 31(4):344–353.

Collins J. (2019). *The Energy Plan*. Vermilion, London.

Collins J & Rollo I. (2014). Practical considerations in elite football. *Sport Sci Exch* 27(133):1–7.

Collins J et al. (2021). UEFA expert group 2020 statement on nutrition in elite football. Current evidence to inform practical recommendations and guide future research. *Br J Sports Med* 55(8):416.

Costello RB et al. (2014). The effectiveness of melatonin for promoting healthy sleep: a rapid evidence assessment of the literature. *Nutr J* 13:106.

Costill DL et al. (1990). Impaired muscle glycogen resynthesis after eccentric exercise. *J Appl Physiol* 69(1):46–50.

Coutts AJ. (2017). Challenges in developing evidence-based practice in high-performance sport. *Int J Sports Physiol Perform* 12(6):717–718.

Currell K et al. (2009). Carbohydrate ingestion improves performance of a new reliable test of soccer performance. *Int J Sport Nutr Exerc Metab* 19(1):34–46.

Curtis L. (2016). Nutritional research may be useful in treating tendon injuries. *Nutrition* 32(6):617–619.

Da Silva AI et al. (2008). Energy expenditure and intensity of physical activity in soccer referees during match play. *J Sports Sci Med* 7(3):327–334.

Da Silva RP et al. (2012). Pre-game hydration status, sweat loss, and fluid intake in elite Brazilian young male soccer players during competition. *J Sports Sci* 30(1):37–42.

Datson N et al. (2017). Match physical performance of elite female soccer players during international competition. *J Strength Cond Res* 31:2379–2387.

De Boer M et al. (2007). Time course of muscular, neural and tendinous adaptations to 23 day unilateral lower-limb suspension in young men. *J Physiol* 583:1079–1091.

Desbrow B et al. (2014). Sports Dietitians Australia position statement: sports nutrition for the adolescent athlete. *Int J Sport Nutr Exerc Metab* 24(5):570–584.

Devlin BL et al. (2016). Dietary intake, body composition and nutrition knowledge of Australian football and soccer players: Implications for sports nutrition professionals in practice. *Int J Sport Nutr Exerc Metab* 6:1–21.

Di Salvo V et al. (2010). Sprinting analysis of elite football players during European Champions League and UEFA Cup matches. *J Sports Sci* 28:1489–1494.

Discreet and Delicious (Performance Chefs) website: https://www.discreetanddelicious.co.uk

Dobrowollski H et al. (2020). Nutrition for female soccer players – recommendations. *Medicina* 56(28):1–17.

Dorling JL & Earnest CP. (2013). Effect of carbohydrate mouth rinsing on multiple sprint performance. *J Int Soc Sports Nutr* 10(1):41.

Doyle JA et al. (1993). Sherman WM, Strauss RL. Effects of eccentric and concentric exercise on muscle glycogen replenishment. *J Appl Physiol* 74(4):1848–1855.

Duffield R et al. (2012). Hydration, sweat and thermoregulatory responses to professional football training in the heat. *J Sports Sci* 30(10):957–965.

Dupont G et al. (2010). Effect of 2 soccer matches in a week on physical performance and injury rate. *Am J Sports Med* 38:1752–1758

Dvorak J et al. (2011). Injuries and illnesses of football players during the 2010 FIFA World Cup. *Br J Sports Med* 45(8):626–630.

Ekblom B. (1986). Applied physiology of soccer. *Sports Med* 3(1):50–60.

Enright K et al. (2015). The effect of concurrent training organisation in youth elite football players. *Eur J Appl Physiol* 115:2367–2381.

Enright K et al. (2017). Implementing concurrent-training and nutritional strategies in professional football: a complex challenge for coaches and practitioners. *J Sci Med Football* 1:65–73.

Ersoy N et al. (2016). Assessment of hydration status of elite young male soccer players with different methods and new approach method of substitute urine strip. *J Int Soc Sports Nutr* 13(1):34

Esco MR et al. (2011). The accuracy of hand-to hand bioelectrical impedance analysis in predicting body composition in college-age female athletes. *J Strength Cond Res* 25(4):1040–1045.

Farup J et al. (2014). Whey protein hydrolysate augments tendon and muscle hypertrophy independent of resistance exercise contraction mode. *Scand J Med Sci Sports* 24(5):788–798.

Fédération Internationale de Football Association (FIFA) (2020). Physical analysis of the FIFA women's world cup France 2019 report.

Fédération Internationale de Football Association (FIFA) website: https://www.fifa.com

Ferguson A. (2013). *Alex Ferguson My Autobiography.* Hodder and Stoughton, London.

Fernandes HS. (2020). Carbohydrate consumption and periodization strategies applied to elite soccer players. *Curr Nutr Rep* 9(4):414–419.

Field A et al. (2020). The demands of the extra-time period of soccer: A systematic review. *J Sport Health Sci* doi: 10.1016/j.jshs.2020.03.008. Online ahead of print.

Food Standards Agency (2018). Food hygiene for your business. Retrieved from https://www.food.gov.uk/business-guidance/food-hygiene-for-your-business.

Football4Football website: https://www.football4football.com

Foskett A et al. (2009). Caffeine enhances cognitive function and skill performance during simulated soccer activity. *Int J Sport Nutr Exerc Metab* 19:410–423.

Fowler P et al. (2015). Effects of northbound long-haul international air travel on sleep quantity and subjective jet lag and wellness in professional Australian soccer players. *Int J Sports Physiol Perform* 10(5):648–654.

Fowler PM et al. (2017). Greater effect of east versus west travel on Jet Lag, sleep, and team sport performance. *Med Sci Sports Exerc* 49(12):2548–2561.

Gabbett TJ et al. (2014). The relationship between workloads, physical performance, injury and illness in adolescent male football players. *Sports Med* 44(7):989–1003.

Ganio MS et al. (2011). Effect of ambient temperature on caffeine ergogenicity during endurance exercise. *Eur J Appl Physiol* 111(6):1135–1146.

Ganio MS et al. (2011). Mild dehydration impairs cognitive performance and mood of men. *Br J Nutr* 106(10):1535–1543.

Gant N et al. (2010). The influence of caffeine and carbohydrate coingestion on simulated soccer performance. *Int J Sport Nutr Exerc Metab* 20:191–197.

Garthe I & Maughan RJ. (2018). Athletes and supplements – prevalence and perspectives. *Int J Sport Nutr Exerc Metab* 28(2):126–138.

Garvican LA et al. (2014). Lower running performance and exacerbated fatigue in soccer played at 1600 m. *Int J Sports Physiol Perf* 9(3):397–404.

Geyer H et al. (2008). Nutritional supplements cross-contaminated and faked with doping substances. *J Mass Spec* 43(7):892–902.

Geyer H et al. (2004). Analysis of non-hormonal nutritional supplements for anabolic-androgenic steroids – Results of an international study. *Int J Sports Med* 25:124–129.

Gibson JC et al. (2011). Nutrition status of junior elite Canadian female soccer athletes. *Int J Sport Nutr Exerc Metab* 21(6):507–514.

Gladden LB. (2004). Lactate metabolism: a new paradigm for the third millennium. *J Physiol* 558(1):5–30.

Gleeson M. (2015). Effects of exercise on immune function. *Sports Sci Exch* 28(151):1–6.

Gleeson M. (2016). Immunological aspects of sport nutrition. *Immunol Cell Biol* 94:117–123.

Gleeson M. (2020). *Eat, Move, Sleep, Repeat.* Meyer & Meyer Sport. Aachen, Germany.

Gleeson M. (2020). *Beating Type 2 Diabetes.* Meyer & Meyer Sport. Aachen, Germany.

Gleeson M. (2020). *The Pick 'n Mix Diet.* Meyer & Meyer Sport. Aachen, Germany.

Gleeson M. et al. (2011). The anti-inflammatory effects of exercise: Mechanisms and implications for the prevention and treatment of disease. *Nat Rev Immunol* 11:607–615.

Gleeson M. et al. (2013). *Exercise Immunology.* Abingdon: Routledge.

Gore CJ et al. (2006). Increased serum erythropoietin but not red cell production after 4 wk of intermittent hypobaric hypoxia (4,000–5,500 m). *J Appl Physiol* 101(5):1386–1393.

Gore CJ et al. (2008). Preparation for football competition at moderate to high altitude. *Scand J Med Sci Sports* 18(S1):85–95.

Grant WB et al. (2020). The benefits of vitamin D supplementation for athletes: better performance and reduced risk of COVID-19. *Nutrients* 12(12): 3741.

Guest NS et al. (2021). International society of sports nutrition position stand: caffeine and exercise performance. *J Int Soc Sports Nutr* 18(1):1.

Gunnarsson TP et al. (2013). Effect of whey protein- and carbohydrate-enriched diet on glycogen resynthesis during the first 48 h after a soccer game. *Scand J Med Sci Sports* 23:508–515.

Haakonssen EC et al. (2015). The effects of a calcium-rich pre-exercise meal on biomarkers of calcium homeostasis in competitive female cyclists: a randomised crossover trial. *PLoS One* 10(5): e0123302.

Hannon MP et al. (2020). Cross-sectional comparison of body composition and resting metabolic rate in Premier League academy soccer players: Implications for growth and maturation. *J Sports Sci* 38(11-12):1326–1334.

Hannon MP et al. (2021). Energy requirements of male academy soccer players from the English Premier League. *Med Sci Sports Exerc* 53(1):200–210.

Hargreaves M & Spriet LL. (2020). Skeletal muscle energy metabolism during exercise. *Nature Metab* 2(9):817–828.

Harley JA et al. (2011). Three-compartment body composition changes in elite rugby league players during a super league season, measured by dual-energy X-ray absorptiometry. *J Strength Cond Res.* 25(4):1024–1029.

Harper LD et al. (2016). Physiological and performance effects of carbohydrate gels consumed prior to the extra-time period of prolonged simulated soccer match play. *J Sci Med Sport* 19(6):509–514.

Harper LD et al. (2016). The effects of 120 minutes of simulated match play on indices of acid-base balance in professional academy soccer players. *J Strength Cond Res* 30(6):1517–1524.

Harris RC et al. (1992). Elevation of creatine in resting and exercised muscle of normal subjects by creatine supplementation. *Clin Sci* 83(3):367–374.

Harris RC et al. (2006). The absorption of orally supplied beta-alanine and its effect on muscle carnosine synthesis in human vastus lateralis. *Amino Acids* 30(3):279–289.

He CS et al. (2013). Influence of vitamin D status on respiratory infection incidence and immune function during 4 months of winter training in endurance sport athletes. *Exerc Immunol Rev* 19:86–101.

He CS et al. (2016). Is there an optimal vitamin D status for immunity in athletes and military personnel? *Exerc Immunol Rev* 22:42–64.

Hector AJ & Phillips S. (2017). Protein recommendations for weight loss in elite athletes: a focus on body composition and performance. *Int J Sport Nutr Exerc Metab* 28:1–26.

Henderson B et al. (2015). Game and training load differences in elite junior Australian football. *J Sports Sci Med* 14(3):494–500.

Herriman M et al. (2017). Dietary supplements and young teens: Misinformation and access provided by retailers. *Pediatrics* 39(2):1257.

Holway FE & Spriet LL. (2011). Sport-specific nutrition: practical strategies for team sports. *J Sports Sci* 29 Suppl 1:S115–125.

Horowitz M. (2014). Heat acclimation, epigenetics, and cytoprotection memory. *Compar Physiol* 4(1):199–230.

Hughes M et al. (2006). Enhanced fracture and soft-tissue healing by means of anabolic dietary supplementation. *J Bone Joint Surg Am* 88(11):2386–2894.

Informed Sport website: https://www.sport.wetestyoutrust.com/

Institute of Medicine (US) Panel on Micronutrients. *(2001), Dietary Reference Intakes for Vitamin A, Vitamin K, Arsenic, Boron, Chromium, Copper, Iodine, Iron, Manganese, Molybdenum, Nickel, Silicon, Vanadium, and Zinc.* Washington, DC: The National Academies Press.

Institute of Performance Nutrition website: https://www.theiopn.com

Intraperforrnance Group website (performance nutrition): https://www.intraperformancegroup.com/performancenutrition

Jackman SR et al. (2010). Branched-chain amino acid ingestion can ameliorate soreness from eccentric exercise. *Med Sci Sports Exerc* 42:962–970.

James Sinclair Performance Nutrition website: https://www.jamessinclairnutrition.com

Jeong T-S et al. (2015). Acute simulated football specific training increases PGC-1 alpha mRNA expression in human skeletal muscle. *J Sports Sci* 33:1493–1503.

Jeukendrup AE & Gleeson M. (2019). *Sport Nutrition.* 3rd edition. Human Kinetics: Champaign, IL.

Judelson DA et al. (2007). Hydration and muscular performance: Does fluid balance affect strength, power and high-intensity endurance? *Sports Med* 37(10):907–921.

Kamimori GH et al. (2002). The rate of absorption and relative bioavailability of caffeine administered in chewing gum versus capsules to normal healthy volunteers. *Int J Pharm* 234(1-2):159–167.

Kasper AM et al. (2020). High prevalence of cannabidiol use within male professional rugby union and league players: a quest for pain relief and enhanced recovery. *Int J Sport Nutr Exerc Metab* 30:315–322.

Kelly V. (2018). Beta-alanine: performance effects, usage and side effects. *Br J Sports Med* 52(5):311–312.

Kenefick RW & Cheuvront SN. (2012). Hydration for recreational sport and physical activity. *Nutr Rev* 70(Suppl 2):S137–142.

Kerr A et al. (2017). Impact of food and fluid intake on technical and biological measurement error in body composition assessment methods in athletes. *Br J Nutr* 117(4):591–601.

Kilding AE et al. (2009). Sweat rate and sweat electrolyte composition in international female soccer players during game specific training. *Int J Sports Med* 30(6):443–447.

Kingsley M et al. (2014). Effects of carbohydrate-hydration strategies on glucose metabolism, sprint performance and hydration during a soccer match simulation in recreational players. *J Sci Med Sport* 17:239–243.

Koehle MS et al. (2014). Canadian Academy of Sport and Exercise Medicine position statement: athletes at high altitude. *Clin J Sport Med* 24(2):120–127.

Koopman R et al. (2007). Nutritional interventions to promote post-exercise muscle protein synthesis. *Sports Med* 37(10):895–900.

Krustrup P et al. (2006). Muscle and blood metabolites during a football game: Implications for sprint performance. *Med Sci Sports Exerc* 38:1165–1174.

Krustrup P et al. (2011). Maximal voluntary contraction force, SR function and glycogen resynthesis during the first 72 h after a high-level competitive soccer game. *Eur J Appl Physiol* 111(12):2987–2995.

Krustrup P et al. (2015). Sodium bicarbonate improves high-intensity intermittent exercise performance in trained young men. *J Int Soc Sports Nutr* 12:25.

Książek A et al. (2020). Assessment of the dietary intake of high-rank professional male football players during a preseason training week. *Int J Environ Res Public Health* 17(22):8567.

Lamon S et al. (2021). The effect of acute sleep deprivation on skeletal muscle protein synthesis and the hormonal environment. *Physiol Rep* 9(1):e14660.

Leatt PB & Jacobs I. (1989). Effect of glucose polymer ingestion on glycogen depletion during a soccer match. *Can J Sport Sci* 14(2):112–116.

Lee JKW et al. (2008) Cold drink ingestion improves exercise endurance capacity in the heat. *Med Sci Sports Exerc* 40:1637–1644.

Leites GT et al. (2016). Energy substrate utilization with and without exogenous carbohydrate intake in boys and men exercising in the heat. *J Appl Physiol* 121(5):1127–1134.

Lin E et al. (1998). Nutritional modulation of immunity and the inflammatory response. *Nutrition* 14(6):545–550.

Lis DM et al. (2015). Exploring the popularity, experiences and beliefs surrounding gluten-free diets in non-coeliac athletes. *Int J Sport Nutr Exerc Metab* 25(1):37–23.

Longland TM et al. (2016). Higher compared with lower dietary protein during an energy deficit combined with intense exercise promotes greater lean mass gain and fat mass loss: a randomised trial. *Am J Clin Nutr* 103:738–746.

Maganaris CN & Maughan RJ. (1998). Creatine supplementation enhances maximum voluntary isometric force and endurance capacity in resistance trained men *Acta Physiol Scand* 163 :279–287.

Malone JJ et al. (2015). Seasonal training-load quantification in elite English premier league football players. *Int J Sports Physiol Perform* 10: 489–497.

Mamerow M et al. (2014). Dietary protein distribution positively influences 24-h muscle protein synthesis in healthy adults. *J Nutr* 144(6):876–880.

Manore MM et al. (2017). Sport nutrition knowledge, behaviors and beliefs of high school soccer players. *Nutrients* 9:E350.

Martin L et al. (2005). Nutritional practices of national female football players: analysis and recommendations. *J Sports Sci Med* 1:130–137.

Matt Gardner Nutrition website: https://www.mattgardnernutrition.com

Matthews NM. (2018). Prohibited contaminants in dietary supplements. *Sports Health* 10(1): 19–30.

Maughan RJ. (1997). Energy and macronutrient intakes of professional football (soccer) players. *Br J Sports Med* 31:45–47.

Maughan RJ. (2005). Contamination of dietary supplements and positive drugs tests in sport. *J Sports Sci* 23:883–889.

Maughan RJ & Gleeson M. (2010). *The Biochemical Basis of Sport Performance.* 2nd edition. Oxford: Oxford University Press.

Maughan RJ & Griffin J. (2003). Caffeine ingestion and fluid balance: a review. *J Human Nutr Dietetics* 16:411–420.

Maughan RJ & Leiper JB. (1995). Sodium intake and post-exercise rehydration in man. *Eur J Appl Physiol* 71(4):311–319.

Maughan RJ et al. (1996). Restoration of fluid balance after exercise-induced dehydration: effects of food and fluid intake. *Eur J Appl Physiol* 73(3-4):317–325.

Maughan RJ et al. (2005). Fluid and electrolyte balance in elite male football (soccer) players training in a cool environment. *J Sports Sci* 23(1):73–79.

Maughan RJ et al. (2012) Achieving optimum sports performance during Ramadan: Some practical recommendations. *J Sports Sci* 30(Suppl 1):S109–S117.

Maughan RJ et al. (2018) IOC consensus statement: dietary supplements and the high-performance athlete. *Br J Sports Med* 52:439–455.

McGregor SJ et al. (1999). The influence of intermittent high-intensity shuttle running and fluid ingestion on the performance of a football skill. *J Sports Sci* 17(11):895–903.

Medina D et al. (2014). Injury prevention and nutrition in football. *Sport Sci Exch* 27(132):1–5.

Mettler S & Zimmermann MB. (2010). Iron excess in recreational marathon runners. *Eur J Clin Nutr* 64(5):490–494.

Meyer F et al. (2012). Fluid balance and dehydration in the young athlete: assessment considerations and effects on health and performance. *Am J Lifestyle Med* 6:489–501.

Meyer T. (2021). The importance of nutrition in football: perspective of a national team's doctor. *Br J Sports Med* 55(8):412–413.

Milanese C et al. (2015). Seasonal DXA-measured body composition changes in professional male soccer players. *J Sports Sci* 33:1219–1228.

Milsom J et al. (2014). Case-Study: Muscle atrophy and hypertrophy in a Premier League soccer player during rehabilitation from ACL Injury. *Int J Sport Nutr Exerc Metab* 24(5):543–52.

Milsom J et al. (2015). Body composition assessment of English Premier League football players: a comparative DXA analysis of first team, U21 and U18 squads. *J Sports Sci* 33:1799–1806.

Mohr M et al. (2011). Caffeine intake improves intense intermittent exercise performance and reduces muscle interstitial potassium accumulation. *J Appl Physiol* 111:1372–1379.

Mohr M & Krustrup P. (2013). Heat stress impairs repeated jump ability after competitive elite soccer games. *J Strength Cond Res* 27(3):683–689.

Moore D et al. (2009). Ingested protein dose response of muscle and albumin protein synthesis after resistance exercise in young men. *Am J Clin Nutr* 89(1):161–168.

Morgans R et al. (2014). An intensive Winter fixture schedule induces a transient fall in salivary IgA in English premier league football players. *Res Sports Med* 22:346–354.

Morton JP et al. (2012). Seasonal variation in vitamin D status in professional soccer players of the English Premier League. *Appl Physiol Nutr Metab* 37(4):798–802.

Morton RW et al. (2015). Nutritional interventions to augment resistance training-induced skeletal muscle hypertrophy. *Front Physiol* 6:245.

Moss SL et al. (2021). Assessment of energy availability and associated risk factors in professional female soccer players. *Eur J Sport Sci* 21(6):861–870.

Mountjoy M et al. (2014). International Olympic Committee Consensus Statement: Beyond the female athlete triad-relative energy deficiency in sport (RED-S). *Br J Sports Med* 48:491–497.

Murphy CH et al. (2015). Considerations for protein intake in managing weight loss in athletes. *Eur J Sport Sci* 15:21–28.

Murray NG et al. (2017). Individual and combined effects of acute and chronic running loads on injury risk in elite Australian footballers. *Scand J Med Sci Sports* 27:990–998.

Muse R & Dowst B. (2019). *Food For Footballers*. Kindle eBook.

Nana A et al. (2016). Importance of Standardised DXA Protocol for Assessing Physique Changes in Athletes. *Int J Sport Nutr Exerc Metab* 26(3):259–267.

Naughton RJ et al. (2016). Daily distribution of carbohydrate, protein and fat intake in elite youth academy soccer players over a 7-day training period. *Int J Sport Nutr. Exerc Metab* 26(5):473–480.

Nédélec M et al. (2013). Recovery in soccer: Part II – Recovery strategies. *Sports Med* 43:9–22.

Nicholas CW et al. (1999). Carbohydrate-electrolyte ingestion during intermittent high-intensity running. *Med Sci Sports Exerc* 31(9):12801286.

Nicholas CW et al. (1995). Influence of ingesting a carbohydrate-electrolyte solution on endurance capacity during intermittent, high-intensity shuttle running. *J Sports Sci* 13(4): 283290.

Nieman DC et al. (2011). Upper respiratory tract infection is reduced in physically fit and active adults. *Br J Sports Med* 45:987–992.

Nieman DC et al. (2007). Quercetin reduces illness but not immune perturbations after intensive exercise. *Med Sci Sports Exerc* 39:1561–1569.

Nilsson LH et al. (1973). Carbohydrate metabolism of the liver in normal man under varying dietary conditions. *Scand J Cin Lab Invest* 32(4):331–337.

Nyakayiru J et al. (2017) Beetroot juice supplementation improves high-intensity intermittent type exercise performance in trained soccer players. *Nutrients* 9(3):314.

Owens DJ et al. (2015). A systems based investigation into vitamin D and skeletal muscle repair, regeneration and hypertrophy. *Am J Physiol Endocrinol Metab* 309(12): E1019–1031.

Owens DJ et al. (2017). Efficacy of high-dose vitamin D supplements for elite athletes. *Med Sci Sports Exerc* 49(2):349–356.

Owens DJ et al. (2018). Vitamin D and the athlete: Current perspectives and new challenges. *Sports Med* 48(Suppl 1):3–16.

Paddon-Jones D et al. (2004). Essential amino acid and carbohydrate supplementation ameliorates muscle protein loss in humans during 28 days bedrest. *J Clin Endocrinol Metab* 89(9):4351–4358.

Pasiakos SM et al. (2014). Effects of protein supplements on muscle damage, soreness and recovery of muscle function and physical performance: a systematic review. *Sports Med* 44(5):655–670.

Peeling P et al. (2007). Effect of iron injections on aerobic-exercise performance of iron depleted female athletes. *Int J Sport Nutr Exerc Metab* 17(3):221–231.

Peeling P et al. (2008). Athletic induced iron deficiency: new insights into the role of inflammation, cytokines and hormones. *Eur J Appl Physiol* 103(4):381–391.

Peternelj TT & Coombes JS. (2011). Antioxidant supplementation during exercise training: beneficial or detrimental? *Sports Med* 41(12):1043–1069.

Pettersen SA et al. (2014). Caffeine supplementation does not affect match activities and fatigue resistance during match play in young football players. *J Sports Sci* 32(20):1958–1965.

Phillips SM. (2014). A brief review of higher dietary protein diets in weight loss: a focus on athletes. *Sports Med* 44 (Suppl 2):S149–153.

Phillips SM. (2016). The impact of protein quality on the promotion of resistance exercise-induced changes in muscle mass. *Nutr Metab* 13:64.

Phillips SM et al. (2011). Carbohydrate ingestion during team games exercise: current knowledge and areas for future investigation. *Sports Med* 41(7):559–585.

Piérard C et al. (2001). Resynchronization of hormonal rhythms after an eastbound flight in humans: effects of slow-release caffeine and melatonin. *Eur J Appl Physiol* 85(1):144–150.

Pyne DB et al. (2015). Probiotics supplementation for athletes - clinical and physiological effects. *Eur J Sport Sci* 15(1):63–72

Ranchordas MK et al. (2017). Practical nutrition recovery strategies for elite soccer players when limited time separates repeated matches. *J Int Soc Sports Nutr* 14(35):1–14.

Randell RK et al. (2021). Physiological characteristics of female soccer players and health and performance considerations: A narrative review. *Sports Med* doi: 10.1007/s40279-021-01458-1. Online ahead of print.

Rawson ES & Persky AM. (2007). Mechanisms of muscular adaptations to creatine supplementation: review article. *Int Sport Med J* 8:43–53.

Reed JL et al. (2014). Nutritional practices associated with low energy availability in Division I female football players. *J Sports Sci* 32(16):1499–1509.

Reilly T & Gregson W. (2006). Special populations: the referee and assistant referee. *J Sports Sci* 24(7):795–801.

Reilly T & Thomas V. (1976). A motion analysis of work rate in different positional roles in professional football match play. *J Human Move Stud* 2:87–97.

Reilly T et al. (2009). Some chronobiological and physiological problems associated with long-distance journeys. *Travel Med Infect Dis* 7(2):88–101.

Res P et al. (2012). Protein ingestion prior to sleep improves post-exercise overnight recovery. *Med Sci Sports Exerc* 44(8):1560–1569.

Riddell MC. (2008). The endocrine response and substrate utilization during exercise in children and adolescents. *J Appl Physiol* 105(2):725–733.

Rittweger J et al. (2006). Bone loss from the human distal tibia epiphysis during 24 days of unilateral lower limb suspension. *J Physiol* 15:331–337.

Roberts AC et al. (1996). Acclimatization to 4,300-m altitude decreases reliance on fat as a substrate. *J Appl Physiol* 81(4):1762–1771.

Roberts PA et al. (2016). Creatine ingestion augments dietary carbohydrate mediated muscle glycogen supercompensation during the initial 24 h of recovery following prolonged exhaustive exercise in humans. *Amino Acids* 48(8):1831–1842.

Roden D. (2021). *Fit For Every Game*. https://www.fitforeverygame.com/

Rodriguez FR et al. (2015). Effects of beta-alanine supplementation on wingate tests in university female football players. *Nutr Hosp* 31(1):430–435.

Rodriguez-Giustiniani P et al. (2019). Ingesting a 12% Carbohydrate-Electrolyte beverage before each half of a soccer match simulation facilitates retention of passing performance and improves high-intensity running capacity in academy players. *Int J Sport Nutr Exerc Metab* 18:1–9.

Rollo I et al. (2015). The influence of carbohydrate mouth rinse on self-selected intermittent running performance. *Int J Sport Nutr Exerc Metab* 25(6):550–558.

Rollo I et al. (2020). Role of sports psychology and sports nutrition in return to play from musculoskeletal injuries in professional soccer: an interdisciplinary approach. *Eur J Sport Sci* doi: 10.1080/17461391.2020.1792558. Online ahead of print.

Rollo I et al. (2021). Fluid balance, sweat Na^+ losses, and carbohydrate intake of elite male soccer players in response to low and high training intensities in cool and hot environments. *Nutrients* 13(2):401.

Romijn JA et al. (1993). Regulation of endogenous fat and carbohydrate metabolism in relation to exercise intensity. *Am J Physiol* 265:E380–E391.

Romijn JA et al. (1995). Relationship between fatty acid delivery and fatty acid oxidation during strenuous exercise. *J Appl Physiol* 79(6):1939–1945.

Ruiz F et al. (2005). Nutritional intake in soccer players of different ages. *J Sports Sci* 23:235–242.

Russell M & Kingsley M. (2014). The efficacy of acute nutritional interventions on soccer skill performance. *Sports Med* 44(7):957–970.

Russell M et al. (2011). Dietary analysis of young professional soccer players in 1 week during the competitive season. *J Strength Cond Res* 25:1–8.

Russell M et al. (2012). Influence of carbohydrate supplementation on skill performance during a soccer match simulation. *J Sci Med Sport* 15(4):348–354.

Russell M et al. (2016). Changes in acceleration and deceleration capacity throughout professional soccer match play. *J Strength Cond Res* 30(10):2839–2844.

Sánchez-Díaz S, et al. (2020). Effects of nutrition education interventions in team sport players. A systematic review. *Nutrients* 12(12):E3664.

Sawka MN et al. (2007). American College of Sports Medicine position stand. Exercise and fluid replacement. *Med Sci Sports Exerc* 39(2)377–390.

Schenk K et al. (2018). Exercise physiology and nutritional perspectives of elite soccer refereeing. *Scand J Med Sci Sports* 28(3):782–793.

Scherr J et al. (2012). Nonalcoholic beer reduces inflammation and incidence of respiratory tract illness. *Med Sci Sports Exerc* 44(1):18–26.

Schwellnus M et al. (2016). How much is too much? (Part **2)** International Olympic Committee consensus statement on load in sport and risk of illness. *Br J Sports Med* 50(17):1043–1052.

Shaw G et al. (2017). Vitamin C-enriched gelatin supplementation before intermittent activity augments collagen synthesis. *Am J Clin Nutr* 105(1):136–143.

Shirreffs SM & Sawka MN. (2011). Fluid and electrolyte needs for training, competition and recovery. *J Sports Sci* 29:539–546.

Shirreffs SM et al. (2005). The sweating response of elite professional soccer players to training in the heat. *Int J Sports Med* 26(2):90–95.

Shirreffs SM et al. (2006). Water and electrolyte needs for football training and match play. *J Sports Sci* 24(7):699–707.

Singh M & Das RR. (2011). Zinc for the common cold. *Cochrane Database Syst Rev* 2:CD001364.

Smith G, et al. (2011). Dietary omega-3 fatty acid supplementation increases the rate of muscle protein synthesis in older adults: a randomised controlled trial. *Am J Clin Nutr* 93(2):402–412.

Snijders T et al. (2015). Protein ingestion before sleep increases muscle mass and strength gains during prolonged resistance-type exercise training in healthy young men. *J Nutr* 145(6):1178–1184.

Snijders T et al. (2019). The impact of pre-sleep protein ingestion on the skeletal muscle adaptive response to exercise in humans: An update. *Front Nutr* 6:17.

Somerville VS et al. (2016). Effect of flavonoids on upper respiratory tract infections and immune function: A systematic review and meta-analysis. *Adv Nutr* 7(3):488–497.

Sonneville KR et al. (2012). Vitamin D, calcium, and dairy intakes and stress fractures among female adolescents. *Arch Pediatr Adolesc Med* 166(7):595–600.

Sousa M et al. (2016). Nutritional supplements use in high-performance athletes is related with lower nutritional inadequacy from food. *J Sports Sci Health* 5(3):368–374.

Sportbite website: http://www.sportbite.live/

Stokes T et al. (2018). Recent perspectives regarding the role of dietary protein for the promotion of muscle hypertrophy with resistance exercise training. *Nutrients* 10:180.

Stølen T et al. (2005). Physiology of soccer: An update. *Sports Med* 35(6):501–536.

Stuart C et al. (1990). Effect of dietary protein on bed-rest-related changes in whole-body-protein synthesis. *Am J Clin Nutr* 52(3):509–514.

Sundgot-Borgen J et al. (2013). How to minimise risks for athletes in weight-sensitive sports. *Br J Sports Med* 47:1012–1022.

Talk Eat Laugh (Rachel Muse) website: https://www.talkeatlaugh.com

Tallis J et al. (2021). The prevalence and practices of caffeine use as an ergogenic aid in English professional soccer. *Biol Sport* 38(4):525–534.

Theron N et al. (2013). Illness and injuries in elite football players--a prospective cohort study during the FIFA Confederations Cup 2009. *Clin J Sport Med* 23(5):379–383.

Thevis M et al. (2013). Adverse analytical findings with clenbuterol among U-17 soccer players attributed to food contamination issues. *Drug Test Analysis* 5:372–376.

Thomas DT et al. (2016). American College of Sports Medicine Joint Position Statement. Nutrition and Athletic Performance. *Med Sci Sports Exerc* 48:543–568.

Timmons BW et al. (2007). Influence of age and pubertal status on substrate utilization during exercise with and without carbohydrate intake in healthy boys. *Appl Physiol Nutr Metab* 32(3):416–425.

Tipton K. (2015). Nutritional support for exercise-induced injuries. *Sports Med* 45:S93–104.

Tobias J. (2021). An investigation into probiotic supplements, the immune system and diet of female footballers. PhD thesis, University of the West of Scotland.

Townsend R et al. (2017). The effect of postexercise carbohydrate and protein ingestion on bone metabolism. *Med Sci Sports Exerc* 49(6):1209–1218.

Training Ground Guru website: https://www.trainingground.guru

Trommelen J & van Loon LJ. (2016). Pre-sleep protein ingestion to improve the skeletal muscle adaptive response to exercise training. *Nutrients* 8(12):763.

Trommelen J et al. (2019). The muscle protein synthetic response to meal ingestion following resistance-type exercise. *Sports Med* 49:185–197.

Trumbo P et al. (2002). Dietary reference intakes for energy, carbohydrate, fiber, fat, fatty acids, cholesterol, protein, and amino acids. *J Am Diet Assoc* 102(11):1621–1630.

Tscholl PM et al. (2008). The use of medication and nutritional supplements during FIFA World Cups 2002 and 2006. *Br J Sports Med* 42:725.

Union of European Football Associations (UEFA) website: https://www.uefa.com

van Loon LJ. (2013). Role of dietary protein in post-exercise muscle reconditioning. *Nestle Nutr Inst Workshop Ser* 75:73–83.

Vardy J. (2016). *Jamie Vardy From Nowhere My Story*. Ebury Press, London.

Varley I et al. (2017). Increased training volume improves bone density and cortical area in adolescent football players. *Int J Sports Med* 38(05):341–346.

Veith R et al. (2007). The urgent need to recommend an intake of vitamin D that is effective. *Am J Clin Nutr* 85(3):649–650.

Vigh-Larsen JF et al. (2021). Muscle glycogen metabolism and high-intensity exercise performance: A narrative review. *Sports Med* doi: 10.1007/s40279-021-01475-0. Online ahead of print.

Vitale KC et al. (2017). Tart cherry juice in athletes: A literature review and commentary. *Curr Sports Med Rep* 16(4):230–239.

Volek JS & Rawson ES. (2004). Scientific basis and practical aspects of creatine supplementation for athletes. *Nutrition* 20(7-8):609–614.

Volek JS et al. (2015). Rethinking fat as a fuel for endurance exercise. *Eur J Sport Sci*, 15(1):13–20.

Wachsmuth N et al. (2013). Changes in blood gas transport of altitude native soccer players near sea-level and sea-level native soccer players at altitude (ISA3600). *Br J Sports Med* 47(Suppl 1):i93–99.

WADA (World Anti-Doping Agency) website: https://www.wada-ama.org/en/

WADA (2021). The World Anti-Doping Code. Available at: https://www.wada-ama.org/sites/default/files/resources/files/2021_wada_code.pdf

Wall B et al (2013). Substantial skeletal muscle loss occurs during only 5 days of disuse. *Acta Physiol Scand* 210(3):600–611.

Wall B et al. (2013). Disuse impairs the muscle protein synthetic response to protein ingestion in healthy men. *J Clin Endocrinol Metab* 98(12):4872–4878.

Wall B et al. (2015). Strategies to maintain skeletal muscle mass in the injured athlete: nutritional considerations and exercise mimetics. *Eur J Sport Sci* 15:53–62.

Wall B et al. (2016). Short-term muscle disuse lower myofibrillar protein synthesis rates and induces anabolic resistance to protein ingestion *Am J Physiol* 310(2):137–147.

Walsh NP. (2018). Recommendations to maintain immune health in athletes. *Eur J Sport Sci* 11:1–12.

Wang H et al. (2020). Effects of field position on fluid balance and electrolyte losses in collegiate women's soccer players. *Medicina* 56:502.

Waterhouse J et al. (2005). Transient changes in the pattern of food intake following a simulated time-zone transition to the east across eight time zones. *Chronobiol Int* 22(2):299–319.

Wenger A. (2020). *Arsène Wenger My Life in Red and White: My Autobiography*. Weidenfeld & Nicolson, London.

Wenger A. (2021). Importance of nutrition in football: the coach's perspective. *Br J Sports Med* 55(8):409.

Weston M et al. (2012). Science and medicine applied to soccer refereeing: an update. *Sports Med* 42(7):615–631.

White A et al. (2018). Match play and performance test responses of soccer goalkeepers: A review of current literature. *Sports Med* 48(11):2497–2516.

Widrick JJ et al. (1992). Time course of glycogen accumulation after eccentric exercise. *J Appl Physiol* 72(5):1999–2004.

Wilk B et al. (2013). Mild to moderate hypohydration reduces boys' high-intensity cycling performance in the heat. *Eur J Appl Physiol* 114:707–713.

Witard O et al. (2014). Myofibrillar muscle protein synthesis rates subsequent to a meal in response to increasing doses of whey protein at rest and after resistance exercise. *Am J Clin Nutr* 99(1):86–95.

Witard OC et al. (2014). High dietary protein restores overreaching induced impairments in leukocyte trafficking and reduces the incidence of upper respiratory tract infection in elite cyclists. *Brain Behav Immun* 39:211–219.

Wu G. (2016). Dietary protein intake and human health. *Food Funct* 7(3):1251–1265.

ABOUT THE AUTHOR

Michael Gleeson is Emeritus Professor at Loughborough University. He retired in March 2016 and was previously Professor of Exercise Biochemistry in the School of Sport, Exercise and Health Sciences of Loughborough University, England. His first degree was in Biochemistry at the University of Birmingham, graduating in 1976. His PhD research was carried out at the University of Central Lancashire in collaboration with Queen's College London, and concerned the effects of diet and exercise training on energy metabolism. Michael carried out postdoctoral research in exercise physiology and metabolism at Salford University for three years and this was followed by three years as a temporary lecturer at the University of Edinburgh. He conducted further research on diet-exercise interactions as a senior research fellow at the University of Aberdeen for three years and then joined Coventry University as a senior lecturer in 1987.

Michael moved to the University of Birmingham in January 1996 where he progressed from senior lecturer to professor in the School of Sport and Exercise Sciences, being awarded a personal chair in exercise biochemistry in 1999. He joined Loughborough University's School of Sport, Exercise and Health Sciences in 2002. Loughborough is renowned for its excellence in sport and sport science. Michael's main research interests have been in the metabolic responses to exercise, sports nutrition and the effects of acute and chronic exercise on the function of the immune system.

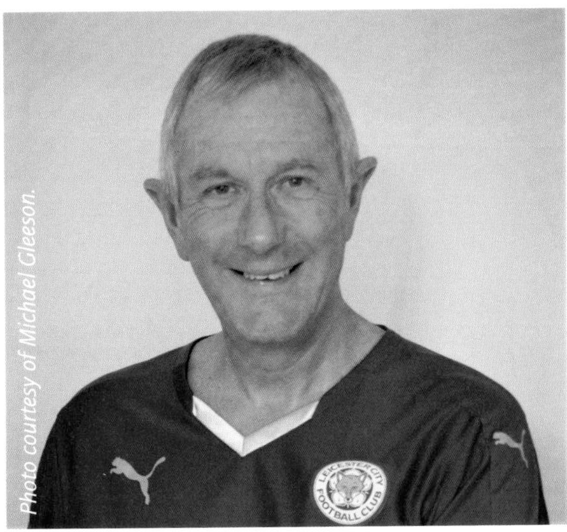

The author wearing his 2015–16 Leicester City shirt (the year that they won the Premier League).

He was the physiology section editor for the *Journal of Sports Sciences* and an associate editor of *Exercise Immunology Review*. He has published over 200 research papers in scientific and medical journals, contributed chapters to over 30 books and has co-authored textbooks entitled *Biochemistry of Exercise and Training* (Oxford University Press 1997), *The Biochemical Basis of Sports Performance* (Oxford University Press 2004 and 2010), *Sport Nutrition* (Human Kinetics 2004, 2010 and 2019), *Immune Function in Sport and Exercise* (Elsevier 2006) and *Exercise Immunology* (Routledge 2013). Michael is a Fellow of the British Association of Sport and Exercise Sciences (BASES) and the European College of Sport Science (ECSS), a BASES accredited exercise physiologist, as well as a past president of the International Society of Exercise and Immunology (ISEI). He has taught thousands of BSc sport science students, hundreds of MSc exercise physiology students and supervised 17 PhD students. He has featured in several national radio and TV programmes in the UK, recorded numerous webinars and podcasts, and his research has attracted interest from local, national and international media.

Michael is still an active science writer and, in the past few years, has contributed to international expert consensus reviews sponsored by the IOC (training load and illness, 2016; training load and injury, 2016), ISEI (immuno-nutrition, 2017), ISSN (probiotics for athletes, 2019; the athlete gut microbiota, 2020) and UEFA (nutrition in elite football, 2020) as well as completing the 3rd edition of his highly popular book *Sport Nutrition* (Human Kinetics, 2019), which he co-authors with Professor Asker Jeukendrup. He has also written a trilogy of new healthy lifestyle guidebooks for the general public: *Eat, Move, Sleep, Repeat*; *Beating Type 2 Diabetes;* and *The Pick'n Mix Diet,* all published in 2020 by Meyer & Meyer Sport. Michael has had a longstanding interest in football and the factors influencing player health and performance. Many of his students now work in sport science support roles at major football clubs, including several in the English Premier League and the MLS. He is a nutrition consultant to Leicester City FC, who became the Premier League Champions in 2016 as 5,000–1 outsiders. He has also worked with other top clubs including Chelsea, Manchester United and Manchester City.